Understanding Gender-Based Violence

Caroline Bradbury-Jones · Louise Isham
Editors

Understanding Gender-Based Violence

An Essential Textbook for Nurses, Healthcare Professionals and Social Workers

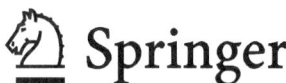 Springer

Editors
Caroline Bradbury-Jones
Institute of Clinical Sciences, College of
Medical and Dental Sciences
University of Birmingham
Birmingham
UK

Louise Isham
Institute of Applied Health Research
University of Birmingham
Birmingham
UK

ISBN 978-3-030-65005-6   ISBN 978-3-030-65006-3   (eBook)
https://doi.org/10.1007/978-3-030-65006-3

This Springer imprint is published by the registered company Springer Nature Switzerland AG
The registered company address is: Gewerbestrasse 11, 6330 Cham, Switzerland

Preface

Identifying and Responding to Violence and Abuse: Why Adopt a Gendered Lens?

Gender-based violence remains a critical and pervasive problem across the world. It refers to violence that occurs as a result of the normative expectations as regards gender, along with the unequal power relationships between genders [1]. Gender-based violence disproportionately affects girls and women, particularly through certain forms of violence such as child marriage, intimate partner violence (IPV), female genital mutilation (FGM), 'honour' killings or trafficking [2]. Most forms of gender-based violence, particularly IPV, are rooted in coercive and controlling behaviours, as recognised only relatively recently in UK policy [3]. The seminal work of Evan Stark (2007) has been influential in bringing this to the fore and as he observed, coercive control is the most common context in which [women] are abused and it is also the most dangerous [4].

Gender-based violence is frequently legitimised by patriarchal (and sometimes misogynistic) cultures, norms and institutions. That is, the violence and abuse that women and girls suffer—and the way it is understood and responded to by others in a given social context—is inextricably linked to other inequalities they experience: for example, absent or diminished economic power, inequality in the eyes of the law, infringements on their bodily autonomy through law and social attitude—that all arise because of their gender. However, gender discrimination does not operate in a vacuum and inequalities rooted in gender biases are often compounded (and sometimes uniquely shaped) by other forms of discrimination and oppression, based on class, race, ethnicity, able-bodied bias and sexuality. This means that some women and girls are much more likely than others to suffer gender-based violence and experience repeat victimisation. They are also less likely to receive timely or effective support from formal support services.

Gender-based violence is often understood to be synonymous with violence against women and in that respect, it can refer to acts of violence directed at a woman, *because* she is a woman. The United Nations defines violence against women as:

Any act of gender-based violence that results in, or is likely to result in, physical, sexual, or mental harm or suffering to women, including threats of such acts, coercion or arbitrary deprivation of liberty, whether occurring in public or in private life (United Nations 1993).

As regards prevalence, the organisation UN Women reports that 35% of women worldwide have experienced either physical and/or sexual IPV by a non-partner (not including sexual harassment) at some point in their lives [5]. However, some studies report the rates to be much higher, with up to 70% of women having experienced physical and/or sexual violence from an intimate partner in their lifetime [6].

The terms 'gender-based violence' and 'violence against women' are frequently used interchangeably. The reason for this interchangeability is recognition that most gender-based violence is perpetrated by men against women. Social constructions of gender, from which gender-based violence arises, are explained by the World Health Organization (WHO) [7] as the phenomenon that people are born female or male, but learn to be girls and boys. In turn, they then grow into women and men. This is attempting to illustrate that gender is socially constructed—it does not exist in itself, it is something that human beings construct as a reality. We would argue that the WHO explanation is too narrow and that it fails to take account of non-binary understandings of sex and gender development where there is blurring of traditional male-female boundaries. It is important to acknowledge that abuse and violence occur in the lives of many individuals, irrespective of gender or sexual identity. Many men and boys across the world are victims of violence and so too are people who identify as lesbian, gay, bisexual, transgender or queer (LGBTQ). However, it is widely acknowledged that most people affected by gender-based violence are women and girls. Moreover, women and girls as victims of violence suffer specific, long-term consequences of gender discrimination in myriad ways [8].

Gender-Based Violence: A Health and Social Problem of Global Scale

Gender-based violence occurs in different forms and it is a problem right across the world. The types of violence may vary between and within countries, but no country is left untouched. A seminal piece of work that continues to be well cited is the multi-country study of Garcia-Moreno and colleagues [9]. This involved ten countries: Bangladesh, Brazil, Ethiopia, Japan, Namibia, Peru, Samoa, Serbia and Montenegro, Thailand, and the United Republic of Tanzania. Just over 24,000 women took part. The reported lifetime prevalence of physical or sexual partner violence, or both, varied from 15 to 71%, which shows a vast difference between countries. Between 4 and 54% of respondents reported physical or sexual partner violence, or both, in the past year which again shows a large differential. The findings confirmed that physical and sexual partner violence against women is widespread. In all settings (except one) women were at far greater risk of physical or sexual violence by a partner than from violence by other people. This illustrates that so-called stranger danger is far less of a risk to women than that which occurs within

a domestic setting. The authors who reported on the study concluded that the variation in prevalence within and between settings shows that violence in not inevitable
and that there is considerable scope for us to collectively lower prevalence rates [9].

According to the WHO [10], no single factor explains why different forms of
violence are more prevalent in some countries and communities than others. They
suggest that there are multiple risk factors associated with both perpetration and
victimisation at individual, relationship, community and societal levels. When contextualising the problem of gender-based violence then, it is really important to bear
this in mind. The same WHO report from 2016 lays out the most prominent forms
of gender-based violence experienced by women, including:

- Violence by intimate partners and by family members;
- Sexual violence (including rape) by non-partners (e.g. acquaintances, friends,
  teachers and strangers);
- Trafficking, including for sexual and economic exploitation;
- Femicide, including intimate partner femicide (i.e. murder of a woman by a cur-
  rent or former partner);
- Murders in the name of honour or because of dowry;
- Sexual harassment in schools, workplaces and public places, and increasingly
  also online.

The specific violations against girls are also reported:

- FGM, which is concentrated in approximately 29 countries in Africa and the
  Middle East but occurs elsewhere, including in countries with diaspora
  communities;
- Child, early and forced marriage, which has a higher prevalence and is increasing
  in some regions (e.g. South and Central Asia, parts of sub-Saharan Africa);
- Sexual abuse and trafficking, which is a higher risk than for boys;
- IPV, which is a risk especially for adolescent girls who are married or are in dat-
  ing relationships [10].

The effects of many forms of gender-based violence are known to be serious and
long term, with negative impacts on health and social well-being. Violence against
women—particularly IPV and sexual violence—is a major public health problem
and a violation of women's human rights. Most of this violence takes the form of
IPV. Violence can negatively affect women's physical, mental, sexual, and reproductive health and may increase the risk of acquiring HIV in some settings [11].
Evidence shows that women who have experienced physical or sexual IPV report
higher rates of depression, having an abortion and acquiring HIV, compared to
women who have not [6]. When it comes to children, 12 million girls under 18 are
married each year and in sub-Saharan Africa—where this harmful practice is most
common—almost four out of 10 young women were married before their 18th
birthday [5]. The impacts as regards reproductive and sexual health are well documented, with attendant risks of giving birth young. Finally, gender-based violence

is lethal. Globally, as many as 38% of murders of women are committed by a male intimate partner [11]. Some data suggest that the figures may be even higher. Out of an estimated 87,000 women worldwide who were intentionally killed in 2017, more than half (50–58%) were killed by intimate partners or family members [12]. This equates to 137 women across the world being killed by a member of their own family every day.

To capture the lifetime risks and consequences of gender-based violence, the WHO [13] advocates a life course approach, which is very much aligned to our own thinking about the problem. The life course approach is congruent with thinking about gender-based violence because it emphasises how as a health determinant, gender cuts across four age stages—the girl child, adolescent girl, adult women and older women. It also means of course that potentially, women and girls face a lifetime of discrimination, violation and abuse. Gender-based violence makes no concessions when it comes to age.

Spotlight: Why Are Some Women and Girls Disproportionally Affected by Gender-Based Violence?

Women from Black, Asian and other racial or minority ethnic backgrounds: Research indicates that women from ethnic or racial minorities (a term that itself reflects a white majority and white privileged position) are at greater risk of experiencing violence than women in the majority ethnic population [14]. Because racial women from minority groups are more likely to experience economic disadvantage and live in environments of deprivation, they are more likely to be exposed to harmful and high-risk behaviours associated with sexual violence perpetration and victimisation [15]. From a cultural and historic perspective, women who are in minority racial and ethnic groups have been routinely subjected to objectification, exoticism and derogatory attitudes on the ground of race and cultural difference and this has contributed to the devaluing and 'othering' of their bodies in Western culture and socieities. In turn, this may contribute to attitudes that de-personify some women and promote the acceptability of violent or abusive behaviour towards them [14]. Research indicates that non-Caucasian women are less likely to seek formal support, in part because of previous experiences of institutional racism and/or feeling that their needs are not meaningfully understood or represented by criminal or healthcare professionals [16].

Disabled women: Disabled women are four times more likely to experience physical and sexual abuse than non-disabled women [17]. They are also more likely to be in a relationship of dependency with the perpetrator, either as a formal or informal caregiver. This can lead to women being targeted because of their perceived physical and social vulnerability; it can also reduce their ability to challenge asymmetric power dynamics that give rise to violence and abuse in caring relationships [18]. Furthermore, because there is a paucity of education and awareness about disabled women's needs following domestic or sexual violence, sometimes underpinned by paternalistic or infantilising attitudes, health and social work professionals may miss opportunities to support this group of women and girls [17].

Older women: The experiences and needs of older women (age 60 years and over) in relation to gender-based violence remain a relatively 'hidden' topic. Although there is evidence that the incidence of sexual violence within intimate partner relationships decreases for this age group in comparison with younger women, this small decrease is not proportionate to the paucity of information about their needs in research and practice. Indeed, in many countries, routine data is still not collected about older women's experiences of IPV and their experience of non-intimate partner sexual assault [19]. Older women report that feelings of shame and anticipatory stigma inhibit them from disclosing sexual and IPV particularly when carried out by a life-long partner or family member [20]. The complex dynamics of love, care and inter-dependency in older age create additional challenges for older women seeking help in relation to a taboo expression of violence and abuse—that perpetrated by people who need and who 'give' care [21, 22]. Help-seeking is further hampered by a lack of specialist, age-sensitive services in most countries.

Disclosure and Help-Seeking: Formal and Informal Routes

Data reported by the United Nations Economic and Social Affairs [23] on the 'world's women' showed that in the majority of countries with available data, less than 40% of the women who experience violence seek help of any type. Among women who do seek help, most turn to family and friends, with very few seeking help from formal institutions such as health and social services. When it comes to accessing support for the police, this figure drops to a mere 10% [23].

These stark figures underscore the need to improve how we think about disclosure and help-seeking. There is growing consensus amongst researchers, practitioners and policy makers about the importance of conceptualising disclosure of violence and abuse as a process rather than a one-off event. This understanding recognises the importance of social and cultural factors shaping individuals' decisions about what information to share, with whom and when. Children, for example, may use emotional and behavioural cues to invite adult exploration rather than talking directly about their experiences of violence and assault, particularly in the initial stages of disclosure. This can help them test how willing an adult is to listen to them and to take concrete actions to help [24]. It is equally important to recognise that adults have different needs and ways of seeking help and developing meaning about their experiences. Processes of disclosure, for example, are shaped by a complex set of behaviours, values and attitudes at the individual, familial, community and social level [25]. Attitudes relating to gender and sexuality shape, for example, belief systems about the ability and right of men to exercise power over women. They also affect the extent to which violence is normalised and sexual violence is explained [26]. For example, in societies which emphasise gender differences and the sanctity of familial relationships and loyalty, there may be less willingness to recognise the harm caused by sexual and domestic violence and a tendency to place responsibility on women to manage or withstand men's sexual behaviour. This can lead people to internalise feelings of blame and social shame. It is also likely to inhibit disclosure and help-seeking processes. These insights are important because they remind us that people share, make sense of and cope with their experiences in different, unique ways [26].

It is also important to remember that while facilitating disclosure of all forms of abuse and violence is important, it is not unproblematic and it is certainly not a panacea. Disclosure needs to be safe and supported and it needs to lead to outcomes that are appropriate and wanted by the person making the disclosure. So for example, taking the issue of IPV, a woman's disclosure does not mean (in most cases) a desire to leave a relationship. Many women chose to disclose their experiences at a particular time to a particular person, with the desire to talk through the problem and explore their safety options. 'Disclosure' does not equate to 'leave'. There are many rational reasons why the woman may want to remain in a relationship, at least for the time, in which case appropriate actions are to support her to stay, while attending to her safety needs and potentially those of her children.

Research Insight
Health Professionals and Women's Disclosures: A 'Dynamic of Silence'
    A qualitative study on IPV by Bradbury-Jones et al. [28] reported that abused women and health professionals all found it difficult to talk about the problem of intimate partner violence. Health professionals struggle to find the right words and are worried about causing offence if they broach the subject and women themselves are extremely reluctant to tell health professionals about their experiences, for fear of being judged, concerns about further violence from their intimate partner and anxieties about what will happen to them, particularly the removal of children. This study highlighted a 'dynamic of silence' between abused women and health professionals that resulted in women feeling silenced and not being able to access professional help, at potentially critical points in their recovery from IPV.

The Role of Health and Social Work Professionals and Systems

The WHO identifies that health and social care systems do not always meet the needs of victim-survivors because they do not consistently recognise the 'multiple entry points' for prevention, intervention and the provision that exist as people transition through these systems at different points in their life [29]. Instead, professional responses have tended to be crisis or forensically focused, concentrating on the clinical care needs of victims in the immediate aftermath of assault; or, the need to protect children or vulnerable adults who are in danger of immediate harm. Underpinned by a strong body of research, the WHO advocates that practitioners adopt a holistic approach to the assessment and treatment of victim-survivors. This should be underpinned by a right-based approach that emphasises the importance of women exercising self-determination about all aspects of their health and having an unconditional right to non-discriminatory care that is confidential and of a high and consistent quality [30]. Care and support should also, the WHO emphasises, be provided in a way that is sensitive to gender issues and inequalities.

A key way of empowering health and social work professionals to take on this role is to educate, train and support them throughout their careers and to provide bespoke guidance depending on their working context. Whilst it is likely that those in specialist roles do receive additional training and support, in the majority of cases professional programmes for nurses, social workers and other healthcare disciplines are tightly packed with content. Professional standards and regulatory bodies stipulate key requirements and outcomes for such programmes and this means that curricula are over-stretched as regards the amount of content that can include. We feel strongly that gender-based violence should be taught on every professional programme for nursing, social work and healthcare students. Moreover, it should not be a one-off session, but rather, a core part of the curriculum, where knowledge is built upon year-on-year as students' progress through their programme. Yet the reality however is that individual programmes often struggle to accommodate even one or two sessions to prepare students for understanding gender-based violence [31]. Empirical research has shown that health and social care students consider themselves to be under-prepared in dealing with gender-based violence and that most curricula do not cover the issue [32, 33]. Irrespective of their interest or commitment to tackle the issue, it is likely that under-prepared and under-confident professionals will miss opportunities to support victim-survivors of gender-based violence.

Rationale and Structure of This Book

This book is written in response to the lack of gender-based violence education for health and social work students. We expect—and hope—that it will also be relevant to a wide range of readers, for example students on post-qualifying health and social care courses, and also some of the faculty/educators teaching on such programmes. We have focused on what we consider to be some of the most pressing gendered issues and the contributors are expert academics and practitioners, working in diverse settings. The book is structured into four parts. The first part considers the 'rise' of gender-based violence and how this once marginalised perspective has become more widely adopted. This section also questions to what extent gender-based violence has become embedded in health and social work training and education and what gaps remain in professionals' understanding and skills. The second part of the book explores some of the expressions, contexts and implications of gender-based violence. Each chapter considers the role of health and social workers and invites the reader to reflect on their work (or future work) across these complex and varied fora. The third part of the collection focuses on one of the most common and insidious forms of gender-based violence that health and social work professionals are likely to encounter: physical, psychological, sexual and financial violence by an intimate partner, who may also be a parent. Finally, the fourth part showcases innovative responses to supporting victim-survivors and challenging systems that contribute to gender inequality. We hope that this section provides insights and examples of what can be achieved when working collaboratively with victim-survivors and colleagues in other disciplines.

Reading This Book: Considering Your Needs and Those Around You

The context of gender-based violence is fraught with ethical and safety issues that surpass those associated with many other areas of clinical and research practice. Moreover, these operate at multiple levels and require consideration of the people we are working and researching with and also our colleagues and the safety of ourselves as practitioners, students, researchers, etc. We think it important to focus here on the ethical and safety issues of those who may be reading the book. The extent of gender-based violence and particularly in one of its forms IPV, is such that we are aware of the likelihood that many readers will have their own personal experiences of the problem. If you feel upset or distressed by engaging with any of the content, take yourself away from it for some time. You are in control as regards how much or how little you read and talking with a trusted person might help. It might be that some students and professionals are living in homes and communities where some form of gender-based violence is an immediate issue. If you feel that someone around you would not want you to be reading this book, please be careful where you place it.

Conclusions

A vision of the WHO [13] is to create a world in which all people are free from all forms of violence and discrimination, their human rights are protected and gender equality and the empowerment of women and girls are the norm. This is an ambitious aim. At a macro level, initiatives by international organisations such as the WHO and UN Women contribute to important frameworks through which strides can be made globally. Nationally, it is incumbent upon governments and policy makers to ensure that tackling all forms of gender-based violence is a priority and that there are laws and policies in place to make sure it happens. These are required to ensure that when it comes to the organisational and individual level, action is possible. We know that many health and social care practitioners are not prepared to deal with gender-based violence. We hope that this book provides some useful insights and information, so that readers are empowered to play their own part in global efforts to tackle gender-based violence.

Birmingham, UK   Caroline Bradbury-Jones
Birmingham, UK   Louise Isham

References

1. Bloom SS. Violence against women and girls: a compendium of monitoring and evaluation indicators. MEASURE Evaluation, Carolina Population Center; 2008. http://www.cpc.unc.edu/measure/tools/gender/violence-against-women-and-girls-compendium-of-indicators. Accessed 4 Apr 2016.
2. Plan International, Gender-based Violence. 2019. https://plan-international.org/ending-violence/gbv-gender-based-violence.
3. Home Office. Controlling or coercive behaviour in an intimate or family relationship: statutory guidance framework. ('Statutory Guidance Framework'). 2015;4.
4. Stark E. Interpersonal violence. Coercive control: how men entrap women in personal life. 2007.
5. UN women, facts and figures: ending violence against women. 2020. http://www.unwomen.org/en/what-we-do/ending-violence-against-women/facts-and-figures.
6. World Health Organization. Global and regional estimates of violence against women: prevalence and health effects of intimate partner violence and non-partner sexual violence. World Health Organization; 2013. https://www.who.int/reproductivehealth/publications/violence/9789241564625/en/.
7. World Health Organization. Gender: definitions. 2017. http://www.euro.who.int/en/health-topics/health-determinants/gender. Accessed 2 May 2017.
8. Health-genderviolence.org. Defining gender-based violence. 2016. http://www.health-genderviolence.org/training-programme-for-health-care-providers/facts-on-gbv/defining-gender-based-violence/21. Accessed 13 Oct 2016.
9. García-Moreno C, Jansen HA, Ellsberg M, Heise L, Watts C. WHO multi-country study on women's health and domestic violence against women. World Health Organization; 2005.
10. World Health Organization. Global plan of action to strengthen the role of the health system within a national multisectoral response to address interpersonal violence, in particular against women and girls, and against children; 2016.
11. World Health Organization. Violence against women. 2017. https://www.who.int/violence_injury_prevention/violence/sexual/en/. Accessed 15 May 2019.
12. United Nations Office on Drugs and Crime. 2019. Global Study on Homicide. https://www.unodc.org/documents/data-and-analysis/gsh/Booklet_5.pdf.
13. World Health Organization Regional Office for Europe. Strategy on women's health and well-being in the WHO European Region. 2016. http://www.euro.who.int/__data/assets/pdf_file/0003/333912/strategy-womens-health-en.pdf.
14. Bryant-Davis T, Chung H, Tillman S. From the margins to the center: ethnic minority women and the mental health effects of sexual assault. Trauma Violence Abuse. 2009;10(4):330–57.
15. Ullman SE. Social support and recovery from sexual assault: a review. Aggress Violent Behav. 1999;4(3):343–58.

16. Wasco SM. Conceptualizing the harm done by rape: applications of trauma theory to experiences of sexual assault. Trauma Violence Abuse. 2003;4(4):309–22.

17. Plummer SB, Findley PA. Women with disabilities' experience with physical and sexual abuse: review of the literature and implications for the field. Trauma Violence Abuse. 2012;13(1):15–29.

18. Saxton M, Curry MA, Powers LE, Maley S, Eckels K, Gross J. "Bring my scooter so I can leave you" a study of disabled women handling abuse by personal assistance providers. Violence Against Women. 2001;7(4):393–417.

19. Bows H. Researching sexual violence against older people: reflecting on the use of freedom of information requests in a feminist study. Femin Rev. 2017;115(1):30–45.

20. Crockett C, Cooper B, Brandl B. Intersectional stigma and late-life intimate-partner and sexual violence: how social workers can bolster safety and healing for older survivors. Br J Soc Work. 2018;48(4):1000–13.

21. Isham L, Bradbury-Jones C, Hewison A. Female family carers' experiences of violent, abusive or harmful behaviour by the older person for whom they care: a case of epistemic injustice?. Sociol Health Illn. 2020;42(1):80–94.

22. Isham, L, Bradbury-Jones, C, Hewison A. "This is still all about love": practitioners' perspectives of working with family carers affected by the harmful behaviour of the older person for whom they care. Br J Soc Work. 2020 (Forthcoming).

23. United Nations Economic and Social Affairs. The world's women 2015, trends and statistics. https://unstats.un.org/unsd/gender/worldswomen.html.

24. Reitsema AM, Grietens H. Is anybody listening? The literature on the dialogical process of child sexual abuse disclosure reviewed. Trauma Violence Abuse. 2016;17(3):330–40.

25. Kennedy AC, Prock KA. "I still feel like I am not normal": a review of the role of stigma and stigmatization among female survivors of child sexual abuse, sexual assault, and intimate partner violence. Trauma Violence Abuse. 2018;19(5):512–27.

26. Flood M, Pease B. Factors influencing attitudes to violence against women. Trauma Violence Abuse. 2009;10(2):125–42.

27. Campbell R, Dworkin E, Cabral G. An ecological model of the impact of sexual assault on women's mental health. Trauma Violence Abuse. 2009;10(3):225–46.

28. Bradbury-Jones C, Taylor J, Kroll T, Duncan F. Domestic abuse awareness and recognition among primary healthcare professionals and abused women: a qualitative investigation. J Clin Nurs. 2014;23(21–22):3057–68.

29. World Health Organization. Understanding and addressing violence against women: intimate partner violence. 2012. https://apps.who.int/iris/bitstream/handle/10665/77432/WHO_RHR_12.36_eng.pdf.

30. World Health Organization. Responding to intimate partner violence and sexual violence against women: WHO clinical and policy guidelines. 2013. http://www.who.int/reproductivehealth/publications/violence/9789241548595/en/.

31. Sammut D, Kuruppu J, Hegarty K, Bradbury-Jones C. Which violence against women educational strategies are effective for prequalifying health-care students?: A systematic review. Trauma Violence Abuse. 2019:1524838019843198.
32. Bradbury-Jones C, Hallett N, Sammut D, Billings H, Hegarty K, Kishchenko S, Kuruppu J, McFeely C, McGarry J, Sheridan J. Gender-based violence: a five-country, cross-sectional survey of health and social care students' experience, knowledge and confidence in dealing with the issue. J Gender Based Violence. 2020.
33. Bradbury-Jones C, Billings H, Hegarty K, Hinsliff-Smith K, Kishchenko S, McFeely S, McGarry J, Sammut D, Sheridan J. Gender based violence: a resource to support students in health and social care. https://bit.ly/2UjoSVL.

Contents

Part III   Spotlight on Intimate Partner Violence

Part IV   Responses and Innovations

About the Editors

Caroline Bradbury-Jones is a registered nurse, midwife and health visitor. She holds a position as Professor of Gender-Based Violence and Health at the University of Birmingham, UK. Her research focuses primarily on violence against women and girls. Her research has been conducted in the UK and in Low and Middle Income Countries, mainly Africa.

Louise Isham is a research fellow at the University of Birmingham and a registered social worker. Her research explores experiences of, and responses to, domestic and sexual violence. Louise's PhD explored women's experiences of violence, abuse and family life in the context of their intimate care relationships.

About the Authors

Juliet Albert is specialist FGM midwife and Trust lead for Female Genital Mutilation at Imperial College Healthcare NHS Trust. She has a Masters in Advanced Practice Midwifery. Her FGM clinic received a Guardian Public Service award in 2011 in ethnicity and diversity. She is currently co-chair of NHS England and NHS Improvement (NHSEI) London Clinical Group and co-runs the Royal College of Midwives FGM Network.

Stuart Allardyce is a Director at the Lucy Faithfull Foundation with responsibilities for Stop It Now! Scotland and research across the UK charity. He has worked as a practitioner and manager with children who have displayed harmful sexual behaviour for over 20 years. He is an honorary research fellow at Strathclyde University and the vice chair of the National Organisation of the Treatment of Abuse.

Kathleen Baird is a registered midwife; she has been a midwife for over 25 years. Kathleen holds the position as professor of midwifery at the University of Technology, Sydney, and is the Director of the Centre of Midwifery, Child and Family Health. Kathleen's research focuses on the health response to domestic and family violence with a focus on pregnancy. Kathleen's PhD explored women's experiences of domestic abuse during pregnancy.

Karen Block is a senior research fellow in the Centre for Health Equity at the University of Melbourne and leads the Migration and Social Cohesion research programme for the Melbourne Social Equity Institute. She conducts research with immigrant and refugee-background young people, women and families focused on social inclusion, health inequalities and gender-based violence.

Ben Donagh is the Children and Young People (CYP) Service Manager at Victim Support. He is a qualified Young Persons Violence Advocate (YPVA) with over 9 years' experience of supporting children and young who have experienced crime and traumatic incidents, predominantly gender-based violence. Ben is currently completing a PhD at the University of Birmingham where his research interests are the experiences of siblings in the context and aftermath of domestic violence and abuse.

Adair Finucane is a yoga educator, Ayurvedic wellness coach and social worker with a background in trauma research. Adair helps healers to fill their own cups, so the work they do in the world can be amplified. She works with women healers, facilitators and teachers of all types to help them feel vital and healthy and strengthen their connection with their intuition.

Renee Fiolet is a registered nurse who works in the School of Nursing and Midwifery at Deakin University, Australia. A scholar in the Safer Families Centre of Research Excellence, Renee's PhD is focusing on Indigenous peoples help-seeking behaviours when experiencing family violence. She has a keen interest in Indigenous health, women and children's health, technology in health care and family violence.

Heather D. Flowe develops theoretically driven procedures that enhance memory retrieval and enable witnesses and victims to achieve their best evidence in criminal proceedings. With practitioners and colleagues from around the world, she is currently investigating methods to improve the accuracy of rape complainant statements and testimony in the US and the UK; working with rape survivors in the Global South to document and preserve memory evidence; and developing novel 3D interactive lineup procedures to increase the reliability and accuracy of eyewitness identification.

Lyndsey Harris is an Associate Professor in Criminology at the University of Lincoln and associate of PraxisCollab. Her research expertise is in domestic abuse and she specialises in qualitative research and coproduction. An ESRC Impact Leader with wide-ranging experience of partnership and stakeholder engagement, Lyndsey chairs Nottingham City's Response to Complexity (R2C) Steering Group, concerned with improving services for survivors of domestic abuse experiencing multiple disadvantage.

Kelsey Hegarty is Professor of Family Violence Prevention at the University of Melbourne and Royal Women's Hospital, Australia. Kelsey is a general practitioner academic and directs the Safer Families Centre of Research Excellence.

Isobel Heywood is a Master of Public Health graduate from the University of Birmingham, UK. Her postgraduate dissertation was the basis for the 'thrivership' study, later published in *BMC Women's Health* Journal. Isobel is passionate about public health and social issues, particularly gender equality and the social determinants of health.

Kathryn Hodges is a registered social worker, with practice experience predominately in the third sector. She is the Director at the Centre for the Study of Modern Slavery at St Mary's University and associate at PraxisCollab. Her research explores the decisions and choices individuals make when seeking help and support, the complexity of help seeking and the relational aspects of care.

Laura L. Jones is a Senior Lecturer in Qualitative and Mixed-Methods Applied Health Research at the University of Birmingham. Her research focusses on undertaking qualitative and mixed-methods research to answer challenging questions around women's and maternal health, and within maternity care. She leads a large UK qualitative study exploring the views of survivors, men and healthcare professionals on improving NHS female genital mutilation service provision.

Wangu Kanja is an affiliated researcher at the University of Birmingham. A human and women's rights activist, she is also the executive director and founder of the Wangu Kanja Foundation. Wangu is the survivor of rape after a carjacking incident in 2002. She is the convener of the survivors of sexual violence in Kenya network, which works to amplify the voices of the survivors to access comprehensive care and support.

Merja Laitinen holds a position as professor of social work at the University of Lapland, Finland. She is also a licensed social worker. Her research interests are related to violence and abuse against women and children from the victim's perspective and research methodology and research ethics among these sensitive topics.

Patricia Logan-Greene is an Associate Professor at the University at Buffalo School of Social Work. Her research examines a broad range of issues related to violence and victimisation, including the lifelong effects of child adversity, legal system responses, gun violence and prevention.

Finn Mackay is a Senior Lecturer in Sociology at the University of the West of England (UWE). Author of *Radical Feminism: Activism in Movement* from Palgrave,

Finn comes from a background in feminist activism and a career in policy and training on domestic violence prevention in education. Finn has worked with the End Violence Against Women Coalition, Women's Aid and Welsh Women's Aid and is proud to still deliver training for practitioners through UWE's social work and nursing programmes.

Elizabeth McLindon is a clinical social worker and researcher at the Women's Hospital and University of Melbourne, Australia. Liz's research has investigated the prevalence, impacts and implications of gender-based violence in the personal lives of health professionals.

Jacky Mulveen is the original founder of WE:ARE (formerly known as the Birmingham Freedom Project). As a survivor of domestic abuse herself, Jacky has dedicated the last 17 years of her life to supporting women through the complex journey from leaving to healing.

Anna Nikupeteri is a postdoctoral researcher at the University of Lapland, Finland, and a licensed social worker. Her research interests are related to violence against women and children from the victim's perspective, especially in the context of post-separation violence and stalking.

Bridget Penhale is a Reader in Mental Health of Older People at the University of East Anglia in the UK and a registered social worker. Her principal research focus concerns elder abuse and adult safeguarding, including gender-based violence against older women; her research interests span domestic violence, mental health of older people, social aspects of dementia, dignity and social care. Bridget's research has largely been undertaken in the UK and Europe.

Sarah R. Rockowitz is a PhD student at the University of Birmingham. Prior to this position, Sarah conducted research on barriers to healthcare access for refugees in Jordan and also lived and worked in Tanzania for a year conducting public health research. Her current research is on medical and legal barriers to post-rape care in Kenya and India.

Simon Sawyer is a registered Advanced Life Support Paramedic in Victoria, Australia, and is a lecturer of Paramedicine at Australian Catholic University. Simon's PhD examined the paramedic response to intimate partner violence and generated the first comprehensive guidelines and education for paramedics in responding to family violence incidents. Simon continues to conduct research with healthcare students and practitioners on how to recognise and respond to family violence.

Mickey Sperlich is a midwife and Assistant Professor at the University at Buffalo School of Social Work. Her research includes developing interventions to address effects of sexual violence and other trauma, particularly for childbearing and early parenting, and examining intergenerational implications of trauma and trauma-informed care across systems.

Claire Sullivan is a lawyer and PhD candidate at the University of Melbourne. She has worked in Australian and UK-based community legal centres in legal and policy/research roles. Claire is interested in the impacts of institutional violence on women and racialised communities and her PhD explores refugee women's experiences of legal responses to gender-based violence.

Siân Thomas is a lecturer at the University of Birmingham and a registered social worker. Her research focuses on gender-based violence, justice responses and child welfare, particularly in the context of forced migration. As a researcher and practitioner in human rights and social work, Siân has worked with survivors of gender-based violence, modern slavery and other rights violations in the UK, Thailand and Turkey.

Cathy Vaughan is an Associate Professor in Gender and Women's Health at the Melbourne School of Population and Global Health, the University of Melbourne. She leads the Community-Engaged Research programme for the Melbourne Social Equity Institute and is Director of the WHO Collaborating Centre for Women's Health hosted by the University. Her research focuses on violence against women and building capacity for violence-related research in Australia, Asia and the Pacific.

Sharron Wareham is a registered social worker with vast experience of working with children and families impacted by child sexual abuse. Sharron has completed research focussing upon Girls and Young Women who display Harmful Sexual Behaviour and Boys and Young Men at risk of Child Sexual Exploitation.

Sanne Weber is a research fellow at the University of Birmingham. Her research explores how post-conflict justice and reconciliation mechanisms can best address and transform gender inequality. She works mostly in Latin America, particularly Colombia and Guatemala. Previously, Sanne worked as a researcher, gender policy advisor and team coordinator for human rights and development organisations in Guatemala.

Peter Yates is a lecturer and programme lead for social work at Edinburgh Napier University. He is a qualified social worker with more than 10 years' experience of child protection. His particular research interests within this field include sibling sexual abuse and victim crossover, and he has published and presented at international conferences on these subjects.

Part I

From the Margins to the Mainstream? Gender-Based Violence in Health and Social Work

Raising Awareness and Improving Responses to Gender-Based Violence: The Contribution of Feminist Thought and Activism

Finn Mackay

1.1 Introduction

There are no responses to sexual violence and domestic abuse which are not feminist informed. Our laws, policy and service sector in the UK are a legacy of feminist work conducted during what is called the second wave of feminism; the period of uprisings of New Left social justice movements that exploded across Western democracies from the late 1960s and into the 1980s. This is just one reason why feminist theory on the causes of GBV is so important to professionals like you. It is your history and, hopefully, it is your future. Without feminist theory, we would not have the understandings we do of crimes like rape, sexual abuse and domestic abuse; in some cases, we would not even have laws against them, or understand them as crimes at all.

Believing that something can be changed is the first step on the path to changing it, and that is an important point that is all too often missed in the field of domestic abuse and sexual violence response services and policy. Healthcare and social work professionals are likely to be in a career characterised by firefighting. As first responders, it is unusual to have time to step back from day-to-day work and reflect on why crimes like sexual abuse, rape and domestic violence are a feature in the lives of so many individuals and families. As a healthcare and social work professional, it is unlikely that you are given adequate support or space to consider the life-changing difference you can make by being someone's first port of call, whether they chose to end up at your door or not. Too often it can feel like these sorts of crimes are just part of the backstory and part of the backdrop of life; too often they will be part of your backstory too. While we all wish there were less of these crimes, it is easy to assume that it was ever thus and ever will be. That is

F. Mackay (✉)
University of the West of England, Bristol, UK
e-mail: Finn.Mackay@uwe.ac.uk

© Springer Nature Switzerland AG 2021
C. Bradbury-Jones, L. Isham (eds.), *Understanding Gender-Based Violence*,
https://doi.org/10.1007/978-3-030-65006-3_1

why it is vital to take time to step back and remind yourself that these crimes are made and not born, to remember that they have causes and thus they can be reduced, or even ended.

1.2   Gender-Based Violence Is Not Inevitable

Without feminist theory, we could not imagine a world without GBV. Feminist theory, and particularly Radical Feminist theory, has given us the promise that commonplace though these crimes may be normal or natural they are not. When we understand GBV as a phenomenon with roots, we can begin to pull them up. That work is not abstract or outside ourselves, it is not something we will do to other people or clients or service users, it is not something we will singularly cure in patients or offenders. This is because the roots of epidemic levels of male sexual violence against women, children and marginalised men do not lie in nature, they grow in the lie that these are men's natural behaviours. They grow not out of the concrete of institutions, but in the hearts and minds of the human beings within them. This is good news, because what is learned can be unlearned. That is the very point of feminism, it is fundamentally a politics of change for the better, teaching us that the way things are is not the way they have to stay.

1.3   Causes and Consequences of Women's Inequality

Everything we know now about these epidemic, everyday forms of violence comes from feminist activists and feminist social scientists. In her analysis of the British feminist movement in the 1970s, Historian Pat Thane [1] points out that one: 'real and lasting achievement of the 'second wave' was to give rape and domestic violence public names, to put the reality of these issues on the public agenda, from which they have never since disappeared—though nor unfortunately have these crimes against women disappeared' (p. 175). Feminist scholars have pioneered research into domestic abuse in same-sex relationships [2], in work with perpetrators [3], on male victims [4], on responses to domestic abuse in Black and global majority communities [5] and on the effects on children of living with domestic abuse [6]. Research centres like the Centre for Gender and Violence Research at the University of Bristol and the Child and Woman Abuse Studies Unit at the London Metropolitan University are important UK hubs for this work, offering a plethora of practical and theoretical insight.

The language that we are all currently familiar with, like that which appears in the 2012 Home Office definition of domestic abuse [7], in the RCN guidance on interpersonal violence [8] or in the 2015 England and Wales legislation on coercive control [9] repeatedly highlight that these are crimes of coercive, controlling and threatening behaviour. The Conservative government's combined strategy [7] on Ending Violence Against Women and Girls (2016–2020) defines that violence against women and girls, or VAWG—in one of the many acronyms that saturate this sector—is a cause and consequence of gender inequality. The strategy promises an ambitious programme to challenge negative gender stereotypes that 'can fuel harmful attitudes towards women which create a fertile environment for VAWG' (p. 15). This sort of language is as commonplace today as politicians in feminist tee shirts, but it never used to be this way.

1.4 What Is the F Word?

Feminism is still a relatively niche movement, even following the phenomenal MeToo movement of 2017 after the hashtag was launched in 2006 by survivor and activist Tarana Burke. Even following the Women's Marches that began in the US in response to the inauguration of Donald Trump in 2017 and which drew around half a million people to the march on Washington alone, with millions taking part across the globe in local protests. Yet, research by the Fawcett Society [10] in 2016 found that while 67% of the British public surveyed would support women having equal rights to men in society, only 7% would openly identify themselves as a feminist. This is such a popular refrain it has practically become a meme—'I'm not a feminist, but'. That there is widespread reluctance to identify with the f-word is likely due to some of the social policing that surrounds the term and which functions to alienate women from one of the oldest and most powerful social justice movements in the world—their own. Homophobia and misogyny are used to discredit and ridicule feminism, because they are so powerful and obviously carry such weight and are very effective weapons. Feminism is associated with lesbianism, as if there is something wrong with lesbianism. Feminism is associated with not shaving one's body hair, as if that is anyone else's business. Feminism is associated with preferring the company of cats, as if that is anything but logical. We know that these associations are common social currency, often used as jokes. This is how a serious political theory and history becomes reduced to a joke or becomes reduced to a discussion about whether you shave your legs or whether you would let a man hold a door open; none of this is coincidental. When considering the contribution of feminist theory to the field of family violence prevention and intervention, it is firstly important to be clear on just what feminism even is. Feminism is a political movement for the liberation of women and society, based on equality for all people. It is not reducible to equality within an unequal world, and it is not struggling for equality with unequal men.

1.5 What Is Patriarchy?

Feminism, like all social justice movements, is revolutionary. It is a radical movement to reduce, end and replace patriarchy as a form of social government [11]. Patriarchy is the term used to describe any society where men as a group overwhelmingly dominate mainstream institutions of power and where this is seen as natural; societies like ours. The Fawcett Society's Women and Power report in 2020 [12] showed that the Westminster parliament is around 70% male; men are three quarters of senior roles in the judiciary; 19 out of every 20 CEOs in FTSE 100 companies are men and around 80% of newspaper editors are men. Women are underrepresented in mainstream positions of power generally, and women from minority groups are even further underrepresented, with Black and global majority women having even more barriers put in their way. Until the 2010 General Election, there were only three Black women MPs, for example, and there are, as yet, no Black or global majority women in the parliaments of the Celtic nations [12]. Black and global majority women in the public eye face horrendous levels of racist and misogynist abuse, which can only further function to punish women for daring to claim positions of power. In the run up to the 2017 General Election, research by Amnesty International found that Hackney MP Diane Abbot alone received just under half of the total of online abuse directed at all the female MPs [13].

While comparatively great strides have been made towards women's equality with men, glacial progress seems to be fought at every step. At Davos in 2018, the World Economic Forum estimated that just on equal pay alone, at the current rate of progress, it would take 202 years for women to reach pay parity with men. Patriarchy is not a concept on some gender studies syllabus, it is just a statistical fact. However, it is important to note that while men as a group dominate mainstream power, not all men are in positions of power nor will feel powerful. Men are affected by the social fractures of racism, homophobia, disability discrimination and social class discrimination, for example. The top of patriarchy does not include all men, it is mainly made up of White wealthy men who come from the minority upper class elite. This is a profoundly unequal structure, and although feminism has fought against sex discrimination within this structure, it has never intended that to be an endpoint. A centuries old political movement has not been striving all this time, losing life and liberty in the process, to simply swap for a few more women from privileged backgrounds at the top of these structures. Feminism is about change, not a changing of the guard.

1.6   What Do Feminists Want?

During the second wave of feminism in the UK, the British Women's Liberation Movement formulated seven demands. These were agreed at annual national conferences from 1971 to 1978. The seven demands still stand as a live womanifesto for feminism, and they are an answer to common questions about what feminism is, what it stands for and what it wants. The demands are as follows:

1. Equal pay
2. Equal education and job opportunities
3. Free contraception and abortion on demand
4. Quality local 24 h free nursery provision
5. Financial and legal independence
6. An end to all discrimination against lesbians and a woman's right to define her own sexuality
7. Freedom from intimidation by threat or use of violence or sexual coercion, regardless of marital status and an end to all laws, assumptions and institutions which perpetuate male dominance and men's aggression towards women

1.7   Gender-Based Violence or Male Violence Against Women and Children?

The seventh demand came after several years of focus on activism against rape and all forms of male violence against women and children, or male VAWC. The first Rape Crisis Centre, for example was opened in London in 1976. The Women's Aid Federation was formally established in 1974 but by that time it was already operating around 40 refuges nationwide. Reclaim the Night, a women's night-time march against all forms of male violence against women, was established across the UK in 1977 by the Leeds Revolutionary Feminist Group. As well as activism, feminists secured changes in law, in the Domestic Violence and Matrimonial Proceedings Act, for example in 1976, and improvements in the Sexual Offences Act 1976. Attention to these forms of violence emerged directly from the practice of Consciousness Raising or CR, which was a staple of women's groups up and down the country. From front rooms to village halls, women all over the UK had started to collectivise their experiences, theorising that incidents of domestic violence, rape and sexual abuse were not isolated individual occurrences but a symptom of women's unequal place in society. 'Throughout the 1970s growing feminist, and also public awareness about the issue of male violence against women, violence specifically directed at women by men, prompted the need for explanation of this phenomenon. Domestic violence and rape were some of the earliest concerns' [14, p. 58].

Feminist scholars in the UK such as Professor Jalna Hanmer, Professor Liz Kelly, Professor Gill Hague and Professor Marianne Hester have gifted some of those explanations. Amazons like these women have and continue to contribute a rich legacy to our understandings of GBV. Feminist theory concluded that male sexual violence against women, children and marginalised men is a fundamental ingredient in the maintenance of patriarchal social governance. The threat and reality of male VAWC is a product of women's inequality and it produces women's inequality. As Professor Hester [14] explains, 'male violence against women, in whatever form—harassment, rape, battering etc.—is a crucial mechanism by which male dominance and control is maintained over women, where, by some men using violence against some women, all women at the same time live with the threat of violence from potentially any man, and all men benefit from the actions of some men' (p. 59).

1.8   Male Violence as a Form of Social Control

The threat and reality of male sexual violence operates as a form of social control, whether one has been individually affected by such crimes or not. In 2018, Plan International published research finding that 66% of girls and young women aged 14–21 years old in the UK had experienced sexual harassment in a public place. Many (46%) did not tell anyone about it, they saw it as a normal part of everyday life. Girls and young women regulate and limit their participation in public space due to the threat and reality of male sexual violence. Women walk a longer route home to avoid underpasses or unlit roads, they save money aside for a taxi rather than spending it all on their night out, they avoid certain kinds of public transport or they try to go home before it gets dark [15]. While young men are more at risk of street violence, from other young men, they usually do not regulate and limit their participation in the public sphere in the same way, this is a profoundly gendered experience. This is one example of what feminist theorists mean when they say that male VAWC operates as a form of social control for all women.

Another way that male VAWC enforces the current social structure is by being the most final and most brutal example of the objectification of women. On average, two women every week in the UK are murdered by a violent male partner or ex-partner. During the lockdown of 2020 in response to the Coronavirus pandemic, many families were physically confined and separated from possible exit strategies and support networks. Existing patterns were exacerbated under such conditions as well as perhaps being used as an excuse by violent men to escalate control. Tragically, the first 3 weeks of lockdown saw an estimated 16 cases of fatal domestic violence perpetrated by men, shining a spotlight on domestic abuse and leading to public demands that the state use hotels to house those fleeing from violent perpetrators; the Conservative government was pressured to agree to extra funds for refuge provision [16]. Although we often hear after such cases that these are isolated incidents, they are obviously far from it. They take place in private but they are facilitated by the state and the public sphere [17]. As scholar Melanie McCarry [18] reminds us, the context matters, and the context is one where women are unequal in law, finances, politics, media and policing. 'Women can be controlled by men because the social, legal and political frameworks within which we live already put men in control' (p. 96). There is a saying that if there is peace and harmony in the home, there will be peace in the nation, but we can also turn this around and consider that where there is violent hierarchy in the society, there will be violent hierarchy in the home.

1.9   A Conducive Context for Male Violence

The body count is the endpoint of women's inequality, and those statistics indicate how far away we are from progress in this field; but behind each of those cases is a process that began much earlier. Professor Liz Kelly has developed the idea of what she calls conducive context, to explain how society enables and facilitates acts that are then treated as aberrant. There is a continuum of male VAWC and it begins with the cultural representation of women and children, particularly girls, as commodities and objects for scrutiny, often sexual objects. From adverts, to children's clothing, to female characters in TV and films, women and girls are routinely sexually objectified. As Professor Hester [19] explains, this is part of the imposition of strict binary gender roles. 'In the contemporary context, this process reduces women to passive heterosexual objects compliant to male needs, though at the same time it also presents women as sexually enticing and potentially threatening, necessitating the reassertion of male control. Women are thus implicated in the process of their own oppression' (p. 11). In a society where women, from a young age, are objectified in media and culture, we should not be surprised when women are treated as just that, as objects, in the streets, in their workplaces and in their homes.

Rape, sexual harassment and sexual assault have long been a site of feminist campaigning. In fact, in the so-called first wave of feminism, the Suffragettes, famous for their use of NVDA or non-violent direct action, were not only working for the right to vote but also for the right to be free from male violence. Suffragette campaigns included demands for women's rights to flee violent husbands, for example and to have custody of their children, to raise the legal age of consent, to stop the exploitation of women in prostitution and for rape in marriage to be a crime. The latter was a particularly lengthy struggle, because it took until 1991 for rape in marriage to finally be recognised as a crime. Rape has for millennia been considered a crime not against women, but against men, a theft of property by one man against another, be that a father, a husband or brother [20, 21]. Our legal system has never adequately responded to this crime or its aftermath. In 2019, the Victim's Commissioner Dame Vera Baird QC demanded an enquiry into the falling rape conviction rate, reporting that convictions had dropped by 21%. While reports continue to rise, no doubt due to public awareness following the MeToo movement and also the historic abuse investigations in the UK, rape convictions continue to fall. The gap between reported rapes and convictions is called the attrition rate and it has never been something to be proud of in the UK [22]. In 2019, the rape conviction rate in England and Wales was around 1.7% [23]. A culture of disbelief surrounds women who report rape. While evidence is often not properly gathered, women's mobile phones and social media meanwhile are heavily scrutinised for images that can be used to discredit the alleged victim, using pseudo-Victorian judgements about so-called provocative behaviour or revealing clothing. Where women know the alleged perpetrator, have accepted drinks or gifts from him or have had sexual contact with him in the past, this is taken to cast doubt on their testimony. Such trends demonstrate ancient stereotypes at work about women's sexual agency and personhood, or lack of it. Women's sexuality is constructed as something owned by men, to be given, groomed or taken. Women who have agreed to sexual activity with one man are seen as in no position to refuse any man, and this is the case with girls also. Girls and women have sometimes been framed as guilty of inciting a man to rape them and these sorts of legal atrocities happen far more often than we would like to think. In 2018, a case in Ireland hit the headlines when a 17-year-old girl was cross-examined about her underwear in court during a rape trial, while the prosecutor suggested that she was lying about the rape due to her having been wearing a thong.

1.10 Believe Her

Going a bit further back in time, in May 1998, a young woman reported that she was raped by an older man she met in a nightclub in Grimsby town centre. After viewing CCTV footage from the inside of the club, which showed the young woman dancing with the alleged perpetrator the police took no further action, stating that this image discredited the allegations made because the dancing was 'in an intimate way' [24]. The man accused of rape had previously been investigated four times over sexual relationships with girls under 16. None of these cases were taken forward. The man was Ian Huntley, and he went on to murder two schoolgirls, Holly Wells and Jessica Chapman, who will be forever aged 10 years old. It is unsettling to think of the lives that could have been saved and the lives left unblighted by violent crime, if police and prosecutors would only believe women the first time. The relationship between men and women has been constructed as one of predator and prey, subject and object, this is deeply entrenched and plays out today in court cases where women are told they naturally wanted and/or deserved rape. There will never be equality between women and men until we tear down these antediluvian stereotypes and together build a relationship based on shared humanity and then make it humane.

1.11   Patriarchy Is Not Nature

This will not be an easy journey because most of us to some extent accept the current status quo and assume it is this way for a reason. As the feminist philosopher bell hooks [25] points out in her work on masculinities, nobody would support rape or domestic homicide, but all of us tolerate the system that creates these crimes. 'I often tell audiences that if we were to go door to door asking if we should end male violence against women, most people would give their unequivocal support. Then if you told them we can only stop male violence against women by ending male domination, by eradicating patriarchy, they would begin to hesitate, to change their position. Despite the many gains of contemporary feminist movement—greater equality for women in the workforce, more tolerance for the relinquishing of rigid gender roles—patriarchy as a system remains intact, and many people continue to believe that it is needed if humans are to survive as a species. This belief seems ironic, given that patriarchal methods of organising nations, especially the insistence on violence as a means of social control, has actually led to the slaughter of millions of people on the planet' (p. 30). In addition, it is a tragic reality that plenty of people do see grey areas in what counts as rape. A third of men surveyed for the End Violence Against Women Coalition in 2018 responded that non-consensual sex could not be classified as rape if the woman had flirted with the man prior; a quarter of people in the survey felt that non-consensual sex was unlikely to be rape in the context of a long-term relationship [26]. Similar confusions lurk behind what counts as excuses or reasons for domestic homicide, reasons which always wend their way back to blaming the victim for causing and/or deserving her own murder. We can see this in the almost clichéd newspaper headlines following family annihilation, which inform us routinely about ordinary family men pushed to the edge by breakdown, extramarital affairs, addiction or bankruptcy [27].

1.12   Un-gendering

Most men do not rape, abuse or murder their female partners and their children. These crimes are overwhelmingly committed by men, but they do not commit them because they are male. There is nothing about being born male that biologically predetermines one to a life of perpetrating sexual violence or intimate partner abuse. Contrary to the accusations of man-hating often thrown at feminists, the very central tenet of all strands of feminism, from radical to liberal, is that all of us can change and that male VAWC is not caused by nature. This is a profound act of faith in men as human beings, from feminists who refuse to believe the lies told about boys who will always be boys. As hooks [25] argues: 'the will to use violence is really not linked to biology but to a set of expectations about the nature of power in a dominator culture' (p. 55). Boys are enculturated into patriarchy via a system of masculinisation that has to work hard to strip them of their innate loving and caring nature. To be emotional is to be human, we should then wonder at the schooling and social pressures which tell boys not to cry, to be tough, to compete with one another at all costs and to use their supposed natural superiority to 'protect' girls who in turn have to stoop as the weaker sex in order for them to define themselves against. If gender came naturally, we would not have to work so hard at it. It is reassuring that despite such conditioning, most men are as humane as the next woman. As feminist psychologist Carol Gilligan [28] notes, this freights great potential and the 'revolutionary insight is that by nature we are coopera-tive, relational beings, and our capacity for mutual understanding is linked to the sur-vival of our species' (p. 56). Within patriarchal society gender, as in masculinity and femininity, are socially constructed as active and passive, dominant and subordinate and all those other dualisms that have scarred our world. Politics in our society fol-lows the masculinist illogic of the law of the bully; the law that might, may not always be right, but still, might will out. The law that those who can, will, and that physical, financial or any other form of power is something that should be used over others for gain, especially less powerful others. We urgently need to move to the opposite model, where power is seen as something that should be shared among, for the benefit of all, especially the most vulnerable.

1.13   Revolutionary Insiders

You have probably been told countless times that you work on the 'frontline'. A strange, militaristic analogy, because you are not at war against poor people, or vulnerable people or abused people. You are, however, part of a struggle against the conditions that perpetrate the violence of poverty and marginalisation against so many in our communities. Enforced poverty does not cause male violence against women and children, but it limits the possible responses, survival strategies and exit plans for those affected. If they manage to leave, poverty and marginalisation limit the healing strategies accessible and the amount of practical options to utilise in rebuilding. Feminist theory from the second wave has given a language about the operation and imposition of gender norms, and it has explained how societal male dominance is maintained through the exercise of power and control, from the most intimate personal relationships to statewide power relationships. Always be a thorn in the side for those forces that acted so unjustly upon every single one of the individuals, children and families that you will work for and with. While successive governments may dream of replacing you with administrative robots or glorified security guards, you must remain and persist. As we live in an imperfect world, you will find that your jobs are imperfect too, underfunded, overstretched and hyper-scrutinised. But, as long as our world is the way it is, and our institutions remain, then brave, bold and passionate people must be in them; playing patriarchy at its own game and winning, winning for all the people who were never meant to thrive, indeed, for all those who were never even meant to survive.

Points for Consideration
Think about what a feminist practice in healthcare and social work would look like. For example:

- Lobby for and practice non-hierarchical ways of working
- Model positive working relationships between the sexes
- Create, use and promote autonomous women's spaces, self-help groups and networks—same with progressive men's groups
- Challenge, highlight and question gender stereotyping of men and women and fathers and mothers
- Do not make gendered assumptions/expectations
- Challenge sexism in yourself, clients and colleagues
- Be aware of and refute woman-blaming, mother-blaming and victim-blaming culture
- Challenge your own prejudices
- Challenge your own stereotyping
- Do not judge irrationality in an irrational, abuse situation

Reflective Exercise

Discuss with colleagues the meanings of feminism and whether or not you would define yourselves as feminists, if not, why not?

References

1. Thane P. Women and the 1970s: towards liberation? In: Black L, Pemberton H, Thane P, editors. Reassessing 1970s Britain. Manchester: Manchester University Press; 2013. p. 167–86.
2. Donovan C, Hester M. Domestic violence and sexuality: what's love got to do with it? Bristol: Policy Press; 2014.
3. Westmarland N, Kelly L. Why extending measurements of 'success' in domestic violence perpetrator programmes matters for social work. Br J Soc Work. 2013;43(6):1092–110.
4. Huntley AL, Potter L, Williamson E, et al. Help-seeking by male victims of domestic violence and abuse (DVA): a systematic review and qualitative evidence synthesis. BMJ Open. 2019;9:e021960. https://doi.org/10.1136/bmjopen-2018-021960. Accessed 20 May 2020.

5. Gill AK, Virdee G. Intersectional interventions to prevent violence against women in black and minority ethnic communities. In: Radford L, Thiara RK, editors. Domestic abuse across the life course: safeguarding and prevention. London: Jessica Kingsley Publishers; 2020.
6. Mullender A, Hague G, Imam U, Kelly L, Malos E, Regan L. Children's perspectives on domestic violence. London: Sage; 2002.
7. Violence against women and girls strategy 2016–2020. HM Government. March 2016. https://assets.publishing.service.gov.uk/government/uploads/system/uploads/attachment_data/file/522166/VAWG_Strategy_FINAL_PUBLICATION_MASTER_vRB.PDF. Accessed 20 May 2020.
8. Royal College of Nursing RCN. Position statement on domestic abuse. 2017. https://www.rcn.org.uk/professional-development/publications/pub-006587. Accessed 13 May 2020.
9. Serious Crime Act. Section 76: controlling or coercive behaviour in an intimate or family relationship. 2015. http://www.legislation.gov.uk/ukpga/2015/9/section/76/enacted. Accessed 2 May 2020.
10. Fawcett Society. We are a nation of hidden feminists. 2016. https://www.fawcettsociety.org.uk/news/we-are-a-nation-of-hidden-feminists. Accessed 4 May 2020.
11. Millett K. Sexual politics. London: Abacus; 1969.
12. Kaur S. Sex and power 2020. London: Fawcett Society; 2020. https://www.fawcettsociety.org.uk/Handlers/Download.ashx?IDMF=bdb30c2d-7b79-4b02-af09-72d0e25545b5. Accessed 13 May 2020.
13. Dhrodia A. Unsocial media: tracking Twitter abuse against women MPs. Amnesty Global Insights. 2017. https://medium.com/@AmnestyInsights/unsocial-media-tracking-twitter-abuse-against-women-mps-fc28aeca498a. Accessed 19 May 2020.
14. Hester M. Lewd women and wicked witches. London: Routledge; 1992.
15. Southgate J, Russell L. Street harassment: it's not ok. Girls' experiences and views. London: Plan International UK; 2018. https://plan-uk.org/file/plan-uk-street-harassment-reportpdf/download?token=CyKwYGSJ. Accessed 19 May 2020.
16. Grierson J. Domestic abuse killings 'more than double' amid Covid-19 lockdown. The Guardian. 15 Apr 2020.
17. Hanmer J. Male violence and the social control of women. In: Feminist Anthology Collective, editor. No turning back: writings from the women's liberation movement, 1975–80. London: Women's Press; 1981. p. 190–5.
18. McCarry M. Views and experiences of young men. Masculinity and gendered interpersonal violence. In: Aghtaie N, Gangoli G, editors. Understanding gender based violence: national and international contexts. London: Routledge; 2015. p. 95–110.
19. Hester M. The dynamics of male domination using the witch craze in 16th and 17th century England as a case study. Women's Stud Int Forum. 1990;13(1–2):9–19.
20. Bourke J. Rape: a history. London: Virago; 2007.
21. Brownmiller S. Against our will. London: Penguin; 1976.
22. Kelly L, Regan L, Lovett J. A gap or a chasm? Attrition in reported rape cases. Home Office Research Study 293. London: Home Office Research, Development and Statistics Directorate; 2005.
23. Dearden L. Only 1.7% of reported rapes prosecuted in England and Wales, new figures show. The Independent. 25 Apr 2019.
24. Smith J. It has never been easier to get away with rape. The Times. 2 Jul 2004. https://www.thetimes.co.uk/article/it-has-never-been-easier-to-get-away-with-rape-tpqjjl6wnmf. Accessed 14 May 2020.
25. hooks b. The will to change: on men, masculinity and love. Washington: Washington Square Press; 2004.
26. EVAW. Attitudes to sexual consent. Research for the end violence against women coalition by YouGov. 2018. https://www.endviolenceagainstwomen.org.uk/wp-content/uploads/1-Attitudes-to-sexual-consent-Research-findings-FINAL.pdf. Accessed 14 May 2020.
27. Beaty Z. Men who kill their wives are not 'jealous husbands', they're murderers. Grazia. 7 Aug 2019.
28. Gilligan C. Joining the resistance. Cambridge: Polity Press; 2011.

Is Gender-Based Violence a Neglected Area of Education and Training? An Analysis of Current Developments and Future Directions

Elizabeth McLindon, Renee Fiolet, and Kelsey Hegarty

2.1 Introduction

Gender-based violence (GBV) is a pervasive social and public health issue that leads to major emotional, physical and social harm [1]. GBV is defined by the World Health Organization (WHO) as 'any behaviour within an intimate relationship that causes physical, psychological or sexual harm to those in that relationship' [2]. Abuse of power against women and children is central to GBV, and types of harm include psychological abuse, physical aggression, forced sexual contact or other threatening or intimidating or controlling behaviours [2]. The term '*survivor*' is used throughout this chapter to refer to women with lived experience of GBV in recognition of their strength and the significant impact of this type of trauma [3]. We focus on GBV against women because gender is the most critical variable in the experience of both surviving and perpetrating GBV; overwhelmingly survivors are women who have been harmed by a trusted male [2].

It is internationally agreed that to reduce GBV and help heal the devastating consequences, a specific response from health and social work professionals is required [4]. Health and social work professionals are both uniquely positioned and specially skilled to address GBV by identifying survivors and engaging them in a timely, evidence-based response that is orientated towards healing and recovery [5]. Importantly, recent evidence suggests that health and social work professionals focused on advocacy and social support can have a positive impact on

E. McLindon (✉) · K. Hegarty
University of Melbourne and Royal Women's Hospital, Parkville, VIC, Australia
e-mail: elizabeth.mclindon@unimelb.edu.au; k.hegarty@unimelb.edu.au

R. Fiolet
School of Nursing and Midwifery at Deakin University, Burwood, VIC, Australia
e-mail: renee.fiolet@deakin.edu.au

© Springer Nature Switzerland AG 2021
C. Bradbury-Jones, L. Isham (eds.), *Understanding Gender-Based Violence*,
https://doi.org/10.1007/978-3-030-65006-3_2

outcomes for women experiencing GBV [6–9]. Preparedness and clinical practice may look different for social workers and other health professionals such as nurses and doctors, because their roles within and outside healthcare are often distinct. Regardless, for all health professionals, including social workers, university education and workplace training is critical to the development of necessary skills for safe and effective survivor care. There is a strong link between education and improved GBV knowledge, attitudes, readiness and clinical skill [10–13]. Training is also an integral component of a whole-of-health-system response to GBV [1].

Historically, GBV was understood as neither a public nor a health issue and was not a component of education and training for health professionals [5]. Several things have changed that landscape. Survivors have broken their silence, talking to friends and professionals, telling their story in court, to politicians and via social and traditional media. Further, advocates have impacted governments around the world to raise awareness, plan for and resource interventions, with significant leadership provided by the WHO [9, 14–16]. GBV is now conceptualised as an urgent public health issue and human rights abuse that must be addressed by the health system [9]. Nevertheless, the international challenge of prioritising a resourced commitment to GBV prevention and response continues [9].

Despite strong advocacy for education and training of health and social work professionals, research continues to suggest low levels of education and training for pre- and post-qualifying health professionals, and inconsistences in the curriculum provided, with programme evaluation rare [17]. Among those working in GBV, professionals with social work degrees are more likely than their colleagues (e.g. psychologists) to rate their degree as having them well prepared, but even then, only 29.5% of social workers say their degree prepared them 'very well' or 'extremely well' [18, p. 10, 19]. Further, there is mounting evidence that nurses, midwives, doctors and other health professionals frequently emerge from university feeling unprepared to deal with GBV [13, 20–23]. For example, recent studies have found that 50% or less of nursing students in Saudi Arabia and Australia have been exposed to GBV content within their degree [24]. The outcomes are no better for medical students, with minimal GBV education offered by most universities [23]. The result is post-qualifying health professionals who are unprepared and lack confidence to address GBV, harbour misconceptions about the issue and exhibit lower readiness to respond [10, 17, 21, 23, 25, 26].

To address this, the WHO has released a health professional training curriculum for the care of women who have experienced GBV [1]. The training content was developed from the previously released clinical policy [4] and practice guidelines [27]. As an excellent contemporary global resource based on the best evidence, WHO's work has been heavily drawn on in the writing of this chapter [1, 4, 27]. WHO have recommended that GBV training should be immediately implemented into pre- and post-qualifying health professional curriculums [1].

2.2   The Difference Between Education and Training

Knowledge, attitudes and skill development are promoted by both education and training, but this chapter sees them as separate concepts. Education often refers to the theory and critical thought underpinning a topic; establishing a purpose for practice. Training is usually more practical learning; active skill development that often occurs in the workplace. Both education and training are important for good clinical care, and one without the other can lead to problems. For example, education without training may result in a gap between a professional's understanding of GBV and feeling confident that they are equipped with the practical tools to draw on in the consulting room. While training without education may mean that the theoretical and/or evidence-based foundations of practice, and the motivation for what is often challenging work, is missing.

2.3   Why Health Professionals and Social Workers?

Health professionals and social workers have important and distinct roles in responding to GBV. Health professionals such as nurses and doctors are at the front line of responding to the health consequences of GBV [27]. Many survivor women will never contact a specialist GBV service but will seek healthcare at different times of their lives, and research suggests that survivor women are, in fact, more likely to seek healthcare and be in contact with healthcare professionals than other women [4]. Further, survivors regularly name health professionals among the people with whom they would feel most comfortable to talk about GBV [4]. Heath professionals are in a position to provide an immediate, or first-line, response to a survivor, and WHO [27] outline this response in their LIVES model (Table 2.1). The basic tenants of the LIVES response includes: demonstrating belief and empathy for a woman's experience, exploring her situation with a focus on both risk and protective factors, understanding and validating that the violence in a survivors' life may be impacting upon her in harmful ways, reassuring against blame, providing offers of practical care, ensuring support is not intrusive of autonomy and facilitating connection with long-term services and resources [4, 7, 27, 28].

Social workers commonly work within health and community settings, and their role is often to provide a more comprehensive response to GBV survivors,

Table 2.1 The WHO LIVES model of first-line GBV support [27]

Listen	Empathetically listen to a survivor without judgement
Inquire	Ask the survivor about her needs, including those that are practical, emotional, physical and social
Validate	Demonstrate that you believe the survivor and reassure her against self-blame
Enhance safety	Explore safety options and collaboratively develop a safety plan
Support	Work with the survivor to connect her with support, information and other services

sometimes over a long period [29]. In high-income countries globally, social workers comprise the largest professional group working in the specialist GBV sector, with an increasing requirement that new workers to the field hold a social work qualification [19]. Social workers in publicly funded health services are someone to whom a first-line responder can refer onsite or externally [4, 27]. However, in rural environments in high-income countries and throughout low-income countries, nurses and doctors are often working in settings where such specialist personnel are not available [4]. Social workers dually focus on understanding safety and well-being across the spectrum of psychosocial impacts using a strength-based perspective, as well as on an individual's social environment, including inequality, injustice and discrimination [30]. The training needs of social workers compared to other health professionals may be different. While all professionals working in health or social support need training to provide a first-line response, social workers and other GBV specialists may require additional education at a pre- and post-qualifying level regarding detailed risk assessment and safety planning, counselling and decision-making and psychosocial interventions with reference to children, parenting, housing, disability, mental health, counselling, cultural issues, financial issues, linkage, interagency collaboration and advocacy [18, 19].

2.3.1 Readiness to Address Gender-Based Violence

To train health and social work professionals, we need to understand holistically what enables them to undertake GBV work. There is a plethora of research about the barriers and facilitators to the uptake of GBV clinical care by health professionals, including social workers, much of which involves discussion of training [13, 26]. Literature on identification shows one-third of women who have experienced GBV ever disclose and an inquiry rate by health professionals of between 10 and 30% [4, 31]. Women face a multitude of barriers when considering whether to disclose GBV, including shame, judgment, disbelief and confidentiality concerns [2]. Health professionals fail to ask their patients and clients about GBV because of insufficient time or skills or feeling overwhelmed by the emotional nature of the work [26]. On the other hand, facilitators to survivor identification include information, screening tools, skills training and support [5, 32]. Recent evidence has also suggested that health professionals' personal exposure to GBV may further enable clinical care of survivor patients [33].

The term '*readiness*' includes concepts of self-efficacy, emotions, motivations and attitudes [34]. '*Preparedness*' often focuses on increasing the knowledge and skills of health and social work professionals through GBV training. Addressing readiness in education and training is more likely to enable health and social work professionals to become practically and emotionally ready for the work [35]. A recent systematic review of 47 qualitative articles exploring health and social work professionals' readiness to address GBV provides some insight into the areas of education and training on which to concentrate [10]. Five themes were identified as enhancing health professional readiness: Having a commitment to GBV; Adopting an advocacy approach; Trusting the relationship; Collaborating with a team; and being supported by the Health system. These themes of Commitment, Advocacy, Trust, Collaboration and Health system support have informed a person-centred health professionals' readiness framework called the CATCH Model (Fig. 2.1) [10].

Table 2.2 paints a picture of what a '*ready*' health professional looks like.

The transtheoretical Stages of Change model identifies five stages of change that can be shifted between: *pre-contemplative, contemplative, preparation, action, maintenance* and *relapsing* [36]. This model is commonly used as a tool to support GBV survivors; however, the CATCH model has been applied to different stages of readiness for GBV clinical work (Table 2.3). Trainers may find it useful in understanding resistance experienced by health and social work professionals (practitioners) for GBV clinical work.

CATCH MODEL Commitment/ Advocacy/ Trust/ Collaboration/ Health system

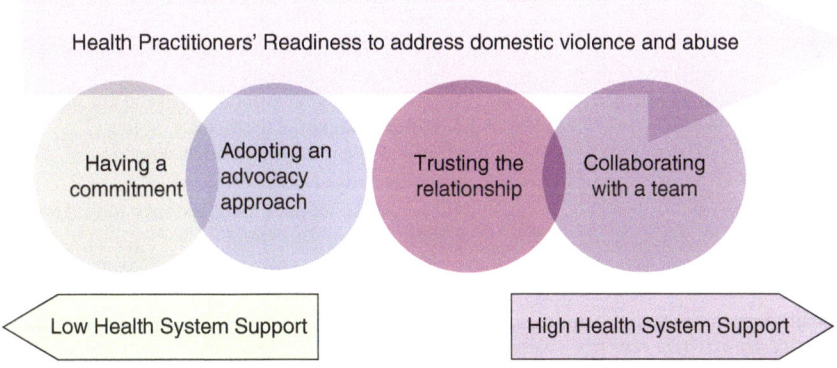

Fig. 2.1 The CATCH model [10, p. 20]. (With permission from: Hegarty, McKibbin, Hameed, Koziol-McLain, Feder, Tarzia & Hooker (2020). Health practitioners' readiness to address domestic violence and abuse: A qualitative meta-synthesis. Plos One, 15(6))

Table 2.2 Portrait of a GBV practice 'ready' health professional [10]

- Motivated to make a difference
- Knows how to respond based on advocacy (see LIVES Table 2.1)
- Feels likely to succeed with a belief that the health setting is a good place to identify and respond to survivor patients
- Has received encouraging feedback
- Works with others
- Is strongly supported with ongoing GBV training, clinical protocols, tools and leadership in the health system
- Feels there is team with whom to collaborate, including specialist GBV social work support if required

Table 2.3 Readiness to address GBV and tailored responses to different stages of change [10, p. 21]

Practitioner stage of change	Response by education/training facilitator
Pre-contemplative Does not think that addressing GBV is their role	**Encourage commitment to the issue** Suggest possibility of a connection between a patient's health issues and GBV and confirm that the health setting is well placed and equipped to address this complex issue
Contemplation Has identified a problem or need to address GBV but remains unsure about whether they are able to undertake the work	**Assess needs of practitioner to provide an advocacy approach with patients** Point out that the workplace is available to support them on their journey towards addressing GBV through available training and resources, e.g. support for survivor staff is in place
Preparation/decision Catalyst for change has arisen (consultation with a patient, attended training, heard a story about personal experience among friends or family)	**Explore issues of clinical experience and level of trust in relationship with patients to undertake this work** Respect the decision about what the practitioner wants to do (asking patients routinely in antenatal care, wearing a lanyard, attending training, documenting better in files, speaking out about GBV to staff as a survivor)
Action Plan devised in the previous stage is put into action	**Ensure collaboration with a team both internally and externally is strong** Offer support to carry out the plan and ensure workplace support is in place e.g. policies, procedures, posters, tools, referral options, secondary consultation
Maintenance Commitment to above actions is firm	**High system support with feedback loops from patients should be strong** Celebrate whatever the practitioner has managed to do and support their actions
Returning Practitioner may feel very frustrated and unable to address GBV as they would like. Reasons include life being stressful, no access to resources, system not supportive	**Engage in advocacy for system support** need to keep engaged even if practitioner is unable to address GBV in their workplace. Reassure that this pattern is common and the practitioner may need to wait until there are higher system supports in place

Using the CATCH and Stages of Change model described above, we now look at a case study to explore training that is tailored to a professionals' level of readiness and Stage of Change (Box 2.1).

2.3.2 Components Necessary for Effective GBV Education and Training

Despite many studies, the best way to train health and social work professionals to enable an evidence-based pathway to survivor safety and well-being is still not completely clear [4, 28, 32, 37]. However, research does show that GBV education and

Box 2.1 Case Study

Fatima graduated from her nursing degree two years ago, and currently works in the antenatal clinic of a busy hospital. She recently attended a brief GBV training session in the emergency department of her hospital. Until now, Fatima does not think she has met any patients who have experienced GBV. However, she has been seeing Laura for more than four months for her regular antenatal appointments, and Fatima has begun to have some concerns over Laura's relationship with her partner, Michael. Michael often answers questions for Laura and has made comments about not allowing Laura to use pain relief during childbirth because he does not want his baby 'born with something wrong with it'. At the most recent appointment Michael was asked to step out of the room, so that Fatima could have a private conversation with Laura, but he refused, saying, 'there's nothing that cannot be said in front of me'. Laura has become disengaged during the sessions, which is a contrast to the very excited young mum Fatima used to see at earlier appointments. Fatima feels that there could be some abuse occurring in Laura's relationship, but she does not feel confident about how to offer Laura appropriate support.

In this case study, Fatima demonstrates personal *commitment* to do the work, which may have been strengthened by her recent attendance at GBV training, but is unsure how to employ an *advocacy* approach with Laura. She may not *trust* that the antenatal care setting is the right place for this work, or she may be unsure about what *collaborative* opportunities there could be for her with the team or what *health system support* there is. In conclusion, Fatima is demonstrating that she is in the contemplative stage of her readiness to address GBV. For Fatima, some of the actions she could choose to take include:

- Exploring what she already knows about providing an appropriate response and determining what her further learning needs are.
- Identifying what resources are available for her to develop her capacity to ask sensitive questions about safety in relationships and provide an informed response to a disclosure of violence—especially useful might be the WHO Clinical Handbook [27].
- Looking for the support offered to her within the workplace (i.e. is there a social work or other colleague available for secondary consultation) and through professional networks.

training can be effective in changing practice with survivors, so what are the critical components? What aspects or principles should training encompass to be successful in improving the care of survivors? The fundamental principle of GBV education and training is to understand GBV and establish a foundation for practice as well as increase a pre- or post-qualifying practitioner's ability to respond helpfully to survivors [13]. Many GBV training models have been evaluated, and a Cochrane Review synthesising all of the randomised control trials (RCTs) and quasi-RCTs about training health professionals to respond to GBV is upcoming [13]. There is broad agreement about topics that must be included in evidence-based GBV education and training and aspects of the facilitation of training that are associated with success, including adopting a consistent approach, having a firm theoretical framework, ensuring an interactive and person-centred approach and longer duration [1].

2.4   Adopting a Consistent Approach to GBV Education and Training: The WHO Training Curriculum

There are likely many thousands of GBV education and training programs for health professionals around the world. However, the WHO [1] training curriculum for post-qualifying health professionals will be spotlighted here [4, 27]. The four objectives of the WHO [1] training are for trainees to demonstrate:

1. General knowledge of GBV as a public health issue.
2. Behaviours consistent with an understanding of the principles of a safe and supportive response to survivors.
3. Clinical skills appropriate to one's profession and specialty.
4. Awareness of how to access resources and support for survivors and oneself.

The curriculum covers 13 sessions delivered across a maximum of two and a half days but can be adjusted depending on the time available [1]. Core competencies cover:

– GBV as a health issue.
– Survivor experiences and how practitioner attitudes affect the care they give.
– The health system response to GBV.
– Practitioner–survivor communication.
– Identification.
– LIVES first-line support.
– Local referral pathways and the legal and policy context.
– Clinical and forensic care for survivors of sexual assault.
– Documentation.
– Health professional self-care.

2.5   Theoretical Framework for Training

Trauma and violence informed care (TVIC) may provide a useful framework for all responses to GBV and, as such, should be integrated into GBV education and training [38]. This is suggested despite the fact that some health professionals will qualify to work in their field with little to no trauma knowledge or training [29]. TVIC is an approach underscored by an awareness that trauma and violence are common and may have a centralising influence in a survivor's life. TVIC prioritises both psychological and physical safety by responding to the diverse and sometimes complex needs of survivors with a focus on autonomy, confidentiality, connection, collaboration and rebuilding a sense of control [38]. Internationally, TVIC has been used as a framework for practice with service users particularly in mental health [39], and it is an approach to guide the operation a system of healthcare [40].

Consistent with TVIC as a lens through which to structure GBV training, training content should address the impact of vicarious or secondary trauma. Vicarious trauma is the impact of exposure to stories by others of abuse and trauma over time [41]. All health and social work professionals are affected by listening to the traumatic stories of their patients and clients and intervening at some of the most difficult and distressing times of life and death [42]. Naming vicarious trauma and its' indicators, as well as suggesting strategies for delaying onset and reducing impact, could enhance training [43] and may even be protective [44].

2.6   Addressing Diversity Through Culturally and Ethically Appropriate Education and Training

To understand the interplay of inequities—such as poverty and race—an intersectional lens can assist in identifying the experiences of those facing multiple forms of oppression, including GBV [45]. It is important, therefore, to apply an intersectional focus to the delivery of education and training on GBV [46]. Many people who experience GBV will be caught at the intersection of race, class, religion, disability and sexuality and may identify one or more oppressive systems (i.e. racism) before gender [45]. Future nurses, doctors, social workers and other health professionals need to be able to address diversity in their responses to GBV and understand the impact of privilege and oppression on those experiencing GBV as well as those who are delivering care [47]. This is particularly important when responding to a social issue that can be experienced by all women, yet is particularly complex and devastating to some cultures or populations where resources may be scarce and structural challenges significant [48].

2.7   Addressing GBV Survivors in the Education and Training Room

A recent study about the prevalence, impacts and implications of GBV against Australian women nurses, doctors, social workers and other allied health professionals found GBV to be common in their lives and associated with greater attendance at pre- and post-qualifying GBV education and training [33, 49]. There is a substantial field of literature investigating the apparent overrepresentation of people who work in mental health, counselling, social work and related therapeutic fields who have their own traumatic history [50–52]. It is likely that there are multiple reasons that the numbers of survivor health professionals attending GBV training may be disproportionally high. These include increased awareness of the prevalence and harm of GBV and the importance of being able to safely and skilfully respond to survivors, and also, knowledge gleaned from training may contribute information or validation about experience [50, 51]. No matter what motivations underscore survivors' attendance, core components of GBV education and training for health and social work professionals should: acknowledge the commonality of trauma among staff; provide strategies for responding to traumatic triggers that occur during the course of routine care (including emotional tools to manage such a response and raise awareness about options for follow-up support); enable discussion of vicarious and cumulative trauma and share local resources for managing personal experience alongside care of patients [41, 43].

2.8   Interactive and Person-Centred Approaches to Learning

A systematic review of educational strategies suggests that interactive educational approaches generate better outcomes than didactic or passive learning methods [12]. WHO [1, p. 2] refer to this as a 'participant-centred approach to learning' whereby trainees are engaged to actively participate wherever possible during training, rather than simply listening to facilitators. Interactive approaches may strengthen a trainee's understanding of how knowledge can be integrated into practice [12]. A person-centred interactive approach includes the use of case studies, guided discussions, role-playing of inquiry and response statements, reflective exercises that encourage trainees to consider the survivor experience and their personal attitudes, challenging the myths and misconceptions they might hold, videos, integration of literature and further reading [1, 53]. A good example of an interactive curriculum is from Canada (see VEGA) [54]. Further, maintaining a practice-focus based on the professional discipline of the trainees is likely to result in better knowledge translation [12, 18].

Key interactive and person-centred training elements in the WHO [1] curriculum focus on:

- Establishing both a safe training space and the expectations of trainees;
- Building on trainee's motivations and strengths (including 'Fear and Motivations in a Hat' exercise—Box 2.2) (see also [53]);
- Understanding trainee's experience and attitudes (including 'Myth or Fact', 'Voting with Your Feet', 'Blanketed by Blame' and 'In Her Shoes' exercises) (see also [36]);
- Active listening (see also [36]);
- Role play (30- or 60-min LIVES practice) and
- Use of survivor's voices ('Case review' exercise) (see also [53]).

Box 2.2 Fear and Motivations in a Hat Interactive Training Exercise [1, p. 15]

- Facilitator starts with two pieces of paper, one is labelled 'fears' and the other 'motivations'.
- On one piece of paper, trainees write something that motivates them to respond to GBV.
- On the other, trainees write one fear they have about responding to GBV.
- Trainees fold the pieces of paper and place into respective boxes.
- Facilitator randomly selects 3–4 responses from the "fears" hat and reads to the group.
- Group then discusses these fears and how they could be overcome.
- Facilitator randomly selects 3–4 "motivations" from the hat and reads to the group.
- Group then discusses the motivations and brainstorms suggestions for how training could build upon these.

2.9 Length of Education and Training

The duration of education and training matters, with longer interventions better able to improve trainee knowledge, attitude and opinions, effecting more sustained practice change [11, 12]. While brief, single session interventions may be effective in changing trainees' knowledge and attitudes, the evidence suggests that this improvement is less likely to be sustained compared with longer educational interventions [12]. A recent study about the associations between health professionals' personal exposure to GBV and their clinical care of survivor patients found that GBV training of eight or more hours, regardless of when it was provided (pre- or post-qualifying) or by whom (university, specialist GBV service or healthcare organisation), was positively associated with all aspects of GBV clinical care, including enquiry, intervention and referral [33]. Further, the relationship between GBV training and clinical care appeared to be graded—the more training a health professional had received (from 1 h upwards), the greater their self-reported clinical care of survivors was in the last 6 months. While we await further evidence on this topic in the upcoming Cochrane Review on GBV training for health professionals, perhaps a rule of thumb is that any GBV education and training at university and in the workplace is better than none, but for sustained change, resources are worth employing towards longer, repeated education and training interventions.

2.10 Evaluation

The purpose of evaluation in education and training is to determine its success (usually in terms of learning-level outcomes based on specific training objectives) as well as to identify areas of improvement [1]. Inconsistent, diverse and insufficient appraisal methods can make it hard to compare training programs, risking poor evaluation that hinders longitudinal follow-up [11, 13]. The literature about GBV education and training evaluation instruments suggests that they commonly assess a combination of trainee knowledge, attitudes and confidence to respond to survivors [13]. WHO [1] recommend that questionnaires be administered to trainees immediately before and after training in addition to regular (3–6 months) intervals, thereafter. Further, their advice is that facilitators record key trainee information and their own reflections as part of quality improvement [1].

2.11 Future Issues and Directions in GBV Education and Training

There is no shortage of challenges to getting adequate GBV education into the tertiary curriculum of all health professionals as well as upskilling the existing health and social work professional workforces. An overflowing list of topics that universities must cover in the pursuit of preparing all health professionals for work compete for ever-decreasing space. Then, once qualified, health and social work professionals are employed in healthcare organisations that are largely driven by demand, where time and resources are in short-supply and things are continually added to the clinical plate but never taken off. Although some studies indicate that health professionals may improve their efficacy in responding to GBV through experience [20], the healthcare profession need practitioners who are ready to respond upon qualification. A future direction for GBV training is bringing in survivor voices through meaningful participation and consultation with those who have lived experience. A valid criticism levelled at health and social services in the United Kingdom, Australia and elsewhere is that they rarely engage women with lived experience of GBV to inform their services [3]. Survivor voices are essential to making organisations responsive to the people they serve; effective and focused on women's and children's needs. Education and training that listens to survivors as informants and facilitators all the way through to co-producers is likely to result in practitioners who are better able to respond to the needs and experiences of women and children in the consulting room.

2.12 Conclusion(s)

Health and social work professionals require education and training to prepare them to respond safely to GBV and provide appropriate survivor care. Drawing on the recommendations of the WHO to Listen, Inquire, Validate, Enhance Safety and Support women who experience GBV (LIVES), this chapter has suggested that education and training can improve health professional GBV awareness, attitudes and skills. Commitment, Advocacy, Trust, Collaboration and Health system support (CATCH) play an important role in preparing health and social work professionals to appropriately respond to GBV, and the health system must be supportive of its workforce to engage in this space.

Current evidence suggests that interactive educational methods produce better learning opportunities than didactic approaches; actively engaging trainees through interactive methods can enhance application to practice. Lengthier interventions are more likely to create practice change compared to short, single session training. Education and training should provide opportunities to acknowledge the commonality of GBV in the lives of health and social work professionals and include strategies to minimise trauma for survivors. Trauma and violence informed case studies and simulations should include representation of diverse populations to encourage an equity informed approach to a sensitive GBV response. This chapter has suggested that GBV education and training should be consistently evaluated for success and potential improvement. Despite the recent movement towards educating health professionals to respond to GBV, challenges such as overloaded curriculums, demand-driven healthcare organisations and a lack of survivor voices threaten the vital healing work that health professionals and social workers strive for every day with survivors. Practitioners who emerge from university having been educated about GBV, and healthcare organisations that commit to ongoing GBV training for their staff, are critical to a whole-of-health-system response to GBV.

Reflective Exercise

To conclude this chapter, we encourage you to engage in a reflective exercise [55] by thinking about:

- WHAT?
  What educational and practice knowledge do you already have about responding to GBV?
- SO WHAT?
  What aspects of GBV and how it relates to your practice do you feel you need more information, resources or support with?
  Thinking back to the 'Fear and Motivations in a Hat' exercise (Box 2.2), *what are your fears and your motivations about responding to survivor patients? How can you access the information, resources and support that you need?*
- NOW WHAT?
  Reflect on your learnings from this book; how will you apply new learnings to your practice?

References

1. World Health Organization. Caring for women subjected to violence: a WHO curriculum for training health-care providers. Geneva: World Health Organization; 2019.
2. Krug E, Dahlberg L, Mercy J, Zwi A, Lozano R. World report on violence and health. Geneva: World Health Organization; 2002.
3. Bond E, Ellis F, McCusker J. I'll be a survivor for the rest of my life. Adult survivors of child sexual abuse and their experience of support services. Suffolk: Survivors in Transition & University of Suffolk; 2018.
4. World Health Organization. Responding to intimate partner violence and sexual violence against women. WHO clinical and policy guidelines. Geneva: World Health Organization; 2013.

5. García-Moreno C, Hegarty K, D'Oliveira A, Koziol-McLain J, Colombini M, Feder G. The health-systems response to violence against women. Lancet. 2015;385:1567–79.

6. Ogbe E, Harmon S, Van den Bergh R, Degomme O. A systematic review of intimate partner violence interventions focused on improving social support and mental health outcomes of survivors. PLoS One. 2020;15(6):e0235177.

7. Ramsay J, Carter Y, Davidson L, Dunne D, Eldridge S, Hegarty K, et al. Advocacy interventions to reduce or eliminate violence and promote the physical and psychosocial well-being of women who experience intimate partner abuse. Cochrane Database Syst Rev. 2009;2009(3).

8. Howarth E, Stimpson L, Barran D, Robinson A. Safety in numbers: summary of findings and recommendations from a multi-site evaluation of independent domestic violence advisors. London: The Henry Smith Charity; 2009.

9. World Health Organization. Global plan of action to strengthen the role of the health system within a national multisectoral response to address interpersonal violence, in particular against women and girls, and against children. Geneva: World Health Organization; 2016.

10. Hegarty K, McKibbin G, Hameed M, Koziol-McLain J, Feder G, Tarzia L, et al. Health practitioners' readiness to address domestic violence and abuse: a qualitative meta-synthesis. PLoS One. 2020;15(6):e0234067.

11. Sawyer S, Coles J, Williams A, Williams B. A systematic review of intimate partner violence educational interventions delivered to allied health care practitioners. Med Educ. 2016;50(11):1107–21.

12. Sammut D, Kuruppu J, Hegarty K, Bradbury-Jones C. Which violence against women educational strategies are effective for prequalifying health-care students? A systematic review. Trauma Violence Abuse. 2019;152483801984319.

13. Kalra N, Di Tanna GL, García-Moreno C. Training healthcare providers to respond to intimate partner violence against women. Cochrane Database Syst Rev. 2017;2017(2):CD012423.

14. Commonwealth of Australia. Fourth action plan—national plan to reduce violence against women and their children 2010–2022. Canberra: Department of Social Services; 2019.

15. Republic of South Africa. National strategic plan on gender-based violence & femicide. Pretoria: Republic of South Africa; 2020.

16. Government of Canada. Setting the stage for a federal strategy against gender-based violence. Ottawa: Government of Canada; 2017.

17. Crombie N, Hooker L, Reisenhofer S. Nurse and midwifery education and intimate partner violence: a scoping review. J Clin Nurs. 2017;26(15–16):2100–25.

18. Cortis N, Blaxland M, Breckenridge J, Valentine K, Mahoney N, Chung D, et al. National survey of workers in the domestic, family and sexual violence sectors. Sydney: Social Policy Research Centre and Gendered Violence Research Network, UNSW; 2018. Contract No.: SPRC Report 5/2018.

19. Wendt S, Natalier K, Seymour K, King D, Macaitis K. Strengthening the domestic and family violence workforce: key questions. Aust Soc Work. 2020;73(2):236–44.

20. Leung TP-Y, Phillips L, Bryant C, Hegarty K. How family doctors perceived their 'readiness' and 'preparedness' to identify and respond to intimate partner abuse: a qualitative study. Fam Pract. 2018;35(4):517–23.

21. Bradbury-Jones C, Broadhurst K. Are we failing to prepare nursing and midwifery students to deal with domestic abuse? Findings from a qualitative study. J Adv Nurs. 2015;71(9):2062–72.

22. Bradbury-Jones C, Hallett N, Sammut D, Billings H, Hegarty K, Kishchenko S, et al. Gender-based violence: a five-country, cross-sectional survey of health and social care students' experience, knowledge and confidence in dealing with the issue. J Gender Based Violence. 2018:1–19.

23. Valpied J, Aprico K, Clewett J, Hegarty K. Are future doctors taught to respond to intimate partner violence? A study of Australian medical schools. J Interpers Violence. 2017;32(16):2419–32.

24. Hutchinson M, Doran F, Brown J, Douglas T, East L, Irwin P, et al. A cross-sectional study of domestic violence instruction in nursing and midwifery programs: out of step with community and student expectations. Nurse Educ Today. 2020;84:104209.

25. Taylor J, Bradbury-Jones C, Kroll T, Duncan F. Health professionals' beliefs about domestic abuse and the issue of disclosure: a critical incident technique study. Health Soc Care Community. 2013;21(5):489–99.
26. Sprague S, Madden K, Simunovic N, Godin K, Pham NK, Bhandari M, et al. Barriers to screening for intimate partner violence. Women Health. 2012;52(6):587–605.
27. World Health Organization. Health care for women subjected to intimate partner violence or sexual violence. A clinical handbook. Geneva: World Health Organization; 2014.
28. Rivas C, Ramsay J, Sadowski L, Davidson L, Dunne D, Eldridge S, et al. Advocacy interventions to reduce or eliminate violence and promote the physical and psychosocial well-being of women who experience intimate partner abuse (Review). Cochrane Database Syst Rev. 2015;2015(12):CD005043.
29. Li Y, Cannon LM, Coolidge EM, Darling-Fisher CS, Pardee M, Kuzma EK. Current state of trauma-informed education in the health sciences: lessons for nursing. J Nurs Educ. 2019;58(2):93–101.
30. Connolly M, Harms L, Maidment J. Social work: contexts and practice. Melbourne: Oxford University Press; 2017.
31. Hegarty K, Feder G, Ramsay J. Identification of partner abuse in health care settings: should health professionals be screening? In: Roberts G, Hegarty K, Feder G, editors. Intimate partner abuse and health professionals new approaches to domestic violence. London: Churchill Livingstone Elsevier; 2006. p. 79–92.
32. O'Doherty LJ, Taft A, Hegarty K, Ramsay J, Davidson LL, Feder G. Screening women for intimate partner violence in healthcare settings: abridged Cochrane systematic review and meta-analysis. Br Med J. 2014;348:1–11.
33. McLindon E, Humphreys C, Hegarty K. Is a clinician's personal history of domestic violence associated with their clinical care of patients: a cross-sectional study. BMJ Open. 2019;9(7):e029276.
34. Prochaska JO, Redding CA, Evers KE. The transtheoretical model and stages of change. In: Glanz K, Rimer B, Viswanath K, editors. Health behaviour and health education theory research and practice. 4th ed. San Francisco: Wiley; 2008. p. 97–118.
35. Short LM, Alpert E, Harris JM Jr, Surprenant ZJ. A tool for measuring physician readiness to manage intimate partner violence. Am J Prev Med. 2006;30(2):173–80.
36. Hegarty K, O'Doherty LJ, Gunn J, Pierce D, Taft AJ. A brief counselling intervention by health professionals utilising the 'readiness to change' concept for women experiencing intimate partner abuse: the weave project. J Fam Stud. 2008;14(2–3):376–88.
37. Feder G, Hutson M, Ramsay J, Taket AR. Women exposed to intimate partner violence. Expectations and experiences when they encounter health care professionals: a meta-analysis of qualitative studies. Arch Intern Med. 2006;166(1):22–37.
38. Browne AJ, Varcoe C, Ford-Gilboe M, Wathen CN, EQUIP Research Team. EQUIP healthcare: an overview of a multi-component intervention to enhance equity-oriented care in primary health care settings. Int J Equity Health 2015;14.
39. Quadara A. Implementing trauma-informed systems of care in health settings: the WITH study. State of knowledge paper. Sydney: Australia's National Research Organisation for Women's Safety Limited (ANROWS); 2015.
40. Harris M, Fallot RD. Trauma-informed inpatient services. New Dir Ment Health Serv. 2001;89:33–46.
41. McCann IL, Pearlman LA. Vicarious traumatization: a framework for understanding the psychological effects of working with victims. J Trauma Stress. 1990;3(1):131–49.
42. Sinclair S, Raffin-Bouchal S, Venturato L, Mijovic-Kondejewski J, Smith-MacDonald L. Compassion fatigue: a meta-narrative review of the healthcare literature. Int J Nurs Stud. 2017;69:9–24.
43. Gates DM, Gillespie GL. Secondary traumatic stress in nurses who care for traumatized women. J Obstet Gynecol Neonat Nurs. 2008;37(2):243–9.
44. Kulkarni S, Bell H, Hartman JL, Herman-Smith RL. Exploring individual and organizational factors contributing to compassion satisfaction, secondary traumatic stress, and burnout in domestic violence service providers. J Soc Soc Work Res. 2013;4(2):114–30.

45. Crenshaw K. Mapping the margins—intersectionality, identity politics, and violence against women of color. Stanford Law Rev. 1991;43(6):1241–99.
46. Bradbury-Jones C, Hallett N, Sammut D, Billings H, Hegarty K, Kishchenko S, et al. Gender-based violence: a five-country, cross-sectional survey of health and social care students' experience, knowledge and confidence in dealing with the issue. J Gender Based Violence. 27 Feb 2020.
47. Fiolet R, Cameron J, Tarzia L, Gallant D, Hameed M, Hooker L, Koziol-McLain J, Glover K, Spangaro J, Hegarty K. Indigenous people's experiences and expectations of health care professionals when accessing care for family violence: a qualitative evidence synthesis. Trauma Violence Abuse. 2020;152483802096187.
48. Fiolet R, Tarzia L, Hameed M, Hegarty K. Indigenous peoples' help-seeking behaviors for family violence: a scoping review. Trauma Violence Abuse. 2019.
49. McLindon E, Humphreys C, Hegarty K. "It happens to clinicians too": an Australian prevalence study of intimate partner and family violence against health professionals. BMC Womens Health. 2018;18:113.
50. Elliott D, Guy J. Mental-health professionals versus non-mental-health professionals—childhood trauma and adult functioning. Prof Psychol Res Pract. 1993;24(1):83–90.
51. Jenkins SR, Mitchell JL, Baird S, Whitfield SR, Meyer HL. The counselor's trauma as counseling motivation: vulnerability or stress inoculation? J Interpers Violence. 2011;26(12):2392–412.
52. Newcomb M, Burton J, Edwards N, Hazelwood Z. How Jung's concept of the wounded healer can guide learning and teaching in social work and human services. Adv Soci Work Welf Educ. 2015;17:55–69.
53. Warshaw C, Taft A, McCosker-Howard H. Educating health professionals: changing attitudes and overcoming barriers. In: Roberts G, Hegarty K, Feder G, editors. Intimate partner abuse and health professionals: new approaches to domestic violence. London: Elsevier; 2006.
54. VEGA. Family violence education resources Canada: VEGA; 2020. https://vegaeducation.mcmaster.ca/?lang=en.
55. Rolfe G, Freshwater D, Jasper M. Critical reflection in nursing and the helping professions: a user's guide. Basingstoke: Palgrave Macmillan; 2001.

Suggested Reading

Cochrane Review. Training healthcare providers to respond to intimate partner violence against women. Cochrane Database Syst Rev. Nov 2020.
Sammut D, Kuruppu J, Hegarty K, Bradbury-Jones C. Which violence against women educational strategies are effective for prequalifying health-care students? A systematic review. Trauma Violence Abuse. 2019;152483801984319.

Additional Resources

World Health Organization. Responding to intimate partner violence and sexual violence against women. WHO clinical and policy guidelines. Geneva: World Health Organization; 2013.
World Health Organization Health care for women subjected to intimate partner violence or sexual violence. A clinical handbook. Geneva, Switzerland: World Health Organization; 2014.
World Health Organization. Caring for women subjected to violence: a WHO curriculum for training health-care providers. Geneva: World Health Organization; 2019.

Part II

Understanding Violence and Abuse in the Context of Gender

Claire Sullivan, Karen Block, and Cathy Vaughan

3.1 Introduction

Refugees and displaced populations often experience gender-based violence in different forms across contexts of conflict, displacement and temporary and permanent resettlement. Gender-based violence (GBV) encompasses 'any harmful act perpetrated against a person based on socially ascribed gender differences between males and females [and] includes acts that inflict physical, sexual or mental harm or suffering, threats of such acts, coercion and other deprivations of liberty' (IASC, [1]). Experiences of GBV can have significant consequences for survivors' mental, physical and sexual/reproductive health, both in the short and long term [2, 3]. In addition to health, well-being domains such as employment, education, access to economic resources and housing may all be affected directly and indirectly by GBV, with such effects exacerbated by the structural inequalities that refugee communities face [4]. It is vital that countries of resettlement recognise and respond to these experiences and take measures to prevent violence where possible. Indeed, service providers working with refugees and displaced people need to be equipped to attend to survivors' past experiences of GBV, as well as violence that begins or continues after resettlement.

3.2 Forced Displacement

Globally, an unprecedented number of people are being forcibly displaced from their homes; an estimated 79.5 million people are currently displaced, including internally displaced people, refugees and asylum seekers [5]. United Nations

C. Sullivan (✉) · K. Block · C. Vaughan
Centre for Health Equity, Melbourne School of Population and Global Health, The University of Melbourne, Parkville, VIC, Australia
e-mail: claire.sullivan@unimelb.edu.au; keblock@unimelb.edu.au; cmvaug@unimelb.edu.au

© Springer Nature Switzerland AG 2021
C. Bradbury-Jones, L. Isham (eds.), *Understanding Gender-Based Violence*,
https://doi.org/10.1007/978-3-030-65006-3_3

High Commissioner for Refugees (UNHCR) reports that in 2019, 317,200 refugees returned to their country of origin, and only 107,800 were resettled permanently in a new country, representing a minute fraction of globally displaced refugees [5]. Many therefore live in precarious locations indefinitely, such as refugee camps or urban settlements, with uncertain prospects. Though the majority of refugees continue to reside in developing countries, a handful of high-income nations offer permanent resettlement programs.

Use of the term 'refugee' is contested due to its narrow legal definition under the Refugee Convention 1951, which fails to capture many people who have been forcibly displaced. We employ the term refugee broadly in this chapter to encompass all those forcibly displaced or forced to migrate, both across and within borders, including asylum seekers unless specified.

The 'refugee journey' includes experiences of conflict, displacement, transit and resettlement. Though the refugee journey is regularly discussed in these terms, it is vital to note that these phases are often not experienced linearly, permanent resettlement is relatively rare and each individual's experience is distinct. BenEzer and Zetter [6] posit that the refugee journey has historically been neglected by scholarship as it has tended to be understood as a transient phase, with researchers preferring to focus on 'the causes and the consequences of exile'. And yet, refugee pathways are often long and arduous, characterised by protracted uncertainty, insecurity and trauma, which can have profound consequences for refugees' future well-being [6]. One such experience which is common throughout the refugee journey and resettlement processes is GBV [7].

3.3   Risk of GBV During the Refugee Journey

Refugees are known to confront particular risks of GBV. Pre-migration factors intersect with the risk posed by migration itself and post-migration factors, to shape refugees' experiences of violence. Physical insecurities inherent in conflict and displacement zones create vulnerabilities to form of GBV, such as rape, trafficking, forced marriage and other forms of exploitation [8]. Sexual violence may be perpetrated against women and men as a tactic of war, with GBV often being the catalyst for families and communities to flee. Due to the comprehensive failure of nation states to ensure refugees' safe passage, protection and resettlement, both those who are required to travel illegally through smuggling channels and those who travel through official humanitarian channels face immense physical insecurities. Protection by formal authorities and informal social systems is often compromised [7]. In the resettlement setting, a confluence of post-migration factors affect refugees' vulnerability to violence, such as separation from social support networks, changing gender roles, trauma and mental health challenges, settlement stressors, and structural inequalities including racism [9, 10].

3.4   Perpetrators and Survivors of GBV Across the Refugee Journey

GBV against refugees may be perpetrated by people in positions of institutional authority (such as members of armed forces, police, humanitarian actors or members of security forces) as well as people in positions of informal power (such as community leaders or members of the host community) [11]. GBV is also commonly perpetrated by people within the personal networks of the refugee, such as intimate partners and family members.

Women and girls are most at risk of experiencing GBV, because of patriarchal positioning of men and women [12]. However, 'gender' should not be conflated with 'women and girls' within discussions of GBV, as this can reproduce binary thinking and fail to account for the complex dimensions of GBV [13, 14]. GBV can also be experienced by men and boys and may be perpetrated against people because of their identity as a lesbian, gay, bisexual, transgender, queer or intersex (LGBTQI) person. The violence that is experienced by men and LGBTQI people across the refugee journey often has gendered underpinnings, regardless of the victim's sex, sexuality or gender, and is based upon toxic masculinities and patriarchal norms. Sexual violence against men often involves processes of 'feminisation' that are tied to traditional ideas about masculinity [15]. Indeed, Carpenter [16] argues that tackling GBV against women and girls in conflict contexts is inextricable from addressing the types of violence that men and boys experience in these contexts.

It is also important to recognise how gender intersects with other social locations to create vulnerabilities to violence [17]. For example, LGBTQI refugees are likely to face additional vulnerabilities to GBV due to stigmatisation, discrimination and lack of access to services, as homophobia intersects with and is produced by gendered inequalities [18, 19]. People may also be particularly targeted by perpetrators of GBV on the basis of disability, age and/or membership of ethnic or religious minority groups throughout the refugee journey due to intersecting power imbalances and circumstances.

3.5   Forms of GBV Violence Experienced from Displacement to Resettlement

GBV can take the form of interpersonal acts of physical, sexual, psychological and economic violence, threats and coercion. It includes rape, sexual abuse and exploitation, forced and early marriage, intimate partner violence, trafficking and female genital cutting. Though not exhaustive, the discussion below focuses on key forms of GBV experienced by refugees, namely sexual violence, intimate partner violence and forced and early marriage, and explores how structural and symbolic violence can be both a form of GBV and reinforce experiences of GBV.

3.5.1 Sexual Violence

Rape, sexual harassment, abuse, threats and exploitation are well-documented forms of GBV that can be experienced by refugees, particularly during conflict, displacement and in transit [20, 21]. A systematic review and meta-analysis conducted in 2013 found that approximately 1 in 5 refugee women had experienced sexual violence in humanitarian settings; however, the authors considered this to be an underestimation of the actual prevalence of sexual violence, due to the significant barriers that victims face to disclosure [21].

Sexual violence can be perpetrated by figures in positions of authority and can include acts that take place under the auspices of their role, such as forced strip searches and other acts of violation [8]. Sexual violence against refugees can be opportunistic interpersonal acts or systematic:

'Sexual violence can be capricious or random—the "spoils of war"—resulting from the breakdown in social and moral systems…. In addition, sexual violence may be systematic, for the purposes of destabilizing populations and destroying bonds within communities and families; advancing ethnic cleansing; expressing hatred for the enemy; or supplying combatants with sexual services' [22].

Survival or transactional sex is also reportedly common in both refugee camps and urban locations, whereby men and women are required to undertake sexual acts in return for money, food, security or to cross borders [23, 24]. Fear of sexual violence has also been found to be a primary consideration and reason for fleeing a country [25]. Refugee women who are single during the refugee journey and in resettlement contexts may be particularly vulnerable to harassment and abuse, perpetrated by people both within and outside of their community. This can place women under pressure to enter unwanted relationships for security [26]. It must also be highlighted that sexual violence or threats of violence in these settings involves dimensions of psychological and other types of physical abuse in addition to sexual abuse.

Risks of sexual violence are exacerbated by the loss of traditional social systems that protect refugees, as well as lack of access to services or authorities. What is more, a lack of legal options for migration can also expose refugees to a greater risk of human trafficking and other forms of sexual violence, as people smuggling routes may be the only option available to displaced people seeking safety and immigration status [27].

3.5.2 Intimate Partner Violence and Family Violence

In addition to violence experienced in public or institutional spaces at the hands of strangers and acquaintances, refugees are at risk of experiencing GBV in the form of intimate partner violence (IPV). The available evidence indicates that refugee women are likely to experience more IPV than prior to forced migration

[25]. Links have been made between exposure to political violence or other types of conflict-related violence and greater exposure to intimate partner violence [28, 29]. Post-traumatic stress disorder, other trauma sequelae and post-migration stressors have been found to be associated with subsequent IPV [30, 31]. In a study exploring the experiences of Mozambican refugee women who were displaced due to conflict, Sideris [32] found that loss of social belonging, tied to the loss of economic roles, kinship systems and social obligations, created contexts and dynamics that increased the risk and consequences of IPV following displacement. In exploring the GBV experiences of displaced women in Colombia, Wirtz et al. [33] similarly found:

'Violence and displacement, often results in trauma, social disruption, experiences of job loss…, poverty, changing gender roles, and general frustration; these factors appear to exacerbate existing levels of IPV that exists in non-conflict settings for these displaced populations'.

Gendered vulnerabilities to violence may also be intensified during different phases of the refugee journey as women and girls may face greater barriers to social and economic participation and accessing services compared to men [18]. However, displacement and resettlement can at times provide women with more economic and social capital than previously enjoyed in their country of origin. While beneficial for women, this can be experienced by men as a loss of power and a point of tension that may trigger violence [34].

The forms of IPV experienced by refugees mirror GBV experienced by other populations, such as physical, psychological, financial, spiritual and sexual abuse, as well as coercive control [9, 33]. The violence may, however, have unique dimensions related to structural circumstances particular to the refugee experience and can involve additional forms of violence such as immigration-related violence (including destruction of identity documents, threats of deportation or cancellation of visa sponsorship) or early and forced marriage. Research suggests that IPV can also be exacerbated where sexual violence experienced in war or displacement is stigmatised within communities [32].

In addition to IPV, GBV can take the form of other types of family violence, including violence perpetrated by parents, children, siblings and in-laws. For example, Vaughan et al.'s [9] research exploring family violence in Australian resettlement settings found that adolescent refugee males were at times using violence against their mothers and siblings. This was sometimes the case within single-parent households where adolescent males were assuming the role of 'head of household' and using violence against their mothers and siblings to control the family. Similarly, some adolescent refugee females reported that they had experienced violence from their fathers, with fathers using violence to control daughters' behaviour in the resettlement context. GBV experienced within refugee families may also include multi-perpetrator violence, whereby more than one family member is responsible for inflicting violence, with some research finding multi-perpetrator violence to be more common within migrant communities [35].

3.5.3   Forced and Early Marriage

Another form of GBV that may be experienced across the refugee experience, including resettlement, is early and forced marriage. Evidence suggests that the Syrian refugee crisis has led to an increase in adolescent girls getting married before the age of 18. One survey conducted in Western Bekaa in Lebanon found that 24% of Syrian refugee girls were married between the ages of 15 and 17 [36]. Paradoxically, this form of GBV often arises out of families' concern for their daughters' safety, as unmarried women and girls may be more vulnerable to GBV and security is sought through marriage. Research with Syrian refugees found that the majority of men in refugee camps or urban settings were concerned about the safety of their partners and daughters [25]. As a result of this insecurity, young women and girls are increasingly vulnerable to early and forced marriage, demonstrating how forms of GBV, such as sexual violence or the threat of sexual violence, can produce other forms of GBV. In addition to concerns about women and girl's physical safety, financial, cultural and immigration pressures can also lead families to arrange marriages for their unmarried daughters in all phases of the refugee journey, including resettlement. Countries of resettlement have implemented various legal responses in recent decades that seek to address forced and early marriage through criminal, immigration and civil protection schemes, many of which have been criticised for focussing on perpetrators rather than addressing the conditions that lead to early/forced marriage [37, 38].

3.5.4   Structural and Symbolic Forms of Violence

It is vital to recognise that GBV is not simply the result of individual agents and intentions, but rather that individuals are embedded within structures that—both directly and indirectly—act upon and constrain their actions, including their use of or exposure to violence [39]. Structural violence here refers to the ways in which institutions, social structures and legal frameworks systemically privilege and oppress people who are located within certain social positions, codified through 'custom, practice, and law, so there need not be an identifiable perpetrator' [40]. Structural violence thereby orders access to power, opportunities, representation and resources [40], including access to safety. Various manifestations of structural violence characterise processes of conflict, displacement and resettlement (such as socio-economic inequalities, inadequate and discriminatory justice systems, nation states' bordering measures and punitive immigration policies) and have gendered dimensions that form and inform GBV.

Structural violence is underpinned by symbolic violence. Sometimes referred to as cultural violence, symbolic violence refers to elements of ideology and discourse that support and validate discrimination and stigma and is mobilised to justify structural as well as interpersonal forms of violence [41]. Gender-based discrimination and gendered attitudes towards men and women are forms of symbolic violence that underpin GBV, intersecting with sexism, racism, classism, ableism, ageism and other oppressive systems of belief. Indeed, although structural and symbolic violence are often gendered, it is also important to understand the operation of GBV through an intersectional lens [17]. In addition to gender, structural and symbolic violence is constituted by race, class, sexuality and other social locations, which interlock with historical sociopolitical conditions, such as colonialism and neoliberalism [42].

As such, refugees may not only experience direct forms of GBV perpetrated by individuals but also through institutions and social structures that discriminate and fail to protect their safety and respond to their needs. Often the violence that is perpetrated by systems and institutions is not experienced as a distinct act. Indeed, the functioning of structural/symbolic violence in producing and reinforcing GBV can be obscured by framing GBV as a confined traumatic event or series of episodes rather than conceptualising GBV as a *continuum of violence*. Understanding GBV through a narrow frame fails to account for the ways in which violence persists and transforms over time, where evolving acts of interpersonal violence interact with varying manifestations of structural/symbolic violence. A continuum of GBV should thus be understood through an 'extended timeframe' which accounts for 'the interwoven spaces and contexts of displacement and resettlement' [14].

Women from refugee backgrounds in research we conducted in an Australian resettlement setting have emphasised how the harm of ongoing IPV experienced in resettlement settings—be it financial, physical, sexual, emotional or reproductive— is often intertwined, temporally and experientially, with institutional systems' failure to protect their safety and meet their material, legal and/or immigration needs [9, 10]. These structural and symbolic failures may persist regardless of whether victims leave violent relationships or choose to stay. We have also found that perpetrators sometimes use threats enabled by structural violence to control and manipulate victims, such as threatening to report victims to immigration authorities [9]. Our findings suggest that refugee victims' fear of punitive institutions in resettlement settings could prevent them from obtaining help, emphasising how structural and interpersonal violence can be interwoven. Indeed, other literature confirms that racialised populations such as refugee communities may be subject to criminalisation, negative immigration consequences and the interference of welfare following disclosure of GBV [43–50].

3.6   Implications for Practitioners Responding to GBV

Service provision in humanitarian settings is not necessarily consistent or well-coordinated, and refugee community members may have little awareness of or trust in services [25]. Indeed, formal assistance services may simply be unavailable or inaccessible throughout certain phases of the refugee journey [33]. Though the evidence-base is limited, interventions aimed at preventing and responding to GBV within humanitarian settings continue to evolve [51–56]. However, contextual considerations that pertain to service provision in humanitarian settings differ from those in the resettlement settings. The remainder of this chapter will focus on the resettlement context in particular and explore factors that act as barriers or facilitators to meeting the needs of refugees who are experiencing or who have experienced GBV and implications for service providers.

3.6.1   Barriers to Help-Seeking in Resettlement Settings

Alongside recognising the particular forms of GBV experienced by refugees, practitioners need an understanding of the key barriers, both individual and structural, that refugees may face when seeking help for GBV in resettlement settings. It must also be borne in mind that refugees are not a homogenous group facing identical barriers, refugees are highly diverse.

Some barriers faced by refugee populations are easily recognisable, such as lack of proficiency in the dominant language and lack of knowledge of the legal and social systems in countries of settlement [57, 58]. Other barriers are complex and function in less predictable ways, such as the potential role of social networks. Evidence suggests that a loss of social belonging and networks can perpetuate experiences of violence, as victims may not have social supports to call upon to address violence or assist them to seek help [4]. In contrast, those who *do* retain strong community networks in resettlement contexts may also face barriers to seeking help. Indeed, victims commonly report stigma surrounding violence and relationship breakdown in their community, which may dissuade them from disclosing violence [59]. Separation from an abusive partner may lead to unwanted social isolation from communities where divorce is not accepted [9]. Many victims are also legitimately concerned that disclosing violence that occurs within their families will further stigmatise and racialise their community in the eyes of the broader public [60–62]. Mason and Pulvirenti [62] highlight the contradictory and multifaceted role that 'community' can play in refugee women's lives, as simultaneously a site of strength and resilience and also one of control, and as such, efforts need to focus on 'protective strategies that help build resilience for the community as a whole [including] resilience against domestic violence'.

Settlement stressors such as lack of employment or economic opportunities have also been found to contribute to or reinforce GBV in resettlement settings [4]. Efforts to address structural and socio-economic inequalities that refugees face are therefore critical. For individual practitioners, this involves paying attention to specific circumstances of individual clients from refugee backgrounds and attempting to 'move beyond a focus on broad social structures to one that comprehends how these structures impact on and are impacted on by local specificities' [32]. As such, a vital aspect of responding to violence within refugee communities is attempting to comprehend the unique barriers, circumstances and risks faced by each individual affected by GBV and provide responsive and flexible supports.

Asylum seekers and those without immigration documentation, for example face particular barriers to seeking help in countries of resettlement [63, 64]. In the context of the hostile environment policy in the United Kingdom, the police have reported victims of violence without settled status to the Home Office for action, as have NGOs providing social services [43, 65]. What is more, victims' asylum applications are often dependent on the perpetrator's application, as one application is regularly drafted in the name of the 'head' of the family, irrespective of the strength of other family members' claims. Asylum seekers and undocumented migrants are also often ineligible for violence-related services in resettlement contexts due to their temporary immigration status [3, 63].

Past experiences of structural and symbolic violence, including experiences of immigration detention, can affect help-seeking options and decision making for those both with and without settled immigration status:

'You know, we say "Oh go to the police." Well I don't think so. It's not safe for them. It hasn't often been safe in their [country of origin] and I don't think there's safety here especially when people have been in detention…so there's less access to safety options for them and the safety options that we just assume [are safe], are not necessarily safe for these people at all' (participant in 9).

The punitive nature of immigration systems within countries of resettlement, and precarity of immigration status, even for those with permanent residency, means that refugees may fear that disclosing violence could lead to the deportation of either themselves or their partner, which may be far from desired [66]. As such, even for those who do have permanent immigration status in their country of resettlement, the immigration ramifications of pursuing certain responses to violence should be considered by practitioners.

3.6.2 Facilitators and Promising Practices in Resettlement Settings

Service providers need to recognise opportunities to provide support at different points across the resettlement experience. Evidence suggests that refugees may not actively or directly seek help for GBV for a number of reasons. People from refugee backgrounds may not conceive of themselves as victims of GBV due to narrow understandings of violence or lack of knowledge of their legal rights (rape within marriage, for example may be normalised) [67]. Alternatively, refugees may have other needs which they prioritise, such as addressing their accommodation, employment, immigration/legal needs or the needs of their children. However, this does not mean that GBV is not a priority; one study found that although newly arrived migrants and refugees reported that they prioritised access to employment and mental health information, they also wanted information regarding family violence to be integrated into the general health information they received [68]. This desire for violence information to be embedded in other health services may be linked to stigma and shame surrounding GBV, noted above. As such, clients from refugee backgrounds may present with various issues that appear unrelated to violence, but which may provide an opportunity to sensitively provide information and assistance regarding GBV where appropriate. Indeed, receiving healthcare or social services are often acceptable forums for refugees to seek help, without risk of stigmatisation [69].

Creating safe spaces in healthcare settings to enable refugees to seek support for GBV experiences is therefore important. Almoshmosh et al. [69] note that safe spaces can be established by practitioners and organisations through several key measures, such as providing clear explanations of the role of the particular service and confidentiality responsibilities; employing qualified interpreters and bicultural workers; recognising different cultural norms; providing adequate time and space for refugees to discuss their experiences in their terms and ensuring opportunities for consultation without other family members present. Trauma-informed approaches have also been found to be important in creating safe spaces for refugees and tend to integrate many of these measures [60, 70]. A trauma-informed approach recognises the impact that trauma has played in refugees' lives and promotes safe and collaborative interactions with clients. Trauma-informed measures include preserving clients' control over interactions to avoid replicating power dynamics inherent in experiences of trauma; supporting clients' autonomy and choices and emphasising their strengths and recognising the interplay of structural factors with trauma experienced by refugees [60].

Creating a safe space for refugees to disclose violence also requires providing culturally responsive services. Research has found that employing a bilingual and bicultural workforce is a key aspect of providing culturally responsive services and building trust with clients from refugee backgrounds [9, 10, 51, 71, 72]. Irrespective of whether there is shared language and culture, bilingual/bicultural employees may share an understanding of the experience of migration with clients from refugee backgrounds, as well as experiences of structural and symbolic violence such as institutional discrimination [9, 10]. Culturally responsive service provision can also involve recognising the victims' cultural understandings of GBV, rather than imposing the values of the practitioner or organisation [73]. In this process, it is vital that refugees' 'culture' is not viewed as fixed or homogenous by service providers; cultural belief systems are evolving and do not operate in a vacuum separate from structural factors. Reified understandings of culture can lead practitioners to assume that GBV is caused by traditional belief systems within refugee communities, which racialises violence and refugee communities, and can act as a further barrier to help-seeking and support [74].

It is also crucial that policymakers and service providers who seek to address GBV in refugee communities listen to refugee communities themselves. Building relationships with refugee communities enhances trust and accessibility of services. Furthermore, ensuring that refugee community organisations and leaders meaningfully participate in the design, planning and implementation of programming concerning GBV response and prevention supports the development of interventions that are tailored to communities' needs and priorities [3, 75].

3.7 Conclusion

Refugees face multiple forms of GBV, which both include and interact with structural/symbolic forms of violence, and manifest in a continuum of violence experienced throughout the refugee journey. Conceptualising GBV as a continuum recognises that the experiences and impacts of GBV are also not temporally confined; victims and their families can experience ongoing GBV and effects across their lifetime and intergenerationally. Practitioners working in this field need to be particularly cognisant of the structural factors which constrain victims' choices in response to GBV and take into account the individual circumstances of each client to avoid homogenising approaches that can serve to racialise refugee communities. Evidence suggests that creating safe spaces for disclosure of violence in health and other settings is key to providing ongoing support across the continuum of GBV, which can be fostered through trauma-informed, culturally responsive care. Approaches and interventions that address GBV that are led by refugee communities themselves are likely to be the most effective. Ultimately, the healing of individuals is tied to the healing of communities, which involves tackling systemic inequalities faced by refugees at all levels within countries of resettlement.

Reflective Questions

How are, or could, principles of trauma-informed care be incorporated into your professional practice?

What systemic barriers might clients from refugee backgrounds face when accessing your service?

What actions can you take as a practitioner to address these? What action might be needed at an organisational level to try to bring about systemic change?

References

1. Inter-Agency Standing Committee (IASC). Guidelines for integrating gender-based violence interventions in humanitarian action: reducing risk, promoting resilience and aiding recovery. 2015. https://gbvguidelines.org/wp/wp-content/uploads/2015/09/2015-IASC-Gender-based-Violence-Guidelines_lo-res.pdf.
2. Ellsberg M, Jansen HA, Heise L, Watts CH, Garcia-Moreno C. Intimate partner violence and women's physical and mental health in the WHO multi-country study on women's health and domestic violence: an observational study. Lancet. 2008;371(9619):1165–72.
3. Keygnaert I, Vettenburg N, Temmerman M. Hidden violence is silent rape: sexual and gender-based violence in refugees, asylum seekers and undocumented migrants in Belgium and the Netherlands. Cult Health Sex. 2012;14(5):505–20.
4. Phillimore J, Pertek S, Alidu L. Sexual and gender-based violence and refugees: the impacts of and on integration domains. 2018. (IRiS Working Paper Series). Report No.: 28/2018. p. 34.
5. UNHCR. Refugee population statistics database. United Nations High Commissioner for Refugees. 2020. [cited 15 Jul 2020]. https://www.unhcr.org/refugee-statistics/.
6. BenEzer G, Zetter R. Searching for directions: conceptual and methodological challenges in researching refugee journeys. J Refug Stud. 2015;28(3):297–318.

7. Freedman J. Sexual and gender-based violence against refugee women: a hidden aspect of the refugee "crisis". Reprod Health Matters. 2016;24(47):18–26.
8. Manjoo R, McRaith C. Gender-based violence and justice in conflict and post-conflict areas. Cornell Int Law J. 2011;44(1):11–32.
9. Vaughan C, Davis E, Murdolo A, Chen J, Murray L, Quiazon R, et al. Promoting community-led responses to violence against immigrant and refugee women in metropolitan and regional Australia. The ASPIRE Project: research report. Sydney: Australia's National Research Organisation for Women's Safety; 2016. Report No.: 07/2016.
10. Vaughan C, Chen J, Block K, Sullivan C, Suha M, Sandhu M, et al. Multicultural and settlement services Supporting women experiencing violence. Sydney: ANROWS; 2020. p. 112. (Research report). Report No.: 11/2020.
11. UNHCR. Sexual and gender based violence (SGBV) prevention and response—UNHCR emergency handbook. 4th ed. Geneva: United Nations High Commissioner for Refugees; 2020. [cited 17 Jun 2020]. https://emergency.unhcr.org/entry/60283/sexual-and-gender-based-violence-sgbv-prevention-and-response.
12. Ward J, Vann B. Gender-based violence in refugee settings. Lancet. 2002;360:s13–4.
13. Moore MW, Barner JR. Sexual minorities in conflict zones: a review of the literature. Aggress Violent Behav. 2017;35:33–7.
14. Ozcurumez S, Akyuz S, Bradby H. The conceptualization problem in research and responses to sexual and gender-based violence in forced migration. J Gend Stud. 2020;21:1–13.
15. Linos N. Rethinking gender-based violence during war: is violence against civilian men a problem worth addressing? Soc Sci Med. 2009;68(8):1548–51.
16. Carpenter RC. Recognizing gender-based violence against civilian men and boys in conflict situations. Secur Dialogue. 2006;37(1):83–103.
17. Crenshaw K. Mapping the margins: intersectionality, identity politics, and violence against women of color. Stanford Law Rev. 1991;43(6):1241–99.
18. Ozcurumez S, Bradby H, Akyuz S. What is the nature of SGBV? Birmingham: University of Birmingham; 2019. p. 33. Report No.: 27/2019.
19. UNHCR. Action against sexual and gender-based violence: an updated strategy. Geneva: United Nations High Commissioner for Refugees; 2011.
20. De Schrijver L, Vander Beken T, Krahé B, Keygnaert I. Prevalence of sexual violence in migrants, applicants for international protection, and refugees in Europe: a critical interpretive synthesis of the evidence. Int J Environ Res Public Health. 2018;15(9):1979.
21. Vu A, Adam A, Wirtz A, Pham K, Rubenstein L, Glass N, et al. The prevalence of sexual violence among female refugees in complex humanitarian emergencies: a systematic review and meta-analysis. PLoS Curr. 2014;6. [cited 22 Jul 2020]. https://www.ncbi.nlm.nih.gov/pmc/articles/PMC4012695/.
22. Ward J. If not now, when? Addressing gender-based violence in refugee, internally displaced, and post-conflict settings: a global overview. New York: Reproductive Health for Refugees Consortium; 2002.
23. Anani G. Dimensions of gender-based violence against Syrian refugees in Lebanon. Forced Migr Rev. 2013;44:75.
24. Sami S, Williams HA, Krause S, Onyango MA, Burton A, Tomczyk B. Responding to the Syrian crisis: the needs of women and girls. Lancet. 2014;383(9923):1179–81.
25. UN Women. 'We just keep silent': gender-based violence amongst Syrian refugees in the Kurdistan Region of Iraq. Kurdistan Region: UN Women; 2014.
26. Bartolomei L, Eckert R, Pittaway E. "What happens there ... follows us here": resettled but still at risk: refugee women and girls in Australia. Refuge Can J Refug. 2014;30(2):45–56.
27. Mandic D. Trafficking and Syrian refugee smuggling: evidence from the Balkan route. Soc Incl Lisbon. 2017;5(2):28–38.
28. Annan J, Brier M. The risk of return: intimate partner violence in Northern Uganda's armed conflict. Soc Sci Med. 2010;70(1):152–9.
29. Gupta J, Acevedo-Garcia D, Hemenway D, Decker MR, Raj A, Silverman JG. Premigration exposure to political violence and perpetration of intimate partner violence among immigrant men in Boston. Am J Public Health. 2009;3:462.

30. Carswell K, Blackburn P, Barker C. The relationship between trauma, post-migration problems and the psychological well-being of refugees and asylum seekers. Int J Soc Psychiatry. 2009;57(2):107–19. [cited 22 Jul 2020]. https://journals.sagepub.com/doi/10.1177/0020764009105699.
31. Wachter K, Gulbas LE. Social support under siege: an analysis of forced migration among women from the Democratic Republic of Congo. Soc Sci Med. 2018;208:107–16.
32. Sideris T. War, gender and culture: Mozambican women refugees. Soc Sci Med. 2003;56(4):713–24.
33. Wirtz AL, Pham K, Glass N, Loochkartt S, Kidane T, Cuspoca D, et al. Gender-based violence in conflict and displacement: qualitative findings from displaced women in Colombia. Confl Health. 2014;8(1):10.
34. Krause U. A continuum of violence? Linking sexual and gender-based violence during conflict, flight, and encampment. Refug Surv Q. 2015;34(4):1–19.
35. Salter M. Multi-perpetrator domestic violence. Trauma Violence Abuse. 2014;15(2):102–12.
36. UNFPA. New study finds child marriage rising among most vulnerable Syrian refugees. United Nations Population Fund. 2017. [cited 24 Aug 2020]. https://www.unfpa.org/news/new-study-finds-child-marriage-rising-among-most-vulnerable-syrian-refugees.
37. Gill A, Anitha S, editors. Forced marriage: introducing a social justice and human rights perspective. London: Zed Books Ltd.; 2012. 142 p.
38. Gill A, Engeland AV. Criminalization or 'multiculturalism without culture'? Comparing British and French approaches to tackling forced marriage. J Soc Welf Fam Law. 2014;36(3):241–59.
39. Heise L. Violence against women: an integrated, ecological framework. Violence Women. 1998;4(3):262–90.
40. Jones C. Levels of racism: a theoretic framework and a Gardner's tale. Am J Public Health. 2000;90(8):121–5.
41. Galtung J. Cultural violence. J Peace Res. 1990;27(3):291–305.
42. Sokoloff N, Dupont I. Domestic violence at the intersections of race, class, and gender—challenges and contributions to understanding violence against marginalized women in diverse communities. Violence Women. 2005;11(1):38–64.
43. Day AS, Gill AK. Applying intersectionality to partnerships between women's organizations and the criminal justice system in relation to domestic violence. Br J Criminol. 2020;60(4):830–50.
44. Holiday YS. Refugees and the misuse of the criminal law. In: Kogovšek Šalamon N, editor. Causes and consequences of migrant criminalization. Cham: Springer; 2020. p. 193–212. . [cited 24 Jul 2020]. (Ius Gentium: Comparative Perspectives on Law and Justice). https://doi.org/10.1007/978-3-030-43732 9_10.
45. INCITE! Statement on gender violence and the prison industrial complex. INCITE!; 2001. [cited 24 Jul 2020]. https://incite-national.org/incite-critical-resistance-statement/.
46. Lewig K, Arney F, Salveron M. Challenges to parenting in a new culture: implications for child and family welfare. Eval Program Plann. 2010;33(3):324–32.
47. Losoncz I. Building safety around children in families from refugee backgrounds: ensuring children's safety requires working in partnership with families and communities. Child Abuse Negl. 2016;51:416–26.
48. Losoncz I. Institutional disrespect: South Sudanese experiences of the structural marginalisation of refugee migrants in Australia. 2019. [cited 20 Oct 2019]. https://doi.org/10.1007/978-981-13-7717-4.
49. Mehrotra GR, Kimball E, Wahab S. The braid that binds us: the impact of neoliberalism, criminalization, and professionalization on domestic violence work. Affilia. 2016;31(2):153–63.
50. Pickering S. The new criminals: refugees and asylum seekers. In: Anthony T, Cunneen C, editors. The critical criminology companion. Leichhardt: Hawkins Press; 2008.
51. Block K, Nasr H, Vaughan C, Sullivan C, Alsaraf S. What responses, approaches to treatment, and other supports are effective in assisting refugees who have experienced sexual and gender-based violence? Birmingham: Institute for Research into Superdiversity; 2018. (IRiS Working Paper Series). Report No.: 30/2019.

52. Glass N, Perrin N, Marsh M, Clough A, Desgroppes A, Kaburu F, et al. Effectiveness of the Communities Care programme on change in social norms associated with gender-based violence (GBV) with residents in intervention compared with control districts in Mogadishu, Somalia. BMJ Open. 2019;9(3):e023819.
53. Marsh M, Purdin S, Navani S. Addressing sexual violence in humanitarian emergencies. Glob Public Health. 2006;1(2):133–46.
54. Noble E, Ward L, French S, Falb K. State of the evidence: a systematic review of approaches to reduce gender-based violence and support the empowerment of adolescent girls in humanitarian settings. Trauma Violence Abuse. 2019;20(3):428–34.
55. Schopper D. Responding to the needs of survivors of sexual violence: do we know what works? Int Rev Red Cross. 2014;96(894):585–600.
56. Wirtz AL, Glass N, Pham K, Perrin N, Rubenstein LS, Singh S, et al. Comprehensive development and testing of the ASIST-GBV, a screening tool for responding to gender-based violence among women in humanitarian settings. Confl Health. 2016;10(1):7.
57. Kulwicki A, Aswad B, Carmona T, Ballout S. Barriers in the utilization of domestic violence services among Arab immigrant women: perceptions of professionals, service providers & community leaders. J Fam Violence. 2010;25(8):727–35.
58. Raj A, Silverman J. Violence against immigrant women: the roles of culture, context, and legal immigrant status on intimate partner violence. Violence Women. 2002;8(3):367–98.
59. Rees S, Pease B. Refugee settlement, safety and wellbeing: exploring domestic and family violence in refugee communities. Victoria: Immigrant Women's Domestic Violence Service; 2006. Report No.: 4.
60. Critelli F, Yalim AC. Improving access to domestic violence services for women of immigrant and refugee status: a trauma-informed perspective. J Ethn Cult Divers Soc Work. 2020;29(1–3):95–113.
61. Larchanché S. Intangible obstacles: health implications of stigmatization, structural violence, and fear among undocumented immigrants in France. Soc Sci Med. 2012;74(6):858–63.
62. Mason G, Pulvirenti M. Former refugees and community resilience: 'papering over' domestic violence. Br J Criminol. 2013;53(3):401–18.
63. Segrave M. Temporary migration and family violence an analysis of victimisation, vulnerability and support. Melbourne: School of Social Sciences, Monash University; 2017. [cited 27 Aug 2019]. http://artsonline.monash.edu.au/gender-and-family-violence/temporary-migration-and-fv.
64. Voolma H. 'I must be silent because of residency': barriers to escaping domestic violence in the context of insecure immigration status in England and Sweden. Violence Women. 2018;24(15):1830–50.
65. Taylor D. Charities referring rough sleepers to immigration enforcement teams. The Guardian. 2017. [cited 30 Jul 2020]. http://www.theguardian.com/society/2017/mar/07/charities-giving-home-office-details-of-rough-sleepers-says-report.
66. Segrave M. How the federal government is migrating responsibility. Monash Lens. 2019. [cited 30 Jul 2020]. https://lens.monash.edu/@politics-society/2019/11/11/1377635?slug=how-australias-migration-system-is-failing-victims-of-gendered-violence.
67. Thomas S, Darkal H, Goodson L. Monitoring and reporting incidents of sexual and gender-based violence across the refugee journey. Birmingham: Institute for Research into Superdiversity; 2019. p. 31. Report No.: 29/2019.
68. Lee SK, Sulaiman-Hill CMR, Thompson SC. Providing health information for culturally and linguistically diverse women: priorities and preferences of new migrants and refugees. Health Promot J Austr. 2013;24(2):98–103.
69. Almoshmosh N, Jefee Bahloul H, Barkil-Oteo A, Hassan G, Kirmayer LJ. Mental health of resettled Syrian refugees: a practical cross-cultural guide for practitioners. J Ment Health Train Educ Pract. 2019;15(1):20–32.
70. Ostrander J, Melville A, Berthold SM. Working with refugees in the U.S.: trauma-informed and structurally competent social work approaches. Adv Soc Work. 2017;18(1):66–79.

71. Bhuyan R, Senturia K. Understanding domestic violence resource utilization and survivor solutions among immigrant and refugee women: introduction to the special issue. J Interpers Violence. 2005;20(8):895–901.
72. Snowden L, Masland M, Ma Y, Ciemens E. Strategies to improve minority access to public mental health services in California: description and preliminary evaluation. J Community Psychol. 2006;34(2):225–35.
73. Atlani L, Rousseau C. The politics of culture in humanitarian aid to women refugees who have experienced sexual violence. Transcult Psychiatry. 2000;37(3):435–49.
74. Burman E, Smailes SL, Chantler K. Culture as a barrier to service provision and delivery: domestic violence services for minoritized women. Crit Soc Policy. 2004;3:332–57.
75. James K. Domestic violence within refugee families: intersecting patriarchal culture and the refugee experience. Aust N Z J Fam Ther. 2010;31(3):275–84.

How Could a Gender-Sensitive Approach Help Us to Identify and Respond to Children Who Have Displayed Harmful Sexual Behaviour?

4

Stuart Allardyce, Peter Yates, and Sharron Wareham

4.1   Introduction

> **Case Study 1: Jerry**
> Jerry (13) and his sister Martha (7) live with their mother in a two-bedroom flat. They moved there a year ago further to their mother separating from their father after he assaulted her. Jerry and Martha share a bedroom. One evening Martha got very upset just before her bedtime and her mother asked what was bothering her. She said that Jerry had asked her to touch 'his peepee' until 'white stuff came out'. He told her that nobody must know about 'their secret game' and if she tells anyone she will have to leave home and live with a different family.

Sexual violence is a profound violation of human dignity that can be deeply traumatising for victims, families and communities [1]. Situations such as Jerry's sexual abuse of his 7-year-old sister as described in Case Study 1 are shocking because of the nature of the exploitation they describe. However, these kinds of scenarios also challenge our conception of childhood as a time of innocence, and especially of sexual innocence.

S. Allardyce (✉)
Lucy Faithfull Foundation, Bromsgrove, UK
e-mail: StuartAllardyce@stopitnow.org.uk

P. Yates
Edinburgh Napier University, Edinburgh, UK
e-mail: P.Yates@napier.ac.uk

S. Wareham
Barnardo's, Ilford, UK
e-mail: sharron.wareham@barnardos.org.uk

© Springer Nature Switzerland AG 2021
C. Bradbury-Jones, L. Isham (eds.), *Understanding Gender-Based Violence*,
https://doi.org/10.1007/978-3-030-65006-3_4

In short, we do not expect children to behave in this way. Nevertheless, situations such as these will unfortunately be familiar to anyone who works in child protection. Between 2012 and 2016, there were 32,452 reports made to police in England and Wales involving alleged sexual offences by children against other children. This represents an average of around 22 initial concerns of child on child sexual abuse every day [2]. Studies in the UK and other jurisdictions suggest that around one-third of sexual crime is perpetrated by children and young people. The largest study of recorded sexual crime to date analysed referrals to law enforcement in 34 US States in 2002 and found that 35.6% of those who committed sexual offences against children were themselves under the age of 18 (n = 13,471) [3].

A range of terms are used in the literature to describe this phenomenon (e.g. 'juvenile sexual offending', 'problematic sexual behaviour', 'peer on peer abuse'). In the UK, 'harmful sexual behaviour' has emerged as the most common umbrella term, defined as:

'Sexual behaviours expressed by children and young people under the age of 18 years old that are developmentally inappropriate, may be harmful towards self or others or be abusive towards another child, young person or adult' [4, p. 13].

As with other forms of child sexual abuse, gendered disparities in the perpetration and experience of harmful sexual behaviour in childhood suggest that it is a form of gendered sexual violence. In Finkelhor et al.'s [3] study, 93% of those who had perpetrated harm were boys and 79% of victims were girls, figures broadly in line with similar studies (e.g. [5, 6]). There is diversity here: some boys sexually abuse other boys, and some abuse both girls *and* boys, while a small proportion of harmful sexual behaviour is carried out by girls, targeting boys, girls, or both. However, the significant over-representation of boys as perpetrators and girls as victims is a striking empirical finding which is rarely analysed or discussed in the relevant literature. This chapter therefore brings a gender lens to a subject often conceptualised by practitioners and researchers in a gender-neutral way.

4.2   Diversity Among Children Who Have Displayed Harmful Sexual Behaviour

Sexual crime incidence figures obscure the fact that harmful sexual behaviour is not a single form of offending behaviour, but rather a heterogeneity of different kinds of behaviours exhibited by different kinds of children in many varied contexts. There are a range of factors that underpin this complexity.

Nature of the behaviour: Although seriousness should never be minimised, harmful sexual behaviours vary in levels of intrusiveness and harm experienced by victims. Children's sexual behaviours that raise concerns for adults may include: sexualised language, sexualised bullying and harassment, exhibitionism and voyeurism, inappropriate sexual touch, sexual assault and even rape. Although media reports commonly depict the most egregious sexual crimes committed by children, around one-third of sexual offences committed by children and young people attract a youth caution or youth conditional caution [7]. Although children do commit serious sexual crimes, a proportion of behaviours that come to the attention of statutory authorities have lower impact in nature involving children misjudging boundaries or contexts in terms of what is appropriate.

Characteristics of individuals who harm: Considerable diversity exists in backgrounds and needs of children who have displayed harmful sexual behaviour, as well as the motivations underpinning behaviour. Although most who come to the attention of statutory services are adolescents, some are prepubescent, with larger proportions of girls identified in cohorts of younger children. Finkelhor and Ormrod [3] found that just 19% of their sample of children were under 12, with 15% of this subgroup being girls. Children and young people with learning disabilities and autism are also over-represented in studies of young people referred to specialist services (e.g. [6]).

Relationship between victim and perpetrator: Regardless of gender, behaviours can target similar-age peers as well as younger children and occasionally adults. Victims are typically known to the perpetrator and can include close family relatives as well as individuals known through social circles, community connections, school or online relationships. Stranger rape or sexual assault offences by adolescents are rare.

Context of the abuse: The vast majority of instances of harmful sexual behaviour take place within domestic spaces such as the family home or the homes of relatives or friends. The most common pattern described in studies of intrafamilial sexual abuse involves an older brother abusing a younger sister. Finkelhor and Ormrod [3] found that nearly 69% of the children and young people in their study sexually abused other children at home, with 12% in school settings. One UK survey found that 29% of 16–18-year-old girls said they had experienced unwanted sexual touching at school [8]. Sexual abuse in public spaces open to the community is much less prevalent and can include public indecency as well as gang-based sexual violence [9, 10]. Online harmful sexual behaviour—including online grooming of younger children by adolescents, sharing of self-produced sexual images without consent and viewing of child sexual exploitation material—is an increasing aspect of recorded sexual crime. In an analysis of online grooming sexual offences in Scotland in 2016–2017, more than 80% of victims were female with a median age of 14, while around 95% of perpetrators were male with a mean age of 18 [11].

Impact of the abuse: There is little research specifically on the impact of abuse by other children in comparison to abuse perpetrated by adults. This issue has been explored in the sibling sexual abuse literature, however, which suggests that sibling sexual abuse is associated with a similar range of consequences to those associated with child sexual abuse in general, and has the potential to be every bit as harmful as abuse by parents [12]. There is therefore no theoretical reason to suppose that child sexual abuse perpetrated by another child or young person should be any less harmful than that perpetrated by an adult. The harm caused to victims may therefore involve physical injury at the time, and a range of other issues that may emerge in childhood or later adulthood, including depression, anxiety, dissociation, low self-esteem and hyper-sexuality [13]; complex post-traumatic stress disorder [14] and even cardiovascular and reproductive disorders [15]. However, impact is mediated by a range of factors including: nature and frequency of the abuse; relationship between victim and abuser; individual factors such as education, interpersonal and emotional competence, coping style, optimism and external attribution of blame and systemic factors such as being believed by adults and support from family and wider social environment [16].

4.3   Differentiating Harmful from Normative Sexual Behaviour

Harmful sexual behaviour is different from sexual exploration and experimentation, which are normal and expected parts of child and adolescent development and help shape sexual identity and an understanding of our relationships with others. Distinguishing between experimental childhood behaviour and inappropriate or abusive behaviour can be a complex task and requires practitioners to have an understanding of healthy normative behaviour and issues of informed consent, power imbalance and exploitation.

Chaffin and Letourneau [17] suggest that if any or all of the following criteria are met, children's sexual behaviour may require more detailed assessment and possible intervention:

- Occurs at a frequency greater than would be developmentally expected;
- Interferes with the child's development;
- Occurs with coercion, intimidation or force;
- Is associated with emotional distress;
- Occurs between children of divergent ages and developmental abilities and/or
- Repeatedly recurs in secrecy after intervention by caregivers.

For practitioners who are not familiar and/or do not routinely work with harmful sexual behaviour, you may find the resources helpful available at https://www.parentsprotect.co.uk/harmful-behaviour-in-young-people-and-children.htm. See also Allardyce and Yates [18] for a more detailed discussion.

4.4   Developmental Perspectives

Unusually for child protection work, in cases of harmful sexual behaviour, the individual who has harmed and the individual who has been harmed are both children. Accordingly, our starting point should be a recognition of their developmental status as children, paying attention to the fact that serious harm may have been caused to the victim, while also avoiding labelling the child who has harmed as a 'mini adult sex offender'. Children and young people represent a distinct population from adults who commit sexual offences, and pathways into—and out of—these behaviours are very different for children compared to adults [19, 20]. The developmental nature of the behaviour is borne out by several key factors that emerge in the literature:

Development disruption: Many children who have displayed harmful sexual behaviour have experienced some form of developmental disruption. In a thematic analysis of 117 cases referred to specialist services in the UK, Balfe and Hackett [21] found most had experienced care-giving environments characterised by chaotic families, erratic living situations, poor family relationships, unstable parental backgrounds, generalised neglect and abuse and school/social problems. Physical abuse and witnessing domestic violence are highlighted in many studies (e.g. [22, 23]), as is sexual victimisation. Seto and Lalumiere's [24] meta-analysis comparing boys known to statutory authorities because of sexual offending with those known for non-sexual offending found that the former group were five times more likely to have experienced sexual abuse than the latter. Girls who have displayed harmful sexual behaviour are more likely than boys to have experienced sexual victimisation. Mathews and Hunter [25], in a comparison of 67 girls and 70 boys who had displayed harmful sexual behaviour, found that girls were twice as likely to have a history of childhood sexual abuse. Furthermore, they tended to have been sexually abused at an earlier age (64% before the age of 5) and were more likely to have been abused by different abusers at various stages in their childhood. Such findings have been replicated in other studies [23, 26, 27].

Age of onset: For boys, early adolescence, particularly the onset of puberty, appears to be a peak time for the onset of harmful sexual behaviours. The Finkelhor and Ormrod [3] study found a significant rise from age 12 years, peaking at 14 years. This spike in early adolescence is well supported by other studies [5, 6] and coincides with a developmental stage where young people are going through a range of physical, cognitive and emotional changes that occur at a time where sexual identity is being forged. Girls tend to have an earlier age of onset than boys, consistent with their histories of sexual abuse.

Developmentally limited nature of abusive behaviour: The majority of boys and girls who have displayed harmful sexual behaviour do not persist with such behaviours into adulthood [28]. Harmful sexual behaviour often coincides with a period of relative immaturity and impulsivity where consequential thinking may be minimal and an appreciation of the seriousness, illegality and impact of their behaviour may be limited. 'Antisocial orientation' or 'antisocial behaviour' in particular have emerged as risk factors for a minority of children whose harmful sexual behaviour in childhood persists into adulthood [29].

4.5   Bringing a Gender Lens to Harmful Sexual Behaviour

Child sexual abuse is a complicated and challenging issue for practitioners, particularly so when the abuse is displayed by a child towards another child. When we add considerations of gender, the complexities are compounded further. However, a dearth of research regarding girls displaying harmful sexual behaviour coupled with limited research into sexual harm experienced by boys means that our understanding of the role of gender in child sexual abuse lacks sophistication and remains ridden with stereotypically gendered attitudes to societal norms and expectations in relation to child development. Even on a very basic level, while we may advocate against the criminalisation of children, within a given offence category and level of severity, boys are more likely to be charged and are more likely to receive a custodial sentence for a sexual offence than girls [23, 30]. There may be variance according to ethnicity, and occasions when girls are treated even more harshly, perhaps because they are seen to act against their gender norm [30]. Nonetheless, in personal correspondence with the authors, the Youth Justice Board for England and Wales confirmed that all children who received a custodial sentence for a sexual offence in 2019 were boys.

There is a marked tendency in both research and practice to see boys in terms of sexual agency, as perpetrators and causing trouble, and to see girls as sexually passive, as victims, and as being troubled. The impact on our responses to both genders is far-reaching. Barnardo [31], for example in a study primarily focused upon improving identification and responses to child sexual exploitation, found that professionals working with children who had displayed harmful sexual behaviour afforded girls more time to build a trusting relationship in order to support an anticipated disclosure of abuse they had experienced. On the other hand, practitioners felt pressured to address 'risky behaviour' in boys to set timescales, with greater emphasis on reducing risk and closing cases. Issues of sexuality and a fear of appearing homophobic prevented many professionals from discussing what was clearly abuse and exploitation of boys by older males. For the boys, it was often their own harmful behaviour that eventually led to a referral to services, rather than their experiences of exploitation. Barnardo's Cymru [32] similarly found that despite abuse histories being significant for both boys and girls referred who had displayed harmful sexual behaviour, symptoms of post-traumatic stress disorder were more often noted in referrals for girls, and the focus of intervention was on their emotional well-being, while for boys the focus remained on behaviour modification. Hallett and Deerfield [33], in a study of 1550 referrals to specialist services in Wales in relation to harmful sexual behaviour as well as child sexual exploitation, similarly note that girls' harmful sexual behaviour is more readily understood by professionals as a response to trauma or abuse. Typically, girls who had displayed harmful sexual behaviour were then referred to services to support their needs as victims.

Such gendered responses are illustrated in the case examples below:

Case Study 2: Nathan

Nathan (15) lives in a residential unit. During a routine check of his mobile phone, residential staff found naked images of a girl that Nathan said was his girlfriend. Staff were concerned that Nathan may have coerced the girl into sending the images, so his phone was confiscated and a professionals meeting held. Nathan maintained that, although he had engaged in mutual sexual behaviour in person with the girl, he was much less happy about sharing images online.

Nathan's girlfriend later confirmed that she had sent him naked pictures of herself and had asked him to send intimate images and videos of himself, which he had felt pressured to send. No further action was taken towards Nathan or his girlfriend. Professionals agreed that the behaviour was experimental, despite Nathan stating he had felt pressured to send the images.

Case Study 3: Lucy

Lucy (14) was referred for support from a specialist service due to concerns of being at risk of sexual exploitation. Lucy was known to go missing, had posted naked images of herself online and had been involved in sexual behaviour at school. Inquiries resulting from the referral established that when Lucy went missing from school she encouraged younger children (from age 11) to go with her and sent them naked images of herself, often causing the children distress. The sexual behaviour at school involved touching same-age boys, raising complaints from the boys and making graphic sexual comments to younger children.

Reflective Exercise

When thinking about your own cases that involve children's sexual behaviour which may be harmful in nature, it is often useful to conduct a thought experiment and switch the sexes of the children involved. Consider:

- Does this change our interpretation of the situation, our feelings towards the children, and our intended response? If so, why?

There was little doubt in Case Study 3 that Lucy was indeed vulnerable to sexual exploitation; however, her behaviour was also harmful to others. If we were to call her Brian, would we bring a different perspective to initial assessment of this situation?

More anecdotally from our own experiences in practice, professionals often ask themselves whether a male or female worker may be better placed to support girls, while this question is rarely asked with respect to boys. An underlying assumption is that girls are likely to have experienced sexual victimisation by a male and that they may feel more comfortable with a female worker. We rarely consider that they may have been abused by a female, nor the potential for positive gender role-modelling by a male worker. For boys the focus is typically their own behaviour rather than their victimisation experiences, and the importance of relationship-building and therefore the gender of the professional are rarely considered.

Whether we take an approach focussed on managing the child's behaviour or on supporting them therapeutically in relation to trauma is unfortunately often dictated by gender rather than the strengths and needs of individual children. A more reflective understanding of gender and its impact on practitioner responses could lead to victimisation experiences and welfare outcomes being given greater prominence in therapeutic work with boys referred for their harmful sexual behaviour. Ensuring that genuine risks presented by girls are not overlooked would also be important. This is not to say, however, that ultimately boys and girls are just the same and can be treated as such. Both Hallett et al.'s [33] and Barnardo's [32] studies, for example found the prevalence of a family history of domestic abuse being nearly identical for girls and boys referred to specialist services. However, the impact of the abuse varied along gender lines. In the Barnardo's study, boys were more likely to internalise the use of aggression, including sexual aggression, as a method of problem-solving or resolving conflict. Girls, on the other hand, appeared more compliant in relationships and were seemingly more tolerant of abuse and control. This highlighted significant areas of intervention for the girls in this study, who may otherwise lack the knowledge of what constitutes a healthy and mutual relationship and be more likely to tolerate abuse and harm (including sexual harm) in future relationships. The study also highlighted, however, that the boys also require education about what constitutes healthy and mutual relationships, including more respectful ways of solving problems and resolving conflict.

4.6   Towards a Sociology of Harmful Sexual Behaviour

Those working with a gendered analysis understand that the over-representation of boys and men as perpetrators and women and girls as victims of sexual violence relates to wider gender inequalities in society, whereby a societal hegemonic masculinity played out at the levels of families and other relationships intersects with an individual at a particular time and place [34]. In short, patriarchal societies are characterised by the articulation of male dominance through a sense of entitlement to sexual access to women and girls. Gender norms that associate manhood with heterosexual prowess and with access to, and control over, the bodies of women, girls and boys contribute to male perpetration of sexual harm [35]. Central to these processes is the strict regulation of women and girls' sexual lives and the simultaneous hyper-sexualisation of their bodies from an early age. Social change over the last century has led to resistance to and disruption of patriarchal orders in society, but gendered socialisation along patriarchal lines continues, and can be seen in modern day attitudes and values in relation to sexual relationships and sexual violence that provide the cultural context of abuse and sexual harm.

Sociological analysis of this nature is relatively absent from the literature on harmful sexual behaviour among children. An exception is found in the work of Messerschmidt [36], who examined a series of detailed life history interviews with 30 White US working class girls and boys aged 15–18 years. Ten had displayed harmful sexual behaviour, 10 had displayed violent non-sexual offending behaviour and 10 had showed no signs of sexual or non-sexual violence. Messerschmidt [37,

p. 207] found these interviews to represent 'detailed accounts of embodied gender interactions in three distinct 'sites': the family, the school and the peer group'. Messerschmidt argues that harmful sexual behaviour is a situated dynamic involving the performing of gender as a form of social control over others. When aged 15, one of the boys in the study sexually abused two girls aged between six and eight, for whom he was babysitting. He argues that one way of understanding this behaviour is within the context of a set of socially constructed assumptions about male sexuality, which legitimised the boy's belief in his 'entitlement' to apply pressure on these girls to have sex. Within a context of a male peer discourse that sexually objectivised girls and valued public boasting about heterosexual sexual exploits, the boy experienced bullying at school and felt unable to connect with female peers to whom he was sexually attracted. Messerschmidt concludes that this boy:

> 'decided to attempt to overcome his lack of masculine resources and thereby diminish the negative masculine feelings and situations through controlling and manipulating behaviour... expressing control and power over younger girls through sexuality' [36, p. 101].

This contrasts with Seto and Lalumiere's [24] finding that problematic sexual scripts concerning consent and coercion did not differentiate adolescent boys who had displayed harmful sexual behaviour from those who had engaged in non-sexual offending, and their conclusion that such scripts held poor explanatory power in the aetiology of harmful sexual behaviour. Messerschmidt, however, drawing on qualitative rather than quantitative methodologies suggests that the concept of hegemonic masculinities allows us to see the interaction between social isolation, problematic sexual scripts and a particular male peer discourse that are the social factors in which this particular boy's abusive behaviour is rooted.

4.7 Interventions for Harmful Sexual Behaviour and Gender

Approaches to interventions with children who had displayed harmful sexual behaviour emerged in the 1980s as an adjunct to clinical practice with adult sex offenders. Over the last 20 years, the emerging evidence has led to an evolution of practice, which recognises the developmental status of children who abuse. Targeted interventions can be highly effective in reducing risk even for those children and young people who are at higher risk of continuing harmful behaviours [29]. These approaches have generally drawn on cognitive behavioural therapy to encourage individuals to consider how attitudes to children, sex, consent and their lack of appreciation of the impact of their behaviours have justified and supported their behaviour [38]. Increasingly, ecological approaches emphasising the role of parents and carers as well as school and the wider environment have been shown to improve outcomes for children [39]. Interventions matched to levels of risk and harm can range from short psychoeducational early intervention programmes through to extensive ecologically orientated community-based interventions and provision within specialist residential and secure settings.

Such approaches tend to be 'gender blind', however, meaning that often socially sanctioned gender stereotypes, victim-blaming attitudes, sexual harassment and rape myths are rarely addressed in intervention programmes. One of the explanations for this is that attitudes and values have not emerged as factors associated with adolescent sexual recidivism, and therefore are not considered to constitute criminogenic needs. However, risk factors such as 'antisocial orientation' may be examples of harmful hyper-masculine norms when viewed through a gender lens [35], and the blind spot may be compounded by an over-reliance of quantitative research and a lack of qualitative orientated studies that explore gender attitudes. Furthermore, interventions need to address welfare needs as well as criminogenic needs and ensure that programmes are holistic enough to address future non-sexual risks (such as intimate partner violence). Children have often had damaging developmental experiences and been affected by aspects of 'toxic masculinity'. Failing to address gender-specific factors in the aetiology of sexual violence may leave the child at risk of other non-sexual forms of gendered violence in adolescence and adulthood. In short, programmes may focus too narrowly on reducing risk of further sexual violence without conceptually grasping that sexual violence may be just one of a range of manifestations of negative patriarchal values and attitudes.

4.8 Future Directions: Harmful Sexual Behaviour Prevention and Gender

The literature on the prevention of harmful sexual behaviour is still in its infancy, and few approaches to preventing child sexual abuse perpetrated by adolescents before it occurs have been evaluated (see [18] for an overview). McKibbin and Humphreys [40] asked 14 young people undertaking intervention programmes in relation to harmful sexual behaviour whether there were any opportunities for adults to intervene that may have prevented their abuse of children. Three prevention strategies emerged: universal education about healthy social relations and sexual behaviour; support for children affected by harm and help for young people so that they are not adversely impacted by access to online pornography.

These empirically defendable prevention goals are compatible with a gendered analysis of sexual violence, but as they stand do not foreground sexual violence as being linked to patriarchal value systems, nor do they recognise that the objectification of women, problematic language and sexist, homophobic or transphobic humour are all part of a continuum of gender-based power relations, which ultimately supports physical and sexual violence at the extreme end of that continuum. This gap in recognising gender becomes even more apparent when reflecting upon the literature on engaging boys in violence prevention, particularly violence against women. Flood [41] provides an overview of such initiatives internationally. In many countries, prevention initiatives address this issue in schools and youth-work settings, requiring boys to consider violence against women and girls as an issue relating to the ways masculinity is articulated in society. Sports coaching settings and institutions such as the military are similarly developing codes to ensure males build respectful cultures. However, as the harmful sexual behaviour literature has not fully engaged with the issue of gender, prevention efforts have developed separately from other initiatives around gender-based violence. This separation means that child sexual abuse and harmful sexual behaviour prevention efforts rarely incorporate approaches that challenge harmful gender norms and, more specifically, harmful masculinities. In a useful summary, Heilman and Barker [35] argue that programmes aimed at child sexual abuse prevention need to:

- 'Investigate and deconstruct the ways in which social norms related to masculinity may lead to the very antisocial tendencies and practices that are linked to the perpetration of child sexual abuse.
- Provide education on what child sexual exploitation is and on how unequal power dynamics operate in intimate and sexual relations.
- Demonstrate the broad, lasting, harmful effects of child sexual exploitation for children of all genders, and insist that it is never justified.
- Foster discussion and exploration of alternative masculinities and sexuality that provide healthy, non-violent ideas of manhood delinked from sexual prowess, dominance and control.
- Ask participants to name, recognise and discuss the exploitative nature of transactional sex and how harmful gender norms inform this dynamic'.

This would extend to universal school-based primary prevention programmes as well as those engaging parents and early intervention programmes for young people and families where such issues are starting to emerge.

4.9   Conclusion

The theoretical and empirical gap in writing about gender in relation to harmful sexual behaviour exemplifies a wider gap in child sexual abuse research. In an overview of the literature on the aetiology of child sexual abuse, Clayton and Jones [42] conclude:

'Noticeably absent from the research is evidence pertaining to community and sociocultural factors. It is important to question critically how different factors interact. For instance, the evidence indicates that girls are more at risk of child sexual abuse, however we do not know what mechanisms are operating to produce this increased risk for girls. Feminist theory hypothesises that culture enforces an unequal social structure that disadvantages women and girls. However, we found no studies exploring the intersections between gender identities and sociocultural constructs'.

The overall conclusion of this chapter is that research and practice in this field needs urgently to take the question of gender more seriously in order to develop approaches to intervention and prevention, which recognise the profoundly gendered nature of this form of sexual violence.

References

1. Kelly L. Surviving sexual violence. New Jersey: Wiley; 2013.
2. McNeish D, Scott S. Key messages from research on children and young people who display harmful sexual behaviour. Barkingside: Barnardo's; 2018.
3. Finkelhor D, Ormrod R, Chaffin M. Juveniles who commit sex offenses against minors. Juvenile justice bulletin. Washington DC: US Government printing office: (1–12).
4. Hackett S, Branigan P, Holmes D. Harmful sexual behaviour framework: an evidence-informed operational framework for children and young people displaying harmful sexual behaviours. 2nd ed. London: NSPCC; 2019.
5. Fox B. What makes a difference? Evaluating the key distinctions and predictors of sexual and non-sexual offending among male and female juvenile offenders. J Crim Psychol. 2017;7:134–50.
6. Hackett S, Phillips J, Masson H, Balfe M. Individual, family and abuse characteristics of 700 British child and adolescent sexual abusers. Child Abuse Rev. 2013;22:232–45.
7. Bateman T. The state of youth justice 2017: an overview of trends and developments. London: National Association for Youth Justice; 2017.
8. Whitfield L, Green S, Krys R. "All day, every day" legal obligations on schools to prevent and respond to sexual harassment and violence against girls. London: End Violence Against Women; 2016.
9. Colombino N, Mercado CC, Levenson J, Jeglic E. Preventing sexual violence: can examination of offense location inform sex crime policy? Int J Law Psychiatry. 2011;34:160–7.
10. Smallbone S, Wortley RK. Child sexual abuse in Queensland: offender characteristics and modus operandi. Brisbane: Queensland Crime Commission and Queensland Police Service; 2000.
11. Justice Analytics Service. Recorded crime in Scotland: other sexual crimes, 2013–14 and 2016–17. Edinburgh: Scottish Government; 2017.
12. Yates P. Sibling sexual abuse: why don't we talk about it? J Clin Nurs. 2017;26(15–16):2482–94.
13. Davidson L, Omar HA. Long-term consequences of childhood sexual abuse. Int J Child Adolesc Health. 2014;7(2):103–7.
14. Kisiel C, Fehrenbach T, Liang L-J, Stolbach B, McClelland G, Griffin G, et al. Examining child sexual abuse in relation to complex patterns of trauma exposure: findings from the National Child Traumatic Stress Network. Psychol Trauma Theory Res Pract Policy. 2014;6(Suppl 1):S29–39.
15. D'Andrea W, Sharma R, Zelechoski AD, Spinazzola J. Physical health problems after single trauma exposure: when stress takes root in the body. J Am Psychiatr Nurses Assoc. 2011;17:378–92.
16. Domhardt M, Münzer A, Fegert JM, Goldbeck L. Resilience in survivors of child sexual abuse: a systematic review of the literature. Trauma Violence Abuse. 2015;16:476–93.
17. Chaffin M, Letourneau E, Silovsky JF. Adults, adolescents, and children who sexually abuse children: a developmental perspective. In: Myers JEB, Berliner L, Briere J, Hendrix CT, Jenny C, Reid TA, editors. The APSAC handbook on child maltreatment. 2nd ed. Thousand Oaks, CA: Sage; 2002.
18. Allardyce S, Yates P. Working with children and young people who have displayed harmful sexual behaviour. Edinburgh: Dunedin; 2018.
19. Lussier P, Blokland A. The adolescence-adulthood transition and Robins's continuity paradox: criminal career patterns of juvenile and adult sex offenders in a prospective longitudinal birth cohort study. J Crim Just. 2014;42:153–63.
20. McKillop N, Brown S, Smallbone S, Pritchard K. Similarities and differences in adolescence-onset versus adulthood-onset sexual abuse incidents. Child Abuse Negl. 2015;46:37.
21. Balfe M, Hackett S, Masson H, Phillips J. The disrupted sociologies of young people with harmful sexual behaviours. J Sex Aggress. 2019;25(2):177–92.

22. Skuse D, Bentovim A, Hodges J, Stevenson J, Andreou C, Lanyado M, et al. Risk factors for development of sexually abusive behaviour in sexually victimised adolescent boys: cross sectional study. Br Med J. 1998;317:175–9.
23. Hickey N, Mccrory E, Farmer E, Vizard E. Comparing the developmental and behavioural characteristics of female and male juveniles who present with sexually abusive behaviour. J Sex Aggress. 2008;14:241–52.
24. Seto MC, Lalumiere ML. What is so special about male adolescent sexual offending? A review and test of explanations through meta-analysis. Psychol Bull. 2010;136(4):526–75.
25. Mathews R, Hunter JA, Vuz J. Juvenile female sexual offenders: clinical characteristics and treatment issues. Sex Abuse. 1997;9:187–99.
26. Hunter JA, Lexier LJ, Goodwin DW, Browne PA, Dennis C. Psychosexual, attitudinal, and developmental characteristics of juvenile female sexual perpetrators in a residential treatment setting. J Child Fam Stud. 1993;2:317–26.
27. Hutton L, Whyte B. Children and young people with harmful sexual behaviours: first analysis of data from a Scottish sample. J Sex Aggress. 2006;12(2):115–25.
28. Caldwell MF. Quantifying the decline in juvenile sexual recidivism rates. Psychology. Public Policy Law. 2016;22(4):414.
29. Worling JR, Langstrom N. Risk of sexual recidivism in adolescents who offend sexually. In: Barbaree HE, Marshall WL, editors. The juvenile sex offender. New York: Guilford Press; 2006.
30. Siegel J, Fix RL. Court outcomes among female juveniles with sexual offences. J Sex Aggress. 2020;26(2):263–73.
31. Barnardo's. Boys2: supporting boys and young men to develop healthy sexual relationships. Barkingside: Barnardo's; 2018.
32. Barnardo's Cymru. Girls talk. Barkingside: Barnardo's; 2015.
33. Hallett S, Deerfield K, Hudson K. The same but different? Exploring the links between gender, trauma, sexual exploitation and harmful sexual behaviours. Child Abuse Rev. 2019;28(6):442–54.
34. Durham A. Young men who have sexually abused: a case study guide. London: Wiley; 2006.
35. Heilman B, Barker G. Masculine norms and violence: making the connections. Washington, DC: Promundo; 2018.
36. Messerschmidt JW. Gender, heterosexuality, and youth violence: the struggle for recognition. Plymouth: Rowman & Littlefield; 2012.
37. Messerschmidt JW. The struggle for hetero-feminine recognition: bullying, embodiment, and reactive sexual offending by adolescent girls. Fem Criminol. 2011;6:203.
38. Sneddon H, Grimshaw DG, Livingstone N, Macdonald G. Cognitive-behavioural therapy (CBT) interventions for young people aged 10 to 18 with harmful sexual behaviour. Cochrane Database Syst Rev. 2020;6(6):CD009829.
39. Borduin CM, Munschy RJ, Wagner DV, Taylor EK. Multisystemic therapy with juvenile sexual offenders: development, validation, and dissemination. In: Boer DP, Eher R, Craig LA, Miner MH, Pfäfflin F, editors. International perspectives on the assessment and treatment of sexual offenders: theory, practice, and research. Chichester: Wiley-Blackwell; 2011. p. 263–85.
40. McKibbin G, Humphreys C, Hamilton B. "Talking about child sexual abuse would have helped me": young people who sexually abused reflect on preventing harmful sexual behavior. Child Abuse Negl. 2017;70:210–21.
41. Flood M. Engaging men and boys in violence prevention. London: Springer; 2018.
42. Clayton E, Jones C, Brown J, Taylor J. The aetiology of child sexual. Child Abuse Rev. 2018;27(3):181–97.

Creating Inner and Outer Safety: Findings from a Research Study on Finnish Women's and Children's Experiences of Post-separation Stalking

5

Anna Nikupeteri and Merja Laitinen

5.1 Introduction: Thinking About Post-separation Stalking as a Form of Violence

Case Study

Katri (female, 42 years) and Heikki (male, 45 years) were married for 14 years. They have three children: Marja (13 years), Mikko (8 years), and Miina (3 years). Katri decided to leave Heikki and moved to a new apartment with the children. Heikki could not understand Katri's decision, and his behaviour, which had already been controlling during their relationship, became increasingly threatening. Following and contacting Katri and the children became an obsession to him.

One day Heikki sent 59 WhatsApp messages to Katri telling her how much he adored and missed her. Katri did not answer. The messages then took on a threatening tone. Heikki said that he would come to their house and harm Katri and the children physically if she wouldn't answer. Once he called her 88 times to have a possibility to talk about their relationship. After this, Heikki sent her flowers with a postcard to say how much he misses her. One night, Heikki appeared outside of Katri's workplace towards the end of her night shift. Katri got a ride home from her work mate because she was afraid of walking home alone. The previous summer, as Katri and the children were driving to the countryside to spend the weekend at the cottage with Katri's sister's family, Heikki was following them by car.

A. Nikupeteri (✉) · M. Laitinen
University of Lapland, Rovaniemi, Finland
e-mail: anna.nikupeteri@ulapland.fi; merja.laitinen@ulapland.fi

© Springer Nature Switzerland AG 2021
C. Bradbury-Jones, L. Isham (eds.), *Understanding Gender-Based Violence*,
https://doi.org/10.1007/978-3-030-65006-3_5

During the past two years, Heikki has terrorised Katri's and the children's relationships in many ways. Heikki has written on his Facebook wall that his ex-partner is selfish and does not let him meet the children. He has also questioned Katri's parental abilities because of her alleged mental problems. Heikki has made several false child abuse allegations about Katri. He has accused her of neglecting the children when she invites men to her home where small children are present, which negatively affects their mental stability. Once the social worker threatened to change the children's custody to the father after having concluded that Katri was attempting to alienate Hannu from his children. Once Heikki came over and helped Marja to fix her laptop when she had problems with it. Heikki has repeatedly told Marja and Mikko that they can call him if they need help. The children have felt confused. They are scared of their father one day and miss him the next.

Once at night Heikki came to the place where the family used to live, knocking on doors and windows, yelling and demanding Katri to let him in. Katri was in panic, Miina and Mikko were crying, and Marja called the police. Often after these kinds of incidents, Marja takes care of Mikko and Miina and calms down their mother. The previous summer, Heikki appeared at Mikko's football training after he got to know his hobby when the photo of his football team had been published on the Internet. Mikko feels uneasy when dad comes to ask questions about mother and he has difficulties to concentrate at school. Miina is often tearful after meeting his dad during the weekends. Marja does not want to invite friends home, because she would be ashamed if dad suddenly came to their house and had a fit of rage in the yard. Marja sees her dad's behaviour as violent and does not want him to be involved in her own or her mother's and siblings' life. Recently, Katri and her children had to move to a new suburb because Heikki got to know their location through their common friends. This was just one relocation among many others. However, they are happy that their new apartment is situated on the third floor of an apartment building that is accessible only with a resident's key.

The composed case example that we present of a Finnish woman and her children reflects the everyday lives of many victims of post-separation stalking. The case example is fictive, but it draws on our present and past research and our understanding of the dynamics of post-separation stalking and its impacts on women and children. The definitions of stalking—or lack of them—vary across legislative contexts and no such definition has been agreed upon in the international research arena, but one widely used definition includes at least two elements: (a) a course of conduct exhibited by the perpetrator; and (b) feelings of fear by the victim [1]. Stalking is a series crime that occurs on more than one occasion [2]. Stalking behaviour can include violent or non-violent acts. It induces fear or other emotional distress in, and causes physical and social harm to the victims [3–7]. Stalking is a major global social and health problem which requires psychosocial and legal approaches at the individual level and in societal interventions [7].

In this chapter, we approach stalking as gender-based violence (GBV) and, as such, as a cultural and relational phenomenon. This means that being victimised to violence, perpetrating violence, and the ways in which stalking is addressed by professionals and other people are complexly interrelated with issues of gender and power [8]. Being a victim of stalking creates additional burden for women as mothers, which emphasises the gendered dimension of professional practices and responses. When using the concept *victim*, we ascribe active agency to women and children instead of seeing them as passive targets. Our choice of this concept is motivated by our wish to stress their right to receive help and support. At the time of conducting the interviews with the women and children for our study, stalking was still ongoing in their lives. All of them had survived under the shadow of stalking and even threat of death. Stalking as a form of gendered violence illustrates that victim and survivor are relational concepts. If stalking ends for one reason or another, it offers both women and children a ground to thrive (read more about thrivership in Chap. 13), whereas, when stalking is an ongoing issue coping with everyday life requires strong agency.

The aim of this chapter is to explore what kind of impact stalking has on women's and children's everyday lives. Based on this, we outline a set of requirements for social workers, and healthcare and other professionals to follow in order to provide help and support to women and children in post-separation stalking situations. The chapter draws on research that started in 2012 and continues as an ongoing research project entitled Children's Knowing Agency in Private, Multi-professional and Societal Settings—the Case of Parental Stalking (CAPS).[1] The learning objectives of this chapter are (1) to understand stalking as a form of gender-based violence that may occur in familial relations; (2) to know the impacts of stalking on its victims and (3) to perceive professional responses both from women and children's viewpoints.

5.2   Finland as a Research Context for Post-separation Stalking

Raising awareness of stalking is an acute issue in Finland. According to an EU-wide survey on violence against women, 18% of women have experienced stalking since the age of 15 by a person known or unknown to them, while the corresponding number in Finland is 24%. The survey also shows that 9% of women over the age of 15 in the EU have been stalked by a previous partner [9]. In the U.S., nearly 16% of women and 5.8% of men report having been stalked at some point in their lifetime [10]. Separating from a partner does not necessarily end violence; rather on the contrary, violence may start or escalate in separation situations [11, p. 183]. Children

---

[1] The project is funded by the Academy of Finland (No. 308470). The webpage of the project: https://www.ulapland.fi/EN/Webpages/CAPS-(2017-2021).

are exposed to stalking in many ways after parents' separation [12, 13]. Separation can be even lethal, both for women [14, 15] and children [13, 16].

More knowledge of post-separation stalking, in particular as experienced by the victims, is needed in order to further develop and strengthen services for the victims. The group of experts on Action against Violence against Women and Domestic Violence (GREVIO) monitoring the implementation of the Istanbul Convention has criticised Finland's policy of gender equality, as it easily shifts towards gender-neutrality in service provision where the gender-specific nature of violence is ignored, and which does not always do justice to women's particular experiences of domestic violence. Many key professionals lack in-depth understanding of the gendered nature of violence, issues of power and control and its impacts on victims [17]. Stalking was criminalised in Finland in 2014 (Criminal Code ch 25 s 7 a) and the law defines a stalker as:

> a person who repeatedly *threatens, observes, contacts* or in another comparable manner unjustifiably stalks another so that this is *conducive towards instilling fear or anxiety* in the person being stalked, shall, unless an equally or a more severe penalty is provided elsewhere in law for the act, be sentenced for stalking to a fine or to imprisonment for at most two years.

Our exploration of post-separation stalking is based on our research projects and collaboration with the professionals of the national Support Centre *Varjo* [Shadow].[2] The Support Center provides services for victims and perpetrators, gives training and consultation for professionals and supports research collaboration on stalking, which has made it possible to conduct research on female and child victims' experiences of post-separation stalking. In this chapter, we have integrated our previous research findings [8, 12, 18–23] and a preliminary analysis of new data on the subject to outline a set of central aspects of women's and children's experiences of being stalked. Our findings are based on various qualitative data sets collected with women and children as well as on official court data (Table 5.1).

Based on joint discussion on our research findings, we first highlight four themes that describe the impacts of post-separation stalking on women and children: (1) Sense of insecurity, fear and threat of death; (2) Changing roles in families and family dynamics; (3) Shrinking of social networks and reduction of social life and (4) Complexities in being acknowledged as a victim and receiving help (Fig. 5.1). Secondly, we highlight three key aspects professionals need to consider when encountering victims of stalking: (1) Understanding the nature of post-separation stalking and recognising the victims' need of various forms of help and support; (2) Multiagency risk assessment with women and children; (3) Creating inner and outer safety for women and children. We need to understand and remain aware of the contextual nature of knowledge of impacts of post-separation stalking. Recognition of stalking as a problem and the responses available to deal with it vary globally as they are connected to cultural and societal structures. Our data and interpretations are related to the context of Finland as a Nordic welfare state, where stalking is

---

[2] Support Center Varjo: https://varjosta.fi/.

Table 5.1   Data on post-separation stalking collected within the projects (2012–2019)

Data set and method	Number of informants/case files	Content of the data
In-depth thematic interviews with women who are stalked by their ex-partner	20 women The women were interviewed individually or together with a professional close to the woman	The women were asked to relate (1) what their everyday life was like as targets of stalking and (2) how the system of professional support had responded to their experiences of stalking
Interviews with children involved in stalking conducted by their biological or stepfather	15 children including 12 girls and 3 boys, aged 4–21 Two of the children were interviewed individually and the rest of them in pairs according to the children's wishes	The children described their experiences of stalking and other violent acts by the (step-)father. They also described their emotions, close relations, supportive resources and need for help
Three therapeutic action groups for children, each consisting of ten sessions The duration of each session was approximately 90 min and it was recorded with a camcorder	13 children including 8 girls and 5 boys, aged 2–12	The themes of the sessions focused on the children's close relations, negative emotions and supportive resources The video material covers the children's discussions, acting, playing and interaction related to the themes. Research data also includes the children's drawings
Case files on court judgements in stalking cases	Collected nationwide, all the district court decisions in stalking cases 2014–2017 ($N = 419$)	Comprehensive data set on legal perspectives on stalking after criminalisation

Fig. 5.1   Conceptual model of impacts of post-separation stalking

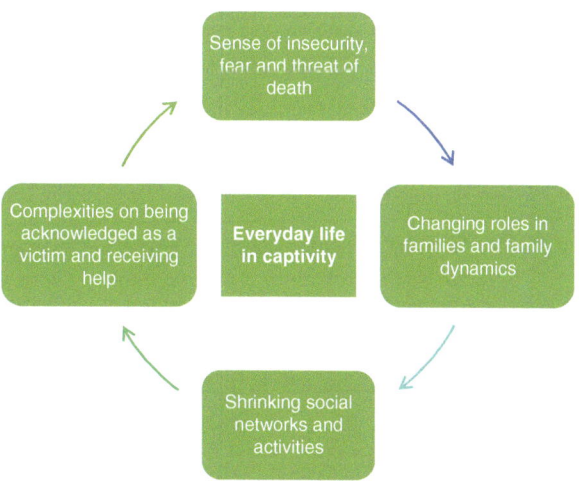

recognised as criminal behaviour and as a form of violence against women. However, descriptions of impacts and the key aspects of professional interventions can be applied also in other, especially Western, countries.

5.3 Impacts of Post-separation Stalking on the Everyday Lives of Women and Children

5.3.1 Sense of Insecurity, Fear and Threat of Death

A study on women's and children's experiences of post-separation stalking shows that a sense of insecurity and fear caused by the behaviour of the woman's former partner—and the children's father—are among the major feelings experienced by those being stalked [18, 23]. This is the case despite the fact that stalking behaviour may include acts which, taken individually, do not constitute illegal behaviour, such as sending flowers. In stalking situations, female and child victims' feelings of insecurity can vary in time and intensity for each individual and across siblings. Being stalked is a pervasive experience, and the victim can sense the omnipresence of the perpetrator [24]. The victim can feel the stalker's acts creating an emotional web of stalking which describes the place- and time-related emotions that tie together the discrete acts and past and potential violent experiences of being stalked. The spectre of stalking describes the state of being stalked—the social reality in which the women and children live—created by the emotions stalking evokes [20].

Women and children exposed to stalking live in a state of continuous alertness for an imminent threat of being attacked. They perceive the stalker's actions as dangerous and coercive [21]. Intrusive actions can lead to psychosocial and physical injuries and, in the most extreme cases, to familicide [23]. Falling victim of stalking changes the meanings of reality. The victim's reality often remains invisible to other people and stalking victims may lose their sense of security, which is a deep socioemotional experience caused by the safety violations inflicted by the perpetrator and uncertainty of the future [18]. The time passing between the moment of signalling the need for safety support and receiving the actual professional response is important, as one child interviewee said:

> Child: Well, let me think about it… If it takes a very long time for the security button to work, then we should have one that works like immediately after you have pressed it, so that you press and they come like in the next second. And then they [professionals] do something useful.

This extract also reveals the omnipresence of stalking as experienced by the victims and the need for concrete actions to prevent it. It is important to notice that victims are exposed to different forms of stalking. Hence, the sense of insecurity, fear and even threat of death are subjective and form a unique ground for the everyday life in emotional captivity.

5.3.2 Changing Roles in Families and Family Dynamics

- Question: Is there anything you have wished?
- Child: I wish they hadn't gotten a divorce or anything like that. We could have stayed in the same home and there would have been no need to go to the shelter or so...

Stalking threatens the social stability of the family by affecting the rights, duties and responsibilities of family members. Stalking socioemotionally and psychosocially affects women's and children's everyday lives, which is particularly manifested through child–parent and sibling relationships. Stalking creates a power play between the family members, where the abuser uses his power, but also the children take and use power in different ways, which affects how they position themselves in relation to the other family members. Children may experience mental ambivalence, suspicion, guilt and mistrust. Their agency can be adapting and withdrawing, vacillating, supportive and constructive, responsible and evaluating and critical and change seeking [19]. Many children exposed to post-separation stalking have ambivalent relationships with their fathers. The small children usually have adaptive, withdrawing and vacillating relationship towards the family members and the family situation at large. The children may experience both negative and positive feelings towards their fathers [25]. Their perceptions of the father depend on the memories of their history with the father as well as on their present life situation, which is marked by negotiations between the mother and the father and the attempts to deal with the stalking.

Stalking inflicted by a child's father creates a close emotional and physical relationship between children and their mother. Children can sense the mother's fear and insecurity and witness her exposure to stalking. As a consequence, the older children may start to take care of, and protect, their mother and younger siblings, thus behaving in a supportive and constructive manner towards them [26]. The older the children are, the more likely they are to perceive the father's behaviour as violent. They may also feel ashamed of their father's behaviour. The older children may start to be critical towards the father's behaviour and demand him to change it. Being stalked makes women change their position and adopt different roles in relation to the former partner and other persons. The victim often tries to pre-empt the next steps the stalker might take and the persons he might use—and these may even be the victim's closest friends—in order to get information on or to establish contact with her. Sometimes keeping in touch with the ex-partner is a way for the victim to prevent dangerous incidents. In cases in which the victim and the perpetrator have common children, the perpetrator may use the children as a means of getting in touch with the ex-partner [13]. The perpetrator utilises the knowledge that the children's suffering hurts their mother the most. Women may have to act against professionals' decisions, for example judicial custody agreements, in order to protect their children. Overall, constant thinking about how to act in the presence of, and contact, other people captivate women and children's everyday lives. Their experiences call for a nuanced understanding of family members' roles and family dynamics as affected by stalking.

5.3.3   Shrinking of Social Networks and Reduction of Social Life

The sense of fear and insecurity caused by post-separation stalking severely constrains women's and children's everyday lives by shrinking their social networks (friends, relatives), by reducing the activities they can participate in and the places they can go. Victims may not have a safe place, because the presence of the woman's ex-partner threatens both public and private places. By shrinking his victims' daily lives, the perpetrator shows that he exercises control over their life. Children's fear of their father's potential presence at school or the feeling that their mother needs to be protected may cause the children to take days off from school. In addition, children may not be willing to invite friends over, because, should the father gain access to their home, the friends would be exposed to his violent behaviour too. Many victims limit their everyday social activities in order to avoid encounters with the stalker, for example in the grocery store, library or workplace. The social and physical isolation may affect the victim's possibilities to obtain education or prevent them from working, thus exacerbating their situation economically as well.

> And yes, I have had a company, which he was very well aware of. I have been working there alone. And then, when I was not there, notes and messages started to appear on my door, saying 'Hi, I am a whore. Services for men available here.' (–) And he also knew the number of my work phone. Which became the main target of his terror. You really can't mute your work phone… (–) The locks at my workplace have been changed, too, because once something was jammed in the keyhole… And there were these times that I couldn't get into my office because a block of concrete had been cast in front of the entrance. (Stalked woman)

Besides being physically present in various places, the perpetrator may use digital technology as part of the acts of stalking. Technology is a tool that effectively creates a sense of the perpetrator's omnipresence, and it may be used to isolate, punish and humiliate the victims [27]. The abuse of technology for such purposes reduces women's and children's possibilities to maintain their social relationships, for example having private conversations in social media. Technological devices, such as spy software installed on mobile phones, also provide a tool for the stalker for monitoring the victim's movements in physical places.

Overall, by making the women and children shrink their social networks and compromise their activities, the woman's former partner, or the children's father, isolates them and strengthens their experience of living in captivity. Female and child victims of post-separation stalking have to consider every situation from the perspective of stalking in order to be able to decide what they can do. And what they want and need is to be able to stay at home without fear of having to escape, and to be able to feel safe when spending time in public places.

5.3.4 Complexities in Being Acknowledged as a Victim and Receiving Help

> For a long time, I tried to make the meetings work. I believed that the children needed to meet their both parents. (−) Anyway, they [professionals] accused me of being resentful, of looking out for my own interests, of trying to take a revenge, or of not wanting the children to meet their father for some other reason. (Stalked woman)

Women and children experience complexities in being acknowledged as victims of stalking by professionals and other people, which may hamper their possibilities of receiving help [5]. The positive, non-violent acts performed by the perpetrator may prevent others from seeing his violent behaviour. The perpetrator's behaviour can include disguised acts, where they perform love and longing for the family and appear as indulging, caring fathers who are concerned of their children's well-being [12, 21]. They may also be jealous of the ex-partner, or reverse the roles and pretend to be the victim, while making the real victim look like the perpetrator. They may exploit helping systems and manipulate professionals as a strategy to control the women's and children's lives [28]. The perpetrator's performances are often targeted at professionals and wider communities (e.g. school staff, relatives, other parents) and may occur alongside his violent behaviour when out of the public eye [21]. Through the performance of love and care and threatening behaviour, the perpetrator hampers his victims' status as victims. The blurred boundaries of stalking behaviour and exercising legal rights, for example the father's right to see his children, can even further victimise the women and children through authorities [13].

As a consequence of this ambivalent behaviour, professionals may view female victims through parental alienation and falsely label as alienating parents who use different strategies, such as not letting the father meet the children in order to distance him from them. Professionals may also view women as un-protective mothers if they are not able to protect the children from the former partner's/children's father's harmful behaviour. When viewed by professionals as overcautious women who exaggerate the ominousness of the ex-partner's behaviour, or as implausible victims because of their active—and ambivalent—strategies used in attempt to cope with the stalking situation and to protect themselves and the children, the professionals prevent the women from receiving help [8]. This captivates the women by creating a reality which does not match their personal perception of their family situation, and thus can even victimise them further. Professionals may make harmful interpretations of the family situation if they lack understanding of the dynamics of gender-based violence. In the worst case, false interpretations may lead to women and children not being recognised as victims of post-separation stalking. Our study emphasises the importance of developing a nuanced understanding of, and valuing, women's and children's subjective views of close relations. In this way, it is possible to maintain family relations that provide protection, are mutually rewarding and enhance the well-being of children and their mothers.

5.4   Helping and Supporting the Victims of Post-separation Stalking

The varied impacts of post-separation stalking as experienced by women and children call for a rethinking of professionals' responses to the stalking victims' need of help and support. We have outlined three requirements that social workers, healthcare and other professionals should consider when offering help and support to women and children exposed to post-separation stalking (Fig. 5.2).

5.4.1   Understanding the Nature of Post-separation Stalking and Recognising the Victims' Need for Various Forms of Help and Support

Understanding the nature of stalking and its devastating consequences to its victims is an important first step for professionals when helping women and children exposed to post-separation stalking. The victims' experiences may challenge professionals to critically analyse the dimensions of power and control between the ex-partner/father, the woman and the children in order to distinguish the different types of violence and to avoid a universal approach to and commonly held beliefs on violence, such as the idea that violence ends at separation [29, 30]. The women's and children's experiences emphasise that the perpetrator's behaviour should be understood as manifold use of power and violence against his ex-partner and children. In terms of this, we highlight the following points in professionals' responses:

- Professionals need to understand the dynamics of gender-based violence in order to interpret stalking cases in a manner that recognises women and children as victims.
- In cases of mothers as victims of stalking, professionals should view the children as victims too. Siblings can have different experiences of the ominousness and harmfulness of the father's behaviour.

Fig. 5.2 Key aspects of professional encounters with victims of post-separation stalking

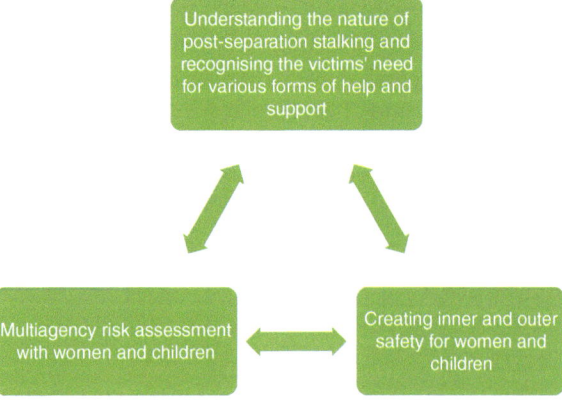

- It is important that professionals are mindful of women and children's own understandings of the ex-partner's/father's behaviour and the family situation. Stalking victims' experiences may not be validated if they are viewed from a strictly legal perspective, or in terms of stereotypical conceptions of domestic violence.
- It is vital that professionals create spaces where they can listen to the children's experiences without the parents' presence.
- Professionals need to critically reflect on their own perceptions of family, parent-hood, motherhood and fatherhood—which may be stereotypical—and the specificity and consequences of separation in the context of domestic violence.
- Professionals need to exercise context- and culture-sensitive practices and strong, moral agency in order to deal with the moral complexities arising from stalking in different situations [22].

5.4.2 Multiagency Risk Assessment with Women and Children

The experience of being stalked is likely to affect victims in various way, thus underlining the need for extensive help by different professionals and collaboration of different agencies, including social and health services, the police, and the criminal justice system [13, 31–33]. A comprehensive and coordinated response to violence after separation and risk analysis can create safety [25]. The risk analysis should be based on the assessment of the perpetrator's coercive and controlling behaviour [34] and the acute risk factors, such as the perpetrator's perceived loss of control over the victim, or the barriers that the victims face when seeking help [33]. Social and healthcare professionals have a key role in evaluating the dynamics of family relations and separation and communicating with the police when estimating the risks. The victim may not be a client of special services for victims of violence, such as shelter or therapy, and thus every encounter with a potential helper matter. It is important that professionals consider the following viewpoints when conducting the risk assessment:

- The perpetrator's non-violent and non-criminalised acts, which nevertheless raise fear and a sense of insecurity in the victims.
- The factors that may cause a risk for the perpetrator's behaviour leading to lethal violence need to be identified systematically and broadly; seeing the risk as multilevel and context related, interwoven in social relationships (e.g. relatives, friends, professionals, proxy-stalkers) and social environments (e.g. work place, school, kindergarten, social media).
- The risk analysis must include ethical and moral evaluation in making sense of the complexity of stalking. There are different kind of systematic risk assessment methods for evaluating the high-risk victims of domestic violence, such as Multi-Agency Risk Assessment Conference (MARAC) [35].

5.4.3   Creating Inner and Outer Safety for Women and Children

One of the most challenging demands facing professionals is the question of how to create security in uncertainty characterising the lives of stalked women and children. Inner safety is connected to the victims' emotions arising from the experience of being stalked and cognition deriving from the omnipresent nature of stalking [6, 21, 24]. Even if the perpetrator has died, the victim may still be afraid of his potential appearance. Outer safety is associated with the victim's physical and social circumstances. By using different strategies, women and children can increase their sense of security and sense of control of the situation. From professionals' viewpoint, it is relevant to acknowledge the victims' coping strategies as a way of responding to the fear in order to make the situation more tolerable, such as going out accompanied by a dog or talking on a mobile phone when carrying rubbish [11, p. 225–238]. Professionals can empower the victims to construct a more secure environment for themselves by planning safety strategies together with them [36]. In creating inner and outer safety, it is central that professionals pay attention to the following perspectives:

- Loved ones, social and health professionals, day care and school staff have a significant role in constructing women's and children's safety, supporting their agency and promoting their recovery [18, 26].
- Work is needed with all parties involved. The perpetrator, too, needs help in order to change his harmful behaviour.
- Safety plans must be made respecting personal experiences; this entails recognising women and children as victims in their own right.
- A digital safety plan is often needed and it includes evaluation of the victim's use of different apps, acting in social media platforms and checking security settings of mobile phones and computers.
- It is important to support the relationship between children and their mothers and strengthen the children's relationship with trusted adults who can create security, including personnel in kindergarten, school and hobbies.
- By considering the factors around the child's well-being and developing the father's parenting skills, it is possible to support safe child–father interactions and reduce children's adjustment problems after the parents' separation [25]. However, it is crucial to notice that every contact with the primary victim can fuel the stalking.
- Professionals need to underscore children's sense of fear and insecurity as crucial factors to be considered in child contact arrangements.
- Professionals have a responsibility to create space for and to sustain joint 'safety talk' as a source of shared knowledge between the children and their mothers that has the potential to enhance security under the shadow of stalking.

The Key Practitional Messages in Encountering Stalked Lives

Identify the multiple manifestations of stalking as violence.
Recognise all victims and gather each victim's experiential knowledge.
Be aware of the multiple impacts of post-separation stalking, which may complicate victims' possibilities to get help.
Approach stalking as a human rights violation which limits the victim's basic personal freedoms [37].
Be aware of the fact that the perpetrator can utilise the victim's friends, relatives and professionals who try to help the victim, as a means to support his stalking behaviour.
Share knowledge with other relevant professionals, with the victim's permission, in order to secure the victims' daily lives. For example, personnel in school and kindergarten should be aware of stalking if there exists a risk that the perpetrator may appear there.
Make physical and digital safety plans with each victim and evaluate the need for restraining orders with the victim(s) and support the women in applying for them—both for themselves and the children.
Make sure that you do not disclose any personal information concerning the victim (e.g. secret address, phone number) when working with the case.
Combine child-centred work and support for both parents in child contact arrangements, if the child meets the perpetrator.

Reflective Exercise

Read the case example of Katri and her children in the beginning of the chapter. From the perspective of your own profession/professional background, ponder the mother's and the children's need of help separately and consider how their needs can be met.

- How would you work with them or what kinds of working methods would you use?
- What kinds of questions do you need to ask from the mother and the children in order to get sufficient information?
- What safety concerns and risks do you recognise and how can they be addressed?
- What options and resources would you provide to the victims?

References

1. Fissel ER, Reyns BW, Fisher BS. Stalking and cyberstalking victimization research: taking stock of key conceptual, definitional, prevalence, and theoretical issues. In: Chan HCO, Sheridan LL, editors. Psycho-criminological approaches to stalking behavior: an international perspective. Wiley series in the psychology of crime, policing and law. New York: Wiley; 2020. p. 11–36.

2. Owens JG. Why definitions matter: stalking victimization in the United States. J Interpers Violence. 2016;31:2196–226. https://doi.org/10.1177/0886260515573577.
3. Mullen PE, Pathé M, Purcell R. Stalkers and their victims. New York: Cambridge University Press; 2000.
4. Davis KE, Coker AL, Sanderson M. Physical and mental health effects of being stalked for men and women. Violence Vict. 2002;17:429–43. https://doi.org/10.1891/vivi.17.4.429.33682.
5. Logan TK, Shannon L, Cole J, Walker R. The impact of differential patterns of physical violence and stalking on mental health and help-seeking among women with protective orders. Violence Against Women. 2006;12:866–86. https://doi.org/10.1177/1077801206292679.
6. Elklit A, Vangsgaard LAG, Olsen ASW, Ali SA. Post-traumatic stress disorder (PTSD) symptoms in secondary stalked children of Danish stalking survivors—a pilot study. Int J Environ Res Public Health. 2019;16:725. https://doi.org/10.3390/ijerph16050725.
7. Chan HCO, Sheridan LL. Psycho-criminological approaches to stalking behavior: an international perspective. Wiley series in the psychology of crime, policing and law. New York: Wiley; 2020.
8. Nikupeteri A. Professionals' critical positionings of women as help-seekers: Finnish women's narratives of help-seeking during post-separation stalking. Qual Soc Work. 2017;16:793–809. https://doi.org/10.1177/1473325016644315.
9. FRA—European Union Agency for Fundamental Rights. Violence against women: an EU-wide survey. Main results. Luxembourg: Publications Office of the European Union; 2014. https://fra.europa.eu/sites/default/files/fra_uploads/fra-2014-vaw-survey-main-results-apr14_en.pdf. Accessed 3 May 2020.
10. Smith SG, Zhang X, Basile KC, Merrick MT, Wang J, Kresnow M, Chen J. National intimate partner and sexual violence survey (NISVS): 2015 data brief—updated release. Atlanta, GA: National Center for Injury Prevention and Control, Centers for Disease Control and Prevention; 2018. https://www.cdc.gov/violenceprevention/pdf/2015data-brief508.pdf. Accessed 3 May 2020.
11. Spitzberg BH, Cupach WR. The dark side of relationship pursuit. From attraction to obsession and stalking. 2nd ed. New York: Routledge; 2014.
12. Nikupeteri A, Laitinen M. Children's everyday lives shadowed by stalking: postseparation stalking narratives of Finnish children and women. Violence Vict. 2015;30:830–45. https://doi.org/10.1891/0886-6708.VV-D-14-00048.
13. Løkkegaard SS, Beck HN, Wolf NM, Elklit A. When daddy stalks mommy: experiences of intimate partner stalking and involvement of social and legal authorities when stalker and victim have children together. Violence Against Women. 2019;25:1759–77. https://doi.org/10.1177/1077801219826738.
14. McFarlane J, Campbell JC, Watson K. Intimate partner stalking and femicide: urgent implications for women's safety. Behav Sci Law. 2002;20:51–68. https://doi.org/10.1002/bsl.477.
15. DeKeseredy WS, Dragiewicz M, Schwartz MD. Abusive endings. Separation and divorce violence against women. Oakland, CA: University of California Press; 2017.
16. Dobash RP, Dobash RE. Who died? The murder of collaterals related to intimate partner conflict. Violence Against Women. 2012;18:662–71. https://doi.org/10.1177/1077801212453984.
17. GREVIO—Group of Experts on Action against Violence against Women and Domestic Violence. GREVIO's (Baseline) Evaluation report on legislative and other measures giving effect to the provisions of the Council of Europe Convention on Preventing and Combating Violence against Women and Domestic Violence (Istanbul Convention): Finland. Council of Europe. https://rm.coe.int/grevio-report-on-finland/168097129d. Accessed 3 May 2020.
18. Nikupeteri A, Tervonen H, Laitinen M. Eroded, lost or reconstructed? Security in Finnish children's experiences of post-separation stalking. Child Abuse Rev. 2015;24:285–96. https://doi.org/10.1002/car.2411.
19. Laitinen M, Nikupeteri A. Ex-partner stalking in Finland: children as knowing agents in parental stalking. In: Sheridan LL, Chan HC, editors. Psycho-criminological approaches to stalking behavior: an international perspective. Wiley series in the psychology of crime, policing and law. New York: Wiley; 2020. p. 55–76.

20. Nikupeteri A. Stalked lives: Finnish women's emotional experiences of post-separation stalking. Nord Soc Work Res. 2017;7:6–17. https://doi.org/10.1080/2156857X.2016.1192055.

21. Katz E, Nikupeteri A, Laitinen M. When coercive control continues to harm children: post-separation fathering, stalking, and domestic violence. Child Abuse Rev. 2020;29:310–24. https://doi.org/10.1002/car.2611.

22. Mikkonen E, Laitinen M, Gupta A, Nikupeteri A, Hurtig J. Cross-national insights into social workers' multi-dimensional moral agency when working with child abuse and neglect. Qual Soc Work. 2020; https://doi.org/10.1177/1473325020902820.

23. Nikupeteri A, Lappi C, Lohiniva-Kerkelä M, Kauppi A, Laitinen M. Potentiaalisesti tappava parisuhde? Erotilanteen uhkaavuus ja uhrien suojaamisen edellytykset sukupuolistuneen väkivallan viitekehyksessä. [Potentially lethal relationship? Threat of separation and protecting victims in the frame of gendered violence]. Oikeus [Finn J Just]. 2017;46:290–309.

24. Humphreys C, Diemer K, Bornemisza A, Spiteri-Staines A, Kaspiew R, Horsfall B. More present than absent: men who use domestic violence and their fathering. Child Fam Soc Work. 2019;24:321–9. https://doi.org/10.1111/cfs.12617.

25. Turhan Z. Safe father–child contact postseparation in situations of intimate partner violence and positive fathering skills: a literature review. Trauma Violence Abuse. 2019; https://doi.org/10.1177/1524838019888554.

26. Katz E. Recovery-promoters: ways in which children and mothers support one another's recoveries from domestic violence. Br J Soc Work. 2015;45(Suppl 1):i153–69. https://doi.org/10.1093/bjsw/bcv091.

27. Woodlock D. The abuse of technology in domestic violence and stalking. Violence Against Women. 2017;23:584–602. https://doi.org/10.1177/1077801216646277.

28. Monk LM. Improving professionals' responses to mothers who become, or are at risk of becoming, separated from their children, in contexts of violence and abuse. Unpublished PhD thesis. Coventry: Coventry University; 2017.

29. Johnson MP. A typology of domestic violence: intimate terrorism, violent resistance, and situational couple violence. Boston: Northeastern University Press; 2008.

30. Haselschwerdt ML, Hardesty JL, Hans JD. Custody evaluators' beliefs about domestic violence allegations during divorce: feminist and family violence perspectives. J Interpers Violence. 2011;26:1694–719. https://doi.org/10.1177/0886260510370599.

31. Stanford S. 'Speaking back' to fear: responding to the moral dilemmas of risk in social work practice. Br J of Soc Work. 2010;40:1065–80. https://doi.org/10.1093/bjsw/bcp156.

32. Stanley N, Miller P, Foster Richardson H, Tomson G. Children's experiences of domestic violence: developing an integrated response from police and child protection services. J Interpers Violence. 2011;26:2372–91. https://doi.org/10.1177/0886260510383030.

33. Sheehan BE, Murphy SD, Moynihan MM, Dudley-Fennessey E, Stapleton JG. Intimate partner homicide. New insights for understanding lethality and risks. Violence Against Women. 2015;21:269–88. https://doi.org/10.1177/1077801214564687.

34. Stark E. Coercive control: how men entrap women in personal life. Oxford: Oxford University Press; 2007.

35. Steel N, Blakeborough L, Nicholas S. Supporting high-risk victims of domestic violence: a review of multi-agency risk assessment conferences (MARACs). Research report 55. London: Home Office; 2011.

36. Miller L, Howell K, Hunter E, Graham-Bermann S. Enhancing safety-planning through evidence-based interventions with preschoolers exposed to intimate partner violence. Child Care Pract. 2012;18:67–82. https://doi.org/10.1080/13575279.2011.621885.

37. Logan TK, Walker R. Partner stalking: psychological dominance or "business as usual"? Trauma Violence Abuse. 2009;10:247–70. https://doi.org/10.1177/1524838009334461.

What Does It Mean to Support Women with 'Complex Needs'? Recognising and Responding to Systems of Power, Oppression and Inequality

6

Kathryn Hodges and Lyndsey Harris

6.1 Introduction

This chapter explores the concept of 'complex needs', how it has been applied in practice and whether there are more thoughtful ways to communicate the complexity of women's lived experiences and better understand the difficulties experienced when seeking help and support. We consider some of the multiple and intersecting lived experiences and the things that happen to women that create precarity and vulnerabilities that increase their risk of exploitation and abuse. Ultimately, there are fatal ramifications for women who are unable to get the help and protection they need. In this chapter, we explore the things that are helpful, or otherwise, for women when they are seeking support and the way they prefer to be met by helping services. The chapter concludes with the Complex Experience Care Model which draws together the decisions and choices made by women when seeking help and support and the steps required by practitioners, services and policymakers to provide women with a safe place to come to and want to return.

K. Hodges (✉)
PraxisCollab and St. Mary's University, Twickenham, UK
e-mail: kathryn.hodges@praxiscollab.com

L. Harris
PraxisCollab and University of Lincoln, Lincoln, UK
e-mail: LyHarris@lincoln.ac.uk

© Springer Nature Switzerland AG 2021
C. Bradbury-Jones, L. Isham (eds.), *Understanding Gender-Based Violence*,
https://doi.org/10.1007/978-3-030-65006-3_6

6.2   Voices of Women

Voices of women and practitioners have been included in this chapter, and the quotes come from two studies. The first study is the evaluation of the R2C project in Nottingham, a project providing wrap around support to victims/survivors of domestic violence and abuse (DVA) who were considered as having complex needs [1, 2]. The evaluation involved participatory action research in both design and dissemination of findings. Through qualitative inquiry the study privilleged the experiences of survivor service users and service providers and explored the efficacy of partnership working and utility of services provided. The second is an in-depth study exploring decisions and choices women experiencing multiple and severe disadvantage make when seeking help and support. Through one-to-one interviews, it heard from 11 women attending a service in an English City who support women involved in prostitution, or who had been trafficked for purposes of sexual exploitation [3, 4]. Voices from study one will be referenced as S1 and those from study two will be referenced as S2.

Case Study: Getting the Right Support and Being Heard
Naomi* had a long history of accessing services but felt unable to keep regular appointments saying that services she was referred to would often not listen to her. This meant Naomi would often be in a cycle of seeking help to leave an abusive domestic intimate partner relationship, then be coerced into retuning by the perpetrator who would exploit her eating disorder to maintain control of her, also subjecting her to emotional, economic, sexual and physical abuse:

> 'A lot of the time, in the past, one of the big reasons why I would return [was] because it felt safer when I was with [perpetrator]. He just took control of my food and everything like that—it just felt kind of life was better when I was with him rather than being in the cycle of the eating and vomiting' (Naomi).

When Naomi was referred into R2C, it was the fourth time she had left the perpetrator and, this time, she had specifically chosen to move out of area to reduce the risk of returning or being found. This was a particularly hard situation as she left behind her child and grandchild. However, she decided it was the right action for her to 'try and break the cycle of returning to him'. At the point of referral, Naomi was housed in a refuge in a neighbouring county, but staff at that refuge had indicated to her that she was ready to move on, and this concerned Naomi as she felt at most risk of returning to the perpetrator. She described:

> 'So when staff at the refuge felt that I was ready to move on, I knew I wasn't and I thought if I get a flat in the city and I didn't know where I wanted to live…I just wasn't ready…I didn't feel I was being heard…it just felt too much at that time'.

Naomi had already been accessing helping services in relation to her mental well-being and an eating disorder. In the past, she had attempted to complete the Freedom Programme. However, the programme left her questioning whether it was 'really us' and 'really describing him', and she returned to the perpetrator.

The regular support from the R2C complex needs specialist domestic abuse worker, included a range of things such as:

- Weekly telephone calls to check on her general well-being and/or face-to-face meetings in a relaxed environment.
- Accompanying Naomi shopping as she was not used to being able to make choices as her shopping budget and finances were controlled by her perpetrator. She gradually built up confidence to buy small household items for her future accommodation.
- When in crisis, Naomi would also contact her support abuse specialist worker and discuss fears and issues specifically related to returning to the perpetrator.
- With Naomi's permission, her wishes and concerns were discussed at multiagency meetings.
- Accompanying Naomi to access housing support and assisting with finding suitable accommodation.

As a result of the support, Naomi stated that she felt she was 'now living'. She described the rapport developed with her support worker:

'I had just had an instant connection time thing. I felt at ease with her and she was bright and cheerful. It wasn't like this was some great big heavy thing. Oh my god like look what's happened to your life and how are you going to get through it? It was just like, "it's in the bag; don't worry about it". You know she made it easy'.

For Naomi, '…moving into a flat on my own in the city made the reality of what has happened to my life real'. Her anxieties were treated seriously and she received support to work towards settled accommodation. Naomi completed the freedom Programme whilst living in the hostel and found it much easier to complete this time with the additional support. Six months after her initial referral into R2C, Naomi said:

'I still occasionally do have like ideas that, "well maybe it could work out", but then I discuss these issues…like yesterday I was worried sick he might have killed himself because [my] family told me someone was looking for me and I thought it was because of a card I'd sent saying that I couldn't have any contact at all anymore for my own recovery'.

Nine months after her referral into R2C, Naomi was in settled accommodation, in a flat of her own. A year later, she was taken off the R2C case load and 2 years on has not returned to the perpetrator.

*Not woman's real name: pseudonym used

6.3   What Do We Mean When We Say 'Complex Needs'?

The language of 'need' has been pivotal since the NHS and Community Care Act 1990. Whilst initially intended to ensure services responded and aligned with individual need, the reality is that the concept of need has become tied up with resource allocation, and cost rationing and control. The concept of need is 'one of the most slippery to define…there is no agreement at a theoretical, policy or practice level on what it means or how it might be measured' [5, p. 1]. Additionally, the term 'complex needs' lacks definition, although it is frequently found in practice language, being used as a descriptor of individuals or groups of individuals [6, 7].

During the evaluation of the R2C project in Nottingham [1, 2], a project set up to increase support for survivors of domestic and sexual abuse who were also identified as experiencing 'complex needs', a broader and more encompassing statement was developed to better describe the experiences of women seeking support. In this project, the term 'complex needs' had been used to refer to those: using substances and/or experiencing mental health problems and/or 'English as a second language' (meaning those for whom English was a foreign language). Harris [2] identified that there were different understandings of the term 'complex needs' across the statutory and voluntary sector in Nottingham. This often meant that some services suitable for survivors experiencing multiple disadvantage became inaccessible when women did not meet defined criteria of eligibility. This led to efforts to reconsider 'complex needs' in the local area in the context of protected characteristics and issues that intersect to disadvantage survivors/victims. Harris [2] argued that when discussing victims/survivors with 'complex needs', this should be understood as:

> Victims/Survivors who experience multiple disadvantage and face barriers and challenges in accessing essential services, and require a person-centred, trauma-informed approach to enhance their safety, well-being and quality of life.

As highlighted, recommendations from the R2C evaluation included viewing multiple disadvantage as the number of things which are working against a survivor. The term 'complex needs' encapsulates and emphasises the responsibility on commissioners, service providers and multi-agency partnerships to recognise how their services might facilitate a person-centred approach to address any wider barriers to essential services. It is recognised this is a difficult task for service providers as service provision in one area may unintentionally have a negative impact upon the survivor in other areas of their life.

Having to seek support from a wide range of providers reflects a failure of helping services to respond to the range and severity of individual experiences [6–8]. Adults facing severe and multiple disadvantage are often living at the very margins of society and are less likely to access helping services or benefit from them when they do, finding it difficult to engage with multiple public services in order to improve their lives [9]. It is essential that practitioners and policymakers understand individuals' lived experience and the environment they interact in, as difficulties faced by individuals cannot be separated from the structure in which they live their lives [5, 10]. More recently this understanding has been reflected in the term 'severe and multiple disadvantage', explaining the things that happen to people as a result of society's actions, or where an individual's experiences exceed a service provider's capability to provide meaningful or effective support [11]. This concept of 'severe and multiple disadvantage' refocuses attention on the impact society has on individuals, and away from individual's engagement with services and their behaviours within that society.

6.4   Intersecting Lived Experiences: The Things That Happen

Women make up the largest proportion of victims of abuse and exploitation in the UK [12–15]. They are more likely to be victims of DVA (83.5%), and a significantly higher proportion of defendants in DVA cases are male (92.1%) [14]. Within prostitution, it is predominately women who sell sex or exchange sex for other goods or services they need (such as accommodation, drugs and so on), and men are the buyers and pimps [16, 17]. This significant gender divide between those who were exploited and the exploiters led Sweden to change its prostitution laws, following agreement that this gendered exploitation fell short of their aim of a gender equal society [18]. Modern Slavery data reports the highly gendered nature of different types of exploitation, where men and boys are more likely to be victims of labour exploitation, and women and girls are more often victims of sexual exploitation and/or domestic servitude [15]. Bindel et al. [19, p. 50] argue that within voluntary and statutory services there is a failure to understand 'the very subtle forms of deception and coercion [that underpin] the abuse of a person's vulnerability'. It is essential that the complex nature of exploitation and the precarity of people's lives are understood to enable women and girls to get the help and support they need, or preferably, that this abuse and exploitation is not experienced in the first place.

The intersecting experiences of women's lives and the things that happen to them shape how they seek help and support. Failing to understand the intersecting nature of women's lived experiences limits women's access to helping services [20]. In order to explore the interdependent nature of women's experiences, it is useful to draw on the concept of intersectionality [21–25]. In recent decades, there has been an increased emphasis on the theory of intersectionality as a way of exploring women's lives, the concept broadly refers to the interaction between multiple forms of oppression [21–23, 26]. Whilst the different approaches of this perspective are not examined in detail here, the term 'intersecting experiences' is used to reflect this awareness and how the 'things that happen' to women are interwoven with systems of power, oppression and social inequalities.

Figure 6.1 illustrates how women's experiences and the things that have happened to them, intersect. It portrays the complexity of women's lives as explored in a recent study [4], mapping the way lived experiences, support needs and ongoing challenges do not exist in isolation and must be considered as an interconnecting picture.

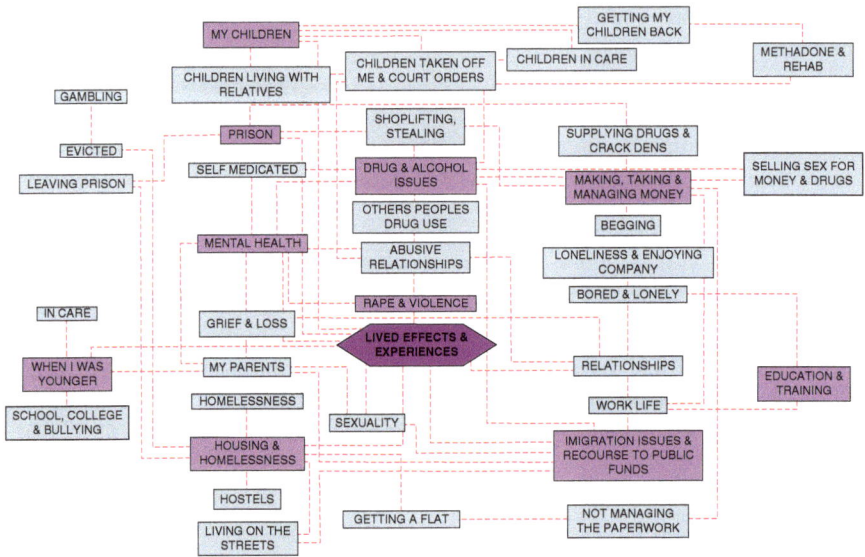

Fig. 6.1 Intersecting lived experiences [4]. (With permission from: Hodges K. An exploration of decision making by women experiencing multiple and complex needs. Anglia Ruskin University; 2018)

In what follows, we have outlined some, although by no means all, of the multiple and intersecting lived experiences which create precarity and vulnerabilities faced by women and girls.

6.5 Childhood, Being Mothers and Support Networks

There is now greater attention on the impact of 'complex trauma' in adulthood associated with childhood abuse and neglect [11]. Poverty, childhood trauma and poor educational experiences can create significant risk that severe and multiple disadvantage will be experienced in later life [27, 28]. Experiences of violence, trauma, childhood abuse or neglect or having been a looked after child in local authority care are considered to increase the risk of being sexually exploited as an adult [17, 29–31]. Additionally, women's roles as mothers must be better taken into account. For women experiencing repeated removal of their children through social services intervention, there is limited support available [32, 33]. Debbie and Anne (S2) talked about the loneliness of this experience:

> My son was taken off me, and my little girl was took into care…I was in such an abusive, abusive domestic violence relationship. I was just such a broken person (Anne, S2).
>
> [I] was just used to having my kids around me and all of a sudden I was a single person again and umm I had a lot to do, because when you go to court you've got so much to do…you're bombarded with appointments…you know…. I really had a lot to do I was very busy, but very lonely (Debbie, S2).

The quote highlights the busyness associated with attending meetings with professionals, and also how this can be accompanied by a deep sense of isolation. Experiences of loss reported by women span from childhood through to adulthood, from parents dying, children passing away and or being removed through safeguarding procedures or 'snatched' by partners [4]. One woman reflected how difficult the child protection meetings were, finding it very difficult to sit there as 13 professionals talked about her and her child, she said she frequently was 'just dying inside for somebody to please, please, please just say something good' [4].

6.6   Poverty, Debt and Housing

Experiences of poverty make women vulnerable to exploitation and abuse. With many women indicating initial involvement in prostitution was driven by the need to fund accommodation, food and other costs associated with supporting children [29, 31, 34]. Traffickers exploit situations of poverty, recruiting victims on false promises of work, trapping women into prostitution and other forms of exploitation [35–38]. Debt and financial issues continue to entrap, with many women unable to complete education or training, impacting on their future employment options [29, 31]. According to the charity Surviving Economic Abuse [39], 95% of women affected by domestic abuse report experiencing economic abuse. This financial abuse is experienced in three main forms: financial control, financial exploitation and financial sabotage [40]. Older women are more likely to have financial problems than older men, particularly if they are separated or divorced [41]. Many women do not disclose financial problems, actively disguising them due to fear and shame, something that is exacerbated when they have been subjected to coercive control and economic abuse by their partners or former husbands [41].

Women's access to safe and secure housing is essential. Women remanded in prison or on a short sentence risk losing their housing, which is particularly significant for women who are primary carers for young children [42]. Loss of accommodation increases the vulnerability of women, increasing isolation and the potential to create harmful dependencies on men [42, 43]. As Judy comments:

> Come out of jail you've got nowhere to go, you end up here, or you end up back in jail, because you've got nowhere to go…and in the end I got sleeping with somebody or got in somewhere which isn't good and putting up with things you shouldn't put up with for a place to stay, sleeping with some old man that's seventy because you'vr got nowhere to go… (Judy, S2).

Additionally, how women are met and responded to by other residents and staff in mixed hostel accommodation can leave women feeling unsafe, increasing their vulnerability when they leave and as a result end up sleeping in the streets, on others' sofas, or in crack houses [a place where crack cocaine is bought and sold] [4, 29]. Women are further exposed to sexual abuse, violence and stigmatisation when living on the streets, often leading them to conceal themselves from those who exploit, but also helping services [44]. It is known that the majority of British nationals who become victims of trafficking had been sleeping rough and/or experienced mental illness or have a learning disability [45, 46]. The priority of finding somewhere to sleep that night can overtake concerns about anything else, which may include attending helping services or programmes of support. Jane (S2) commented 'your head is just not focused enough to concentrate on other things, cause you're always worried, what about tonight?'.

6.7 Involvement in Criminal Activity and the Criminal Justice System

Women's involvement in the criminal justice system creates further disadvantage and brings attention to the cumulative impact of the multiplicity and interlocking nature of women's lived experiences [11]. Most acquisitive crime committed by women is to provide for children, and whilst numbers of women in prison has steadily increased this has not been reflected in the nature of the offences committed requiring a custodial sentencing [43, 47, 48]. There is an association between victimisation and criminality. Significant numbers of women have criminal records resulting from acts of survival, as a result of involvement in prostitution, illicit drug use or acquisitive crimes such as theft; the far-reaching impact of this making changes in their lives is more difficult when trying to find employment [49]. Additionally, DVA is also recognised as playing a major part in female offending [50], with at least 60% of female offenders who have been supervised in the community or in custody reporting that they have experienced domestic abuse [51].

6.8 Substance Use

Drug and alcohol use is reportedly high amongst those involved in prostitution [29, 31, 52], with initial involvement in prostitution providing a way to support drug use. Frequently, ongoing use of substances is a way to self-medicate and manage the psychological impact of prostitution, with continued involvement paying for this use and often for the drug use of a partner [19, 53]. However, the wider experiences and histories of those involved in prostitution must be appreciated, as it is too simplistic to assume that drug use is the key motivator for involvement in prostitution [52]. DVA survivors are also at a higher risk of substance use, alongside substantial evidence demonstrating significant use amongst perpetrators [54–57]. Whilst there have been several efforts made to explore the experiences of survivors who use substances and also experienced mental ill-health [58], it is impossible to separate cause and effect [57]. The intersecting and cyclical nature of the abuse experienced is captured by Feder's foreword to Complicated Matters:

The experience of domestic or sexual violence can lead to mental health problems and substance abuse. In turn, people struggling with mental health problems and substance abuse are more vulnerable to further violence [58].

6.9   Trauma and Mental Well-Being

A range of mental health diagnosis, including anxiety and depression, psychosis, Post Traumatic Stress Disorder (PTSD) and eating disorders, are strongly related to having experienced violence and abuse. Serious mental illness influences the likelihood of being in unsafe environments and increasing vulnerability to violent victimisation [59]. Individuals disassociate from their experiences as a way of protecting themselves from the emotional impact of trauma, but in doing so they also disassociate from cues of danger risking further victimisation in the future [60, 61]. Experiencing violence and abuse has a significant long-term impact on individuals' mental health and well-being, and childhood abuse and trauma adds to this complex picture of mental health [62]. Whilst, survivors of domestic and sexual abuse are considered at the highest risk of repeat victimisation [63], they also experience the barrier of being percieved to be 'problematic people' or a 'social problem' [64].

In the R2C study, a nurse talked about a survivor at a refuge. She commented that the survivors was, 'caught in limbo because she's not quite ready for the crisis team, but she's not quite just for talking therapies either, so she is kind of caught in that situation'. All practitioners highlighted the lack of suitable mental health support for women survivors identified as having complex needs, with minimal provision of psychological therapies in general, and even less available to survivors. One practitioner explained:

> They would be assessed as not suitable for the service, because their needs are too high. If their needs are not currently high but they had history of risk it is possible that they might get 20 sessions with Step 4 Psychological Therapies, but they have to have no active drug taking, no active self-harm, their risk has to be really low. Or, you can go through to the CATS service [Clinical and Assessment Treatment Services] but you have to have a diagnosis of mental health disorder, so if you've been somebody who has been repeatedly abused…if you don't have a diagnosis by a psychiatrist you can't get that help…if you have a primary drug problem, then mental health services will say well it's because she's got a drug problem and if she stopped her drug taking then she wouldn't have these issues (Health Shop).

6.10   Complexity and Multiplicity

There are a range of dynamics that shaper women's lived experiences and related support needs. Amongst others, the impact of age, class, ethnicity, education, disability, language and the interplay with the wider social structures on women's life experience and their access to help and support. The Duluth Power and Control Model can help to surface some of the additional barriers that survivors experience (Fig. 6.2). This diagram brings attention to the way perpetrators exploit facets of

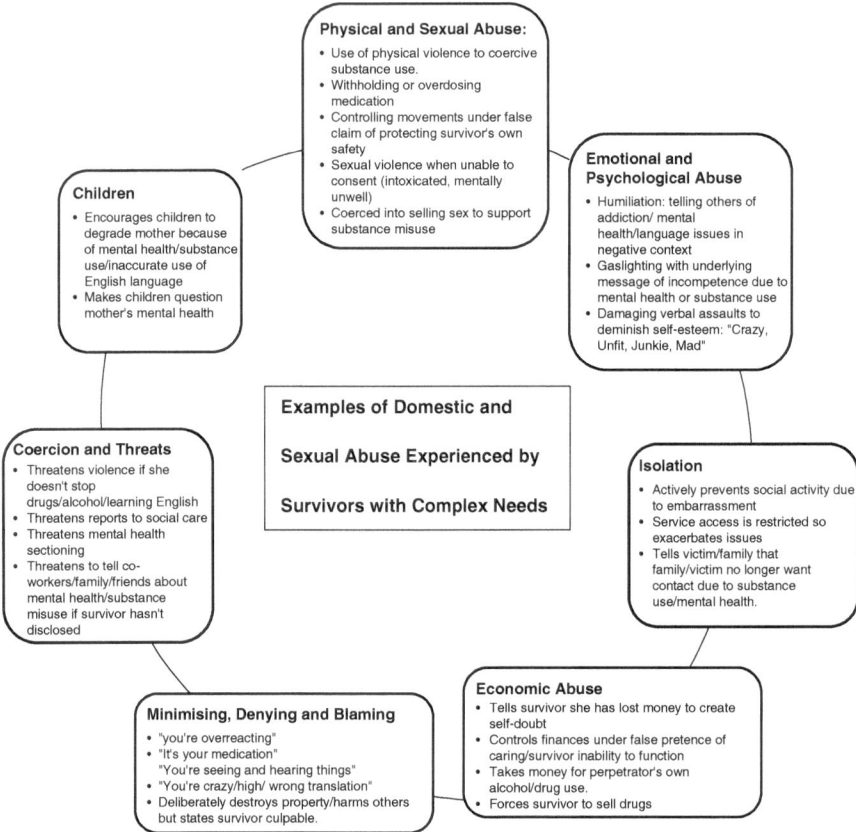

Fig. 6.2 Examples of domestic and sexual abuse experienced by survivors with complex needs. (Adapted from AVA [58]. With permission from Harris, L and Hodges K. (2019) 'Responding to Complexity: Improving Service Provision for Survivors of Domestic Abuse with "Complex Needs"'. Journal of Gender Based Violence)

women's lives such as substance use, mental ill health and language barriers to further enhance their coercive control. This can lead to further isolation and discrimination from statutory agencies and create difficulties in accessing help and support [1].

6.11 Meeting Women

There are fatal ramifications for women who are unable to get the help and protection they need. Service providers remarked on the barriers they had witnessed when trying to support survivors of DVA considered to have complex needs, which included women being portrayed as non-compliant or 'too complex' to house or engage with available services.

'…I can think of one particular woman—all day on the phone trying to find refuge space and we kept getting the same reply that the woman's needs were too high and she would put other women at risk or she would put other children at risk because of her drug taking or mental health issues, and then she was killed. Literally that happened on the Friday [trying to find refuge] and I came back into work on the Monday and she was killed. I can think of 6–7 women that we know have been killed at the point of trying to say "I am not safe and I need to go [into refuge]" but their needs were "too high" for those services.' (Health Shop, S1)

It is essential that women are able to access help and support, so vulnerabilities to exploitation and abuse can be limited. However, vulnerability to exploitation and abuse can stem from the way that services are provided and how women are expected to access support. There is a 'high prevalence of institutional misunderstanding' remaining about the needs and experiences of women, even though there is extensive and clear research (much of it government funded) setting out approaches and methods that would improve women's position [42, p. 16]. Here we explore the things that are helpful, or otherwise, for women when they are seeking support, the way they prefer to be met by helping services, and how this informs decisions and choices made about seeking help and support and returning to services.

6.12 Know That You Have a 'Need'

Women talk about the things that happen to them, but they rarely refer to the language of need used in policy and practice [3]. Numerous factors prevent women being able to attend services, but before being able to access a service for help and support, individuals have to know that their experience is considered a need, understand they are entitled to relevant support and that this support is available. This requires professionals delivering or developing services to understand how women frame the things that have happened to them and then be clear about the way support services can help.

6.13 Support Is Available

The next challenge for some women in seeking help and support is knowing services are there to help and that you have the right to access the service. Rachel (S2) commented that whilst she had been able to ask for help, there were times when she struggled to do so; however, there were other times when she was unaware of available support. She felt that professionals and support services 'need to try and identify and suggest to you that I think you could do with this'. Jane (S2) spoke to a number of shelter places and everywhere was full: 'the refuge was full; the council will get back to you in eight or something weeks'. Gaps in helping provision are also evident when services close down or are time limited and only available for a number of weeks or months. The practical and often coercive demands of service attendance can be very difficult for women [65]. Angela was required to attend probation appointments, but felt they offered her little.

Sometimes I used to turn up there and it was like "hi how are you and how you feeling, here's your next appointment" and that was it…although I was homeless my probation officer didn't do nothing all [and] she kept saying was probation hasn't got the resources to provide you with housing or accommodate you with housing, there's nothing I can do, but make sure you turn up for your next appointment or I'll breach you (Angela, S2).

Corston [42] reported on the number of women in prison who had breached community treatment order/programmes, which in the main had been developed and delivered based on the needs of the male majority, frequently at odds with the experiences and needs of women. Policymakers and commissioners have to fully explore and understand the things that happen to women and their corresponding support needs and priorities before devising systems of support. Otherwise, there is a risk of creating additional barriers and further harm. It is essential that effective support is well researched, available and is helpful.

6.14   Getting There

Many services operate on a conditional basis, yet the conditions are often very hard to fulfil for women whose everyday lives are already challenging and complex. As part of a drug rehabilitation programme, Jane (S2) had to attend multiple appointments across a city and she talked about how she struggled with this,

I was like on the bus here there here, there, every day and eventually I was just…cause mentally I was in a bad way, from my domestic violence and my drinking and my drugs and everything I was just a mess … my head was like a washing machine on spin… you've got to try and concentrate, go to [an] art lesson then go to … this alcohol talk then go to…. And everything is different parts of the city you know, you've got to go from there to there to there (Jane, S2).

Practitioners in the R2C study talked about the way they felt some survivors were perceived by other helping services; often other services would comment about a lack of 'compliance' with the help on offer.

'I think the main challenges are around how this client group are perceived by other services: I think there is still the concept of deserving and undeserving victims' (Opportunity Nottingham, S1).
   'The survivors themselves are often deemed as non-compliant because they are non-compliant, we know this, but there are reasons for why they are non-compliant and that can often be that big sort of stumbling block [to accessing services]' (HHT, S1).

6.15   Histories of Trauma Are Understood

Previous experiences of trauma and unsuccessful attempts at help-seeking must be understood as the context in which women seek support, and also in the way they should be met in services. When providing support to women with intersecting lived experiences, it is essential to integrate relationship-based practice approaches of trauma-informed care (see Chap. 12 for a detailed analysis of trauma-informed approaches). These approaches emphasise the importance of practitioners understanding the impact of previous trauma on help-seeking and responding accordingly.

Women 'read' professional caregivers' behaviour and decide if they are going to help, leaving services or not returning where they feel the response is negative or unhelpful [3]. This decision frequently and unintentionally disadvantages women and increases the risks they face [29]. Women decide if staff and services are trustworthy by noticing body language and assessing whether people seem to care [3].

> The way like they used to speak to you like it's just, like the vibe I used to get off her, you know, and when she would speak to me she'd never look me in the eye or just wee things like that (Anne, S2).
> The way…their body language…isn't it, body language I don't know…I can't put it in words… but it's just that feeling… of safety… hope… help… that you're going… that you're looking for… (Jane, S2).
> They are talking to me… smiling at me, asking how I am, how my son is… (Tina, S2).

Practitioners, service providers and policymakers need to explore and put into practice the literature promoting relationship-based approaches and trauma-informed care [60] and McCluskey's [66] theory of 'goal-corrected empathic attunement'. These approaches emphasise the importance of practitioners understanding the impact of previous trauma on help-seeking and responding accordingly.

6.16   Complexity of Service Provision

Helping services frequently respond to single needs or problems, and women with multiple and intersecting lived experiences are expected to attend different services that respond to the various facets of their lives. Services are not only siloed in the issues to which they will respond, such as addictions, mental health, DVA or housing, but there are variances in access criteria, qualifications and experience of staff. Ultimately this can be confusing and impenetrable for those seeking help and support. Taking the next step to attend a service is difficult without active support from staff at helping services, as Tess (S2) commented,

> I never actually went there because I found it really hard to organise myself and I just needed someone to take me to be honest. I only ever went to things when people told me go here and they went with me…

Additionally, the geographical location of a service can prevent women from accessing support, and this is particularly problematic for health and housing services, where often local connections are required to access support. For some, it is the challenge of physically getting to the location, for others it is about going to an area where they feel unsafe. Sandy (S2) did not go to mental health appointments because they were in an area where she had past experiences she wanted to avoid; she said, 'I just didn't turn up… just couldn't do it'. Accompanying women to appointments is an essential element of effective service delivery. For many women, being 'sign-posted' to a service is little help, it fails to understand the impact of the things that have happened to them on their experience of care-seeking. When services are commissioned, accompanying women to appointments should be considered an essential activity.

6.17   Feeling Safe

A sense of safety is created through other actions than just the practical management of a space. A place of safety involved, 'people that will listen to you and do what they say they are going to do' (Tina, S2). Safety is felt in women-only services [2, 67]. Judy (S2) said that a women-only setting enabled women to talk more freely; she felt that men 'dominated things' at other services. This was echoed in the evaluation of The Whole System Approach (WSA) for women offenders and women at risk of offending in Greater Manchester (introduced in September 2014) which found that:

> … women also reveal benefits from engaging with the women's centres. These include improved feelings about their self in terms of feeling valued, less shame and guilt and improved confidence; improvements in health, both mental health and physical health from reducing alcohol or drug use and reduced isolation; and developing practical skills through education, employment or volunteering opportunities [67].

However, the reality is that creating a safe space is neither simple nor one-dimensional. Symptoms of trauma arise from violence and abuse experienced in the past where a safe environment has been absent, therefore creating a place of safety for women is essential to promote better outcomes and quality of support. For many, it is a priority to recover from trauma before addressing other concerns in their lives, and relational and trauma-informed care approaches establish principles to improve responses for those seeking help and support [68].

6.18   Complex Experience Care Model

This model (Fig. 6.3) was developed from Hodges (S2) [4] research. It serves as a way of presenting the study findings and contextualising them in light of the study recommendations. It is a tool to help professionals understand the interconnecting nature of multiple and serve disadvantage, the priorities of women when help seeking and the responsibilities of those who respond. The model is also a framework for those providing services to support the planning and development of better services for women. The model illustrates aspects of the decisions and choices made by women when seeking help, and the steps required by services and policymakers to improve support and provide women with a safe place to come to and want to return. Underpinning this model is the individual's experience of trauma, consistently reported by women with intersecting lived experiences, making this model transferable into different settings.

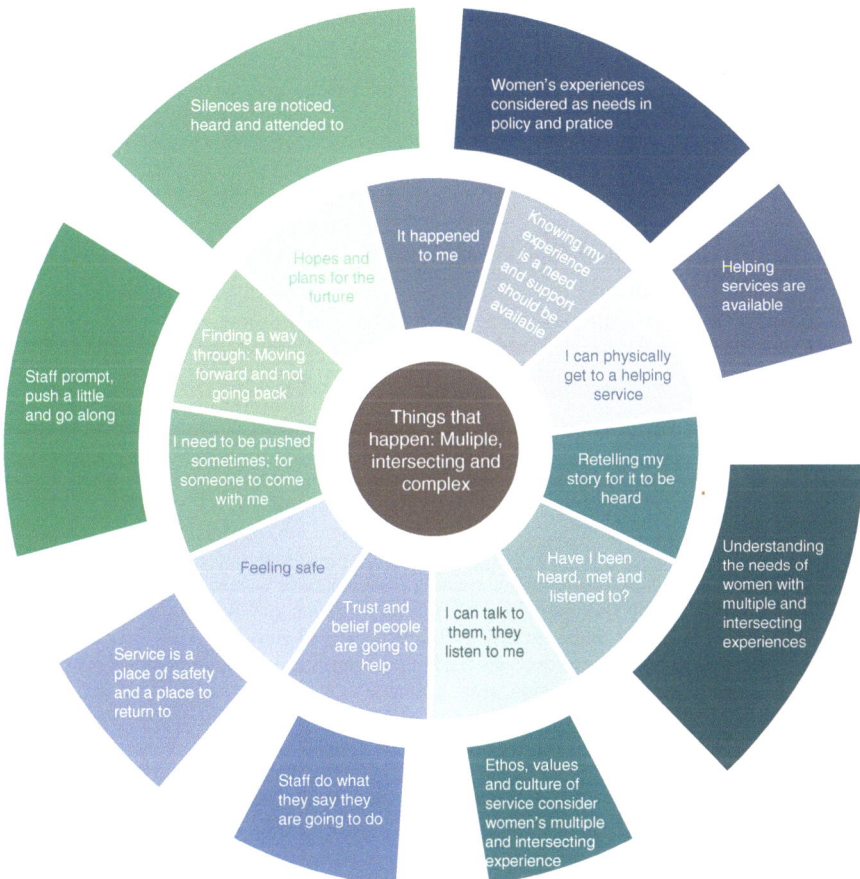

Fig. 6.3 Hodges and Burch (2019) Complex Experience Care Model (CECM)

The centre of the diagram reflects that things happen to individuals, and that these can create multiple, intersecting and complex experiences and related support needs. The middle ring illustrates aspects of decisions and choices made when seeking help and support. The outer ring brings attention to the responses required by policymakers, service commissioners and providers, alongside support staff and volunteers.

6.19   Conclusion

It is imperative that women with multiple and intersecting lived experiences and associated support needs are able to access help and support to limit their vulnerability to exploitation and abuse. A significant barrier to getting help stems from the way services are provided and how individuals are expected to access support [3]. In identifying ways to improve responses to abuse and exploitation, it is essential that practitioners, service providers and policymakers understand how individuals with multiple and intersecting experiences seek help and develop support which meets women in a way that enables them to feel safe.

Reflective Questions

- What will you do differently when 'meeting' women in the course of your work?
- What changes do you think your service, or the services you commission, need to make to become or remain a place where women know they can come to, feel safe, and are effectively supported to reduce the precarity in their lives?
- How could you use the CECM to inform your practice?

References

1. Harris L, Hodges K. Responding to complexity: improving service provision for survivors of domestic abuse with 'complex needs'. J Gend-Based Violence. 2019;3(2):167–84.
2. Harris L. Response to complexity (R2C): final evaluation. Nottingham: The University of Nottingham; 2016.
3. Hodges K, Burch S. Multiple and intersecting experiences of women in prostitution: improving access to helping services. Dign J Sex Exploit Violence. 2019;4(2). https://digitalcommons.uri.edu/cgi/viewcontent.cgi?article=1139&context=dignity.
4. Hodges K. An exploration of decision making by women experiencing multiple and complex needs. Cambridge: Anglia Ruskin University; 2018.
5. Godfrey M, Callaghan G. Exploring unmet need: the challenge of a user-centred response. York: York Pub. Services for the Joseph Rowntree Foundation; 2000.
6. Rosengard A, Laing I, Ridley J, Hunter S. A literature review on multiple and complex needs. 2007. [cited 24 Apr 2017]. http://mcnevaluation.co.uk/download/public/observatory/resource-type/research-evaluation/2007%20scottish%20executive%20lit%20review%20on%20multiple%20and%20complex%20needs.pdf.
7. Rankin J, Regan S. Meeting complex needs: the future of social care. London: IPPR: Turning Point; 2004.
8. Keene J. Clients with complex needs: interprofessional practice: Keene/clients. Oxford: Blackwell Science Ltd; 2001. [cited 23 Jun 2017]. http://doi.wiley.com/10.1002/9780470690352.
9. Cabinet Office. Reaching out: an action plan on social exclusion. London: HMSO; 2006.
10. Neale J. Gender and illicit drug use. Br J Soc Work. 2004;34(6):851–70.
11. Bramley G, Fitzpatrick S, Edwards J, Ford D, Johnsen S, Sosenko F, et al. Hard edges: mapping severe and multiple disadvantage. London: Lankelly Chase Foundation; 2015. [cited 23 Jun 2017]. http://lankellychase.org.uk/wp-content/uploads/2015/07/Hard-Edges-Mapping-SMD-2015.pdf.
12. Department of Health. Responding to domestic abuse: a resource for health professionals. London: Department of Health; 2017.
13. Hester M. Who does what to whom? Gender and domestic violence perpetrators in English police records. Eur J Criminol. 2013;10(5):623–37.
14. CPS. Violence against women and girls report 2017–18. CPS; 2018. [cited 5 Mar 2019]. https://www.cps.gov.uk/sites/default/files/documents/publications/cps-vawg-report-2018.pdf.
15. NCA. National referral mechanism statistics—end of year summary 2017. NCA; 2018. [cited 5 Mar 2019]. http://www.nationalcrimeagency.gov.uk/publications/national-referral-mechanism-statistics/2017-nrm-statistics/884-nrm-annual-report-2017/file.
16. O'Connor M. The sex economy (The gendered economy). Newcastle upon Tyne: Agenda Publishing; 2018. 128 p.

17. Coy M. Introduction: prostitution, harm and gender inequality. In: Coy M, editor. Prostitution, harm and gender inequality: theory, research and policy. Abingdon: Ashgate Publishing; 2016.

18. Ekberg G. The Swedish law that prohibits the purchase of sexual services: best practices for prevention of prostitution and trafficking in human beings. Violence Women. 2004;10(10):1187–218.

19. Bindel J, Brown L, Easton H, Matthews R, Reynolds L. Breaking down the barriers: a study of how women exit prostitution. London: Eaves; 2012.

20. Thiara RK, Hague G, Mullender A. Losing out on both counts: disabled women and domestic violence. Disabil Soc. 2011;26(6):757–71.

21. Walby S, Armstrong J, Strid S. Intersectionality: multiple inequalities in social theory. Sociology. 2012;46(2):224–40.

22. Hancock A-M. When multiplication doesn't equal quick addition. Perspect Polit. 2007;5(1):63–79.

23. McCall L. The complexity of intersectionality. Signs J Women Cult Soc. 2005;30(3):1771–800.

24. Crenshaw KW. Mapping the margins: intersectionality, identity politics, and violence against women of color (women of color at the center: selections from the third national conference on women of color and the law). Stanford Law Rev. 1991;43(6):1241–99.

25. Crenshaw K. Demarginalizing the intersection of race and sex: a black feminist critique of antidiscrimination doctrine, feminist theory and antiracist politics. 1989;(1), Article 8. Univ Chic Leg Forum.

26. Yuval-Davis N. Intersectionality and feminist politics. Eur J Womens Stud. 2006;13(3):193–209.

27. Fitzpatrick S, Bramley G, Johnsen S. Pathways into multiple exclusion homelessness in seven UK cities. Urban Stud. 2013;50(1):148–68.

28. McDonagh T. Tackling homeless exclusions: understanding complex lives. York: Joseph Rowntree Foundation; 2011.

29. Matthews R, Bindel J, Young L, Easton H. Exiting prostitution a study in female desistance. Basingstoke: Palgrave Macmillan; 2014.

30. Coy M. Young women, local authority care and selling sex: findings from research. Br J Soc Work. 2008;38(7):1408–24.

31. Hester M, Westmarland N. Tackling street prostitution: towards a holistic approach. London: DU; 2004. http://dro.dur.ac.uk/2557/.

32. McCracken K, Priest S, Torchia K, Parry W, Stanley N. Evaluation of pause: research report. Department for Education; 2017. [cited 31 Aug 2017]. https://www.gov.uk/government/uploads/system/uploads/attachment_data/file/625374/Evaluation_of_Pause.pdf.

33. Broadhurst K, Alrouh B, Yeend E, Harwin J, Shaw M, Pilling M, et al. Connecting events in time to identify a hidden population: birth mothers and their children in recurrent care proceedings in England. Br J Soc Work. 2015;45(8):2241 60.

34. Dalla RL. Night moves: a qualitative investigation of street-level sex work. Psychol Women Q. 2002;26(1):63–73.

35. Shapiro M, Hughes DM. Decriminalized prostitution: impunity for violence and exploitation. Wake For Law Rev. 2017;52:29.

36. Hales L, Gelsthorpe L. The criminalisation of migrant women. Cambridge: University of Cambridge; 2012. 119 p.

37. Lee M. Trafficking and global crime control. London: Sage; 2011. [cited 5 Oct 2017]. http://knowledge.sagepub.com/view/trafficking-and-global-crime-control/SAGE.xml.

38. Lehti M, Aromaa K. Trafficking for sexual exploitation. Crime Justice. 2006;34(1):133–227.

39. Surviving Economic Abuse. Statistics on financial and economic abuse. 2020. [cited 17 Aug 2020]. https://survivingeconomicabuse.org/wp-content/uploads/2020/03/Statistics-on-economic-abuse.pdf.

40. Postmus JL, Plummer S-B, McMahon S, Murshid NS, Kim MS. Understanding economic abuse in the lives of survivors. J Interpers Violence. 2012;27(3):411–30.

41. Purdam K, Prattley J. Financial debt amongst older women in the United Kingdom—shame, abuse and resilience. Ageing Soc. 2020;21:1–23.

42. Corston J. The Corston report. London: Home Office; 2007. [cited 23 Jun 2017]. http://www.justice.gov.uk/publications/docs/corston-report-march-2007.pdf.
43. Prison Reform Trust, Women in Prison. Home truths: housing for women in the criminal justice system. Prison Reform Trust; 2016. [cited 9 Oct 2017]. http://www.womeninprison.org.uk/perch/resources/final-report-by-prt-and-wip-home-truths.pdf.
44. Bretherton J, Pleace N. Women and rough sleeping: a critical review of current research and methodology. York: University of York; 2018.
45. Keast M. Understanding and responding to modern slavery within the homelessness sector. London: Homeless Link; 2017. [cited 26 Nov 2018]. https://www.antislaverycommissioner.co.uk/media/1115/understanding-and-responding-to-modern-slavery-within-the-homelessness-sector.pdf.
46. Homeless Link. Trafficking and forced labour: guidance for frontline homelessness services. London: Homeless Link; 2016. [cited 26 Nov 2018]. https://www.homeless.org.uk/sites/default/files/site-attachments/Trafficking%20and%20Forced%20Labour%20guidance%20-%20May%202016.pdf.
47. Worrall A, Gelsthorpe L. 'What works' with women offenders: the past 30 years. Probat J. 2009;56(4):329–45.
48. Fawcett Society. Women and the criminal justice system. London: Fawcett Society; 2004.
49. Harvey H, Brown L, Young L. 'I'm no criminal': examining the impact of prostitution-specific criminal records on women seeking to exit prostitution. London: Nia; 2017.
50. Rugmay J. When victims become offenders: in search of coherence in policy and practice. Fam Intim Partn Violence Q. 2010;3(1):47–64.
51. Ministry of Justice. Female offender strategy. Ministry of Justice; 2018. [cited 8 Oct 2018]. https://assets.publishing.service.gov.uk/government/uploads/system/uploads/attachment_data/file/719819/female-offender-strategy.pdf.
52. Brown L. Cycles of harm: problematic alcohol use amongst women involved in prostitution. London: Alcohol Research UK; 2013. [cited 23 Jun 2017]. http://alcoholresearchuk.org/downloads/finalReports/FinalReport_0108.pdf.
53. Young AM, Boyd C, Hubbell A. Prostitution, drug use, and coping with psychological distress. J Drug Issues. 2000;30(4):789–800.
54. Fox S, Galvani S. Substance use and domestic abuse: essential information for social workers. BASW. 2020. [cited 17 Aug 2020]. https://e-space.mmu.ac.uk/625366/1/1811127%20Substance%20use%20and%20domestic%20abuse%20pocket%20guide%20final.pdf.
55. Fox S. "They said if you come you can't drink. I thought, I can't stop." Exploring the journeys to support among women who experience co-occurring substance use and domestic abuse. Manchester: Manchester Metropolitan; 2018. [cited 5 Jun 2020]. https://e-space.mmu.ac.uk/622567/1/Sarah%20Fox%20PhD%20Thesis.pdf.
56. Scott S, McManus S. Hidden hurt: violence, abuse and disadvantage in the lives of women. Agenda; 2016. [cited 10 Oct 2017]. http://weareagenda.org/wp-content/uploads/2015/11/Hidden-Hurt-full-report1.pdf.
57. Trevillion K, Oram S, Feder G, Howard LM. Experiences of domestic violence and mental disorders: a systematic review and meta-analysis. PLoS One. 2012;7(12):1–12.
58. AVA. Complicated matters: a toolkit addressing domestic and sexual violence, substance use and mental ill-health. London: AVA; 2013. [cited 17 Aug 2020]. https://avaproject.org.uk/wp/wp-content/uploads/2013/05/AVA-Toolkit-2018reprint.pdf.
59. Howard L, Trevillion K, Agnew-Davies R. Domestic violence and mental health. Int Rev Psychiatry. 2010;22(5):525–34.
60. Van der Kolk BA. The body keeps the score: brain, mind and body in the healing of trauma. New York: Penguin Books; 2015. 445 p.
61. Ross CA, Farley M, Schwartz HL. Dissociation among women in prostitution. In: Farley M, editor. Prostitution, trafficking and traumatic stress. Binghamton, NY: Haworth Maltreatment & Trauma Press; 2003.

62. Scott S, Williams J, McNaughton Nicholls C, McManus S, Brown A, Harvey S, et al. Violence, abuse and mental health in England (REVA Briefing 1). 2015. p. 13. www.natcen.ac.uk/rev-abriefing1.
63. Holly J. Mapping the maze: services for women experiencing multiple disadvantage in England and Wales. AVA & Agenda. 2017. [cited 8 Sep 2017]. http://weareagenda.org/wp-content/uploads/2017/09/Mapping-the-Maze-final-report-for-publication.pdf.
64. Cook D. Criminal and social justice. London: Sage; 2006.
65. Rummery K. Partnership working and tackling violence against women. In: Violence against women: current theory and practice in domestic abuse, sexual violence and exploitation. London: Jessica Kingsley; 2013. p. 213.
66. McCluskey U. To be met as a person: the dynamics of attachment in professional encounters. London: Karnac; 2005.
67. Kinsella R, O'Keeffe C, Lowthian J, Clarke B, Ellison M. Evaluation of the whole system approach for women offenders: interim report. Sheffield: Sheffield Hallam University; 2015.
68. Sweeney A, Filson B, Kennedy A, Collinson L, Gillard S. A paradigm shift: relationships in trauma-informed mental health services. BJPsych Adv. 2018;24(5):319–33.

Challenging Social Norms and Legal Responses to Rape and Sexual Violence: Insights from a Practice–Research Partnership in Kenya

Sarah R. Rockowitz, Wangu Kanja, and Heather D. Flowe

7.1   Introduction

Sexual violence (SV) is one of the world's most widespread non-communicable diseases [1] and human rights abuses [2]. The World Health Organization (WHO) defines SV as any sexual act or attempt to obtain a sexual act, unwanted sexual comments or advances, acts to traffic or acts directed against a person's sexuality using coercion by anyone no matter their relationship to the victim and in any setting, including home and work [3]. SV around the world is set against a backdrop of impunity, power imbalance and lack of respect for human dignity. Recent analyses of the World Values Survey, for instance, indicate that people hold some sort of bias against women (e.g. men are superior leaders, men are better in business, it is acceptable for a man to beat his wife) in 69 out of the 75 countries surveyed, and that these biases are growing [4]. Pervasive negative beliefs about women, such as rape myths—which are stereotypical and false notions about the crime, victims and perpetrators—cause and sustain inadequate responses to SV by societies, communities, families and individuals and enable cycles of violence to continue [5]. SV impedes sustainable development, and has devastating effects on survivors and their families, and far-reaching social, economic and intergenerational impacts. Thus, duty bearers (including police, courts of law and healthcare workers) and researchers must work in partnership as well as be led by affected communities in the development and delivery of SV prevention, protection and response measures.

Over 11 million women in Kenya have experienced SV as children and/or adults [6]. Gender inequality is widespread in Kenya, which ranks 142 out of 189 countries

S. R. Rockowitz (✉) · H. D. Flowe
University of Birmingham, Birmingham, UK
e-mail: SXR1005@student.bham.ac.uk; H.Flowe@bham.ac.uk

W. Kanja
Wanju Kanja Foundation, Nairobi, Kenya

Box 7.1 The Wangu Kanja Foundation

The Wangu Kanja Foundation (WKF) is a non-profit organization founded in 2005 that focuses on promoting prevention, protection and response towards ending Sexual Violence. WKF envisages a society that is safe and free from all forms of violence. The Wangu Kanja Foundation convenes the Survivors of Sexual Violence in Kenya Network.

The Survivors of Sexual Violence in Kenya Movement brings together a unified voice of the survivors to address all forms of sexual violence and to amplify their voices across the country. The movement is anchored within the already existing community structures for purposes of ensuring innovation and sustainability.

More information can be found at wangukanjafoundation.org

on the Gender Inequality Index [4]. Despite the widespread occurrence of SV in Kenya, we lack systematic data on its nature (e.g. crime hot spots, perpetrator characteristics, crime reporting) and the effectiveness of interventions to prevent and respond to its occurrence. In Kenya, survivors infrequently report rape to the police, and among those who do, their cases are unlikely to be thoroughly investigated, correctly documented and successfully prosecuted.

To understand and address the complexities of SV in Kenya, fair and equitable practice-driven research partnerships are essential. A practice–research partnership is defined by having a common purpose, complimentary skills and effective communication processes across the team [7]. Fair and equitable partnerships are characterised by putting poverty first (by continually questioning whether and how the research contributes to the alleviation of poverty), by having transparency in the administration, budget and conduct of the research, and by sharing research outcomes and benefits, not only with all members of the research team but also with the communities and individuals who are affected by SV [8]. Alongside this, an intersectional feminist lens that examines and challenges power is essential for more ethical and equitable research and impact [9]. In this chapter, we describe the context and aims of a practice–research partnership in Kenya on SV between the Wangu Kanja Foundation (see Box 7.1) and academics specializing in public health, forensic psychology and human memory. In what follows, we outline the historical context of sexual violence in Kenya and summarise research on experiences of SV across the life course, the legal response to SV and research we are undertaking to improve the efficacy of SV response, prevention and protection.

7.2   The Kenyan Context

Kenya is in East Africa, bordering Tanzania, Ethiopia, South Sudan, Somalia and Uganda. As of 2019, Kenya is home to nearly 48 million people living across 47 counties [10]. The number of men and women is nearly equal in Kenya, with there being 98.1 males per 100 females (ibid). Despite the sex ratio being very close, Kenya has a very high ranking on the Gender Inequality Index, placing 134 out of 162 countries evaluated and having a Gender Inequality Index value of 0.545, while countries like the United Kingdom and United States have values of 0.119 and 0.182, respectively [4]. Nairobi City is the most populous county and has a population of over four million people (ibid). Kenya has a social and historical context that is rooted in colonial rule and patriarchal domination [11]. In the years directly preceding British colonialism, when European travellers arrived in Kenya as the face of British commerce, members of European caravans were frequently accused of sexually abusing local Kenyan women [12]. British colonialism then arrived, with the East Africa Protectorate formed in the late nineteenth century, which eventually evolved into the Colony and Protectorate of Kenya, otherwise known as British Kenya, which was part of the British Empire from 1920 to 1963. Colonial forces instituted economic and social structures that disrupted existing kinship relations [11]. Colonial rule also came with a shift in women's roles. Prior to colonial intervention, Kenyan women were responsible for farming the family land and selling farm produce [11]. During post-colonial intervention, land was redistributed and women became unable to produce and sell food, making them economically dependent on men and leading to a heightened culture of domestic patriarchy backed by colonial social norms [11]. This impunity and lack of respect for human rights have contributed to the SV that prevails today.

The long and continuing history of SV in Kenya is also partially attributable to gendered identities and unequal power dynamics that have arisen from decades of armed resistance as a response to colonial oppression and racial domination [13]. The Mau Mau Uprising occurred towards the end of Britain's colonial rule in Kenya. It was an 8-year war between local Kenyans of varying ethnic groups, local European settlers, and the British army [14]. During this time, British-sponsored government forces, especially the police, committed grave human rights abuses against Kenyans, including rape and other forms of sexual assault [14].

The trend of increased sexual violence during political upheaval has continued to present day. Victims in Kenya are often targeted on the basis of their actual or perceived ethnic, religious, political or clan affiliations [15]. Sexual violence is employed as a tactic of ethnic hatred, even ethnic cleansing, and continues to be a weapon of war. It is one of the least reported crimes, with many survivors living in fear of rejection, as communities are more likely to punish the victim than the perpetrator. According to the population-based 2014 Demographic and Health Survey (DHS), 40.7% of women have experienced physical and/or sexual intimate partner violence at least once in their lifetime. Further, 26% of women have experienced physical and/or sexual intimate partner violence in the last 12 months [15]. In collecting this data, the DHS used a modified version of the Conflict Tactics Scale, asking women if they had experienced violence, such as getting pushed, shaken or slapped, getting choked or burned, or getting physically forced to perform sexual acts unwillingly at the hands of a spouse or partner [15]. The DHS uses this approach to ensure the operational definition of violence is clear to respondents. However, this serves to exclude other types of violent acts and may mean that the DHS data underestimates the prevalence of intimate partner violence.

Spikes in sexual violence occur during major political events in Kenya, such as the 2007–2008 and 2017 post-election periods. The 2007–2008 post-election period was especially severe. Women and girls were subject to rape, genital mutilation and physical abuse, sometimes leading to death, as well as extreme sexual harassment, psychological torture and forced divorce and marital separation [13]. One Nairobi hospital noted that during the post-election crisis, there were three times as many women who had suffered sexual violence compared to other periods [13]. Much of this post-election violence is based on ethnic affiliation, and when ethnic violence breaks out, entire subsets of the population move into internally displaced person (IDP) camps, with ensuing sexual violence [11]. In more than half of the post-election sexual violence incidents, the perpetrators worked for the police and state services [14]. Survivors often will not report these incidences due to fear of reprisal [14]. Although the sexual violence concerning the election was well-documented, the government has failed to implement a reparation program and women continue to live with lasting trauma [16]. Additionally, there were reports that the police demanded fees to investigate cases, which precluded survivors from reporting them [16]. Further, the police failed to follow up on the cases that were reported [16]. This knowledge provides scope for improving criminal investigation techniques and providing access to justice. Thus, few, if any, survivors have experienced justice.

Reflective Exercise 1

1. Why is it so important to understand the social and historical context of a topic before beginning research?
2. How might Kenya's past and contemporary history affect formal and informal responses to sexual violence?
3. How might Kenya's history with colonialism influence their willingness to partner with Western organizations?

7.3 Life Course Perspectives and SV Impacts in Kenya

In Kenya, like other patriarchal contexts around the world [2], SV affects people across all stages of life, and largely women and girls. Nearly 41% of women in Kenya have ever experienced lifetime physical and/or sexual intimate partner violence, with nearly 26% reporting having experienced it in the last 12 months [15]. For men, 6% have ever experienced sexual violence and 2% had experienced it in the last 12 months [15]. For comparison, in the United States, 25% of women and 11% of men have ever experienced lifetime physical and/or sexual intimate partner violence, and in England and Wales approximately 30% of women and 15% of men had experienced intimate violence since the age of 16 [17, 18].

Research across low-and middle-income countries has shown that young adult women (aged 20–24 years) have a higher risk of violence than older women, with adolescents (aged 15–19 years) showing comparable risk when compared to young adult women [19]. In Kenya, childhood sexual violence (before age 18) has been experienced by a third of females and nearly a fifth of males according to the most recent population-based survey [20]. This survey was conducted with two age groups: 18–24-year olds with lifetime experience of violence and 13–17-year olds who had experienced violence in the 12 months prior to the survey [20]. Questions on the survey were based on questions from previous international and national surveys such as the Kenya DHS, the Youth Risk Behaviour Survey, the Hopkins Symptoms Checklist and the WHO multi-country study on Women's Health and Domestic Violence against Women [20]. For females in Kenya, the data suggest that 18% experience their first incident of sexual violence by the age of 13, 39% while they are 14–15 years old and 43% when they are 16–17 years old [20]. 24.3% of females also noted that they had experienced unwilling first sexual intercourse prior to age 18 [20]. Sexual violence is often not the only type of violence that female victims in Kenya experience before they are 18 years old, with only 5.5% of females reporting that they experienced sexual violence alone [20]. Among females surveyed in Kenya, 11.8% experienced sexual violence and physical violence, 1.5% experienced sexual violence and emotional violence and 12.8% experienced sexual, physical and emotional violence [20]. Some of the main reasons for the pervasiveness of violence of any type against children, especially girls, are that Kenyan society tends to resolve conflict through physical violence, women are inferior in Kenya's patriarchal society and violence is seen as an appropriate means of social control [21]. Compared to research on SV in women and girls, there is relatively little research on violence against boys in Kenya. Findings from the Kenya Demographic Health Survey in 2010 showed no nationally representative estimates of violence against boys or men in Kenya; however, the 2010 Violence Against Children in Kenya study found that 18% of males experienced sexual violence before age 18, as compared to 32% for females [20].

Overall, the research suggests survivors presenting for medical treatment or reporting cases to the police are young in Kenya. For example, the average age of females seen by a one-stop centre (OSC) in Kenya was 14 years old [22]. Adolescents seem to be at an especially heightened risk for physical and sexual intimate partner violence, defined as any act that results in or may result in physical, sexual or psychological harm or suffering, perhaps owing to their young age and lack of experience with relationships [22]. In up to 42% of cases, a young girl's introduction to sexuality, which public health researchers term *sexual debut* [23], is through coercion, be it via force, gift giving, flattery, pestering, threatening to have sex with other girls or simply letting the man do what he wants [23]. This early and coerced sexual initiation has been connected to issues adolescent girls experience later in life, including violence, controlling partners and continued sexual coercion [24]. According to the ecological model [25], individual experiences are part of a larger dynamic system (see Fig. 7.1). While sexual violence takes place between two (or more) individuals, it is able to do so because of the emotionally unstable or violent interpersonal relationships that exist in a community with poor law enforcement and justice responses that are made possible by the gender inequality and cultural

Fig. 7.1 The ecological model of sexual violence. (Adapted from Krug et al., World report on violence and health, World Health Organization, 2002)

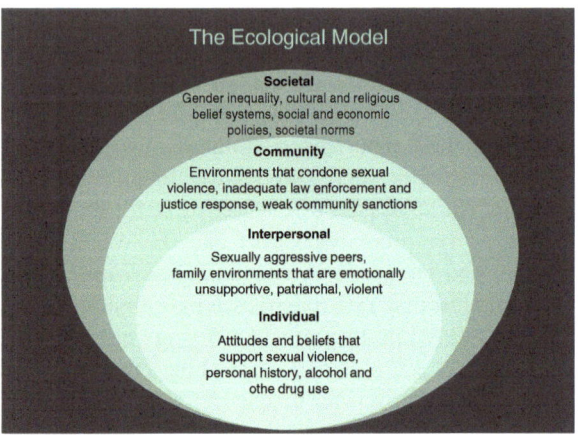

systems that exist on a societal level. Therefore, it is important to consider the cyclical nature of violence and lasting impact of trauma and target interventions at all levels.

Reflective Exercise 2

The ecological model is a popular framework in health and social care and has been used widely to understand the complexity of GBV and its impacts. But how helpful is the model in understanding SV? From what you have read so far in this chapter about the Kenyan context, does the model assist in your understanding of the issue?

Longitudinal and cross-sectional studies in Kenya as well as other countries document the short- and long-term impacts of SV morbidity on health [26]. While there is little research on long-term health impacts of SV in Kenya specifically, research shows that women in Kenya as well as in other countries around the globe who suffer SV are over 1.40 times more likely to have a premature birth, 1.52 times more likely to acquire HIV/AIDS and 4.54 times more likely to die by suicide [27]. Other well-documented harmful effects associated with SV include: death and disability arising from physical injury, damage to sexual and reproductive health, chronic diseases, mental health conditions and health-harming behaviours, such as misuse of alcohol and other drugs [27].

In other global women's health research conducted outside of Kenya, women who had ever experienced physical or sexual partner violence were significantly more likely to report having poor or very poor health than women who had never experienced partner violence [2]. Additionally, previous experience of physical or emotional intimate partner violence and home violence are risk factors for being raped in the future [28]. These findings are in line with other research on cycles of violence showing that people who have experienced violence in the past are at a heightened risk of experiencing it again [28]. Children who witness or suffer SV are more likely than their counterparts to have behavioural problems, poor health and developmental outcomes, and perpetrate intimate partner violence as adults [20, 29, 30]. The human health and social burdens of SV negatively impact educational, social and economic participation, as well as family resilience. Sexual violence is such a significant event in one's life that even after adjusting for age, educational attainment and marital status, intimate partner violence is significantly associated with lasting impacts on women's physical, mental, sexual and reproductive well-being [2]. The human suffering caused by SV is compounded for women and girls in low- and middle-income countries such as Kenya and in displaced, conflict-ridden and rural communities, where the prevalence is high and the response is inadequate. SV morbidity, mortality and its effects on economic and social well-being are major obstacles to the Sustainable Development Goals (SDG), particularly SDG5, which concerns gender equality and the empowerment of women. These findings are in keeping with research conducted in Kenya [15, 27] as well as our experience in working with adult and child SV survivors in Kenya. Thus, SV is an urgent global health problem requiring interdisciplinary research to develop effective responses and interventions.

7.4   SV Response and Intervention

Rape is defined in Kenya as an intentional and unlawful 'act which causes penetration with his or her genital organs; the other person does not consent to the penetration; or the consent is obtained by force or by means of threats or intimidation of any kind' [31, p. 5]. If a survivor reports sexual violence to the authorities, there will be a number of stages of documentation and medico-legal evidence collection before the case can proceed to court. Survivors may first present at a police station where their testimony will be taken by an officer at a gender desk. Gender desks were established to receive, investigate and refer cases to other stakeholders (e.g. to health providers, psycho-social support service providers, NGOs and the courts). After reporting to the police, survivors will be referred to the hospital for a medical examination. Survivors could also seek medical assistance first and the hospital will complete a medical examination and treat them before referring the survivor to the police.

When a survivor attends the hospital for a forensic medical examination, the health practitioner conducting the examination will complete the Post Rape Care and P3 documents to outline any injuries to the victim, and any biological or other specimens the examiner may have collected [32]. Completion of these documents is mandatory for a police investigation, which will include sending specimens for analysis at government facilities. This is a lengthy process for a survivor and can have economic consequences both for individual survivors and society as a whole due to missed work and diverted resources as survivors are charged to collect the necessary documentation required to proceed with a prosecution [33, 34]. Additionally, police and medical facilities are under-resourced. Survivors may be asked to provide expenses for the equipment that is necessary for collecting medico-legal evidence. For example, Wangamati and colleagues [32] found that a child victim was asked to provide money for gloves to conduct her medical examination. These experiences may deter survivors of SV from attempting to access justice, particularly considering the financial and time restrictions survivors face.

The research evidence base on SV in low- and middle-income countries is largely focused on the delivery of healthcare services and case management, albeit few studies have been conducted in Kenya. Research suggests that the poor collection and preservation of medico-legal evidence is a significant factor impeding prosecutions [35]. Health providers and the police receive inadequate training regarding how to properly document crimes on official forms [35]. Providing training to healthcare providers and police personnel on the legal requirements for properly documenting a case has been shown to be effective in increasing the number of forms completed correctly over the course of the intervention [35]. Inadequate infrastructure combined with the development of the standardised form led to the creation of MediCapt, an app that was co-developed by Physicians for Human Rights [36]. MediCapt comprises an Android app, which can be used by the medical sector, and a web-based app that can be accessed by law enforcement and the judiciary. It enables electronically systematising and preserving medico-legal evidence, which is essential in prosecuting sexual violence in Kenya. MediCapt provides a secure channel to submit evidence to the police and courts from the health clinic. However, even with improvements in medico-legal evidence documentation and transmission, attitudes held by police and prosecutors that condone sexual violence discourage survivors from reporting and limit successful adjudication [37]. Further, there is a lack of awareness about the illegality of sexual violence, and citizens need more knowledge about how to report sexual violence crimes to the police (see Situational Analysis and the Legal Framework on Sexual and Gender-Based Violence in Kenya: Challenges and Opportunities, Kenya Law, 2014).

In some locations, sexual violence is dealt with by customary structures, making it less likely that crimes are brought to the attention of the police and judiciary [38]. A limited number of studies have been undertaken to develop or assess interventions aimed at improving the criminal justice response to sexual violence. The limited research that does exist suggests system-wide changes may be required to impact the rate of successful prosecutions. Few cases normally make it to court, and even fewer result in a conviction [39]. Case attrition throughout the legal proceedings is common. Many SV cases are not reported, are not prosecuted or are settled financially out of court [32]. For instance, out of 1052 cases handled by the Wangu Kanja Foundation, 130 were reported to the police, 40 proceeded to court and fewer than 15 cases were concluded. These low numbers underscore the host of challenges survivors face when they try to access justice (Fig. 7.2).

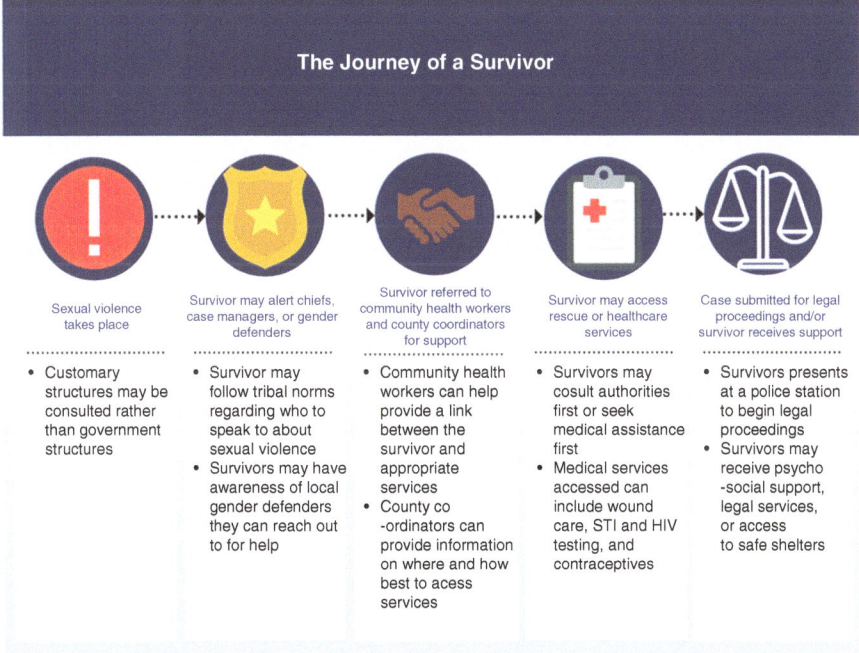

Fig. 7.2 The journey of a survivor

7.5 Special Issues That Arise in Disclosing Sexual Violence in Kenya

There are a number of avenues through which sexual violence survivors may disclose. The route through which a survivor discloses depends on a host of factors, such as their socioeconomic status, geographic location and the wider cultural context [38]. In Kenya, survivors of sexual violence tend to disclose to community health volunteers, human rights defenders, religious institutions and family members, as influenced by culture, tradition, religion and relationships. The majority of men and women do not disclose to anyone or go to health facilities due to fear of separation or being abandoned by their significant other. Figure 7.2 is a schematic of the case referral pathway in Kenya. There are obstacles along the pathway that can prevent survivors from accessing post-rape care services and justice. Survivors may feel threatened and stigmatised and be reluctant to tell the authorities about the violation. Additionally, health centres may be poorly equipped and personnel may not have had adequate training in post-rape care or in forensic medicine. Clinics may also be difficult to access due to distance or a lack of transportation, or be completely out of reach during times of national insecurity (e.g., post-election violence). There may be delays in service delivery, which can threaten the collection and availability of medical evidence. Survivors may also be charged to receive services, which is cost prohibitive and limits access for many. For example, although the forms should be free to access, sometimes there are charges for photocopying and handling. All things considered, further work remains to be done to ensure survivors receive the psychosocial support, clinical care and security that they need and to facilitate criminal investigations.

The Kenyan government has taken steps to improve how sexual assault cases are handled, especially by creating the *National Guidelines on Management of Sexual Violence in Kenya*. These guidelines were updated most recently in 2014 and were created to give information on managing sexual violence in Kenya from clinical, justice and societal approaches. Despite this, there still remains a multitude of barriers that prevent sexual assault survivors from accessing adequate care. One issue is that creating these guidelines did nothing to alter societal perspectives on sexual assault and women's health. For example, although the guidelines clearly state that women should have access to 'termination of pregnancy and post abortion care in the event of pregnancy from rape' [40, p. 78], many health providers still criminalise provision of abortion services to minors on religious grounds or believe that abortion should only be offered if there is risk to the mother [41]. Additionally, Kenya remains a patriarchal and inequitable society that tolerates both blatant and subtle violence against women, such as degrading jokes or demeaning glances.

7.6   Ethics, Sensitivities and Complexities of Working with Survivors

Like all research with SV survivors around the world, working with SV survivors in Kenya raises significant ethical and safety considerations for the survivor, their family and close contacts, as well as for practitioners and researchers [42, 43]. Focusing on the survivor-centred approach, which places the rights of survivors at the centre of the response, considers the needs and vulnerabilities of survivors and complements the human rights-based approach. Some considerations include survivors being vulnerable to traumatic stress reactions, retribution by the perpetrator, who may be a spouse or other person known to the survivor, stigmatisation and social rejection by his or her family and/or community. Furthermore, a level of cultural competence is needed to ensure that responses by practitioners and researchers are cognizant of the context in which the SV took place. SV can look different depending on factors such as social, religious, historical and cultural context, and it is important to consider these when working with survivors.

Researchers should take care not to engage in research with survivors who are in a crisis state or if there is any reason to believe that research participation will compromise the survivor's safety or mental health or cause anyone harm. Research data also should not be personally identifiable or traceable back to individual participants. Research participants should be given information about post-rape care services and medico-legal resources in the event that the survivor wishes to obtain medical care, access social services or legally report the incident. Practitioners and

Table 7.1 Key points in working with survivors

• Using the survivor-centred approach is the best way to ensure the safety and well-being of the survivor in a human rights context
• It is important to consider a survivor's safety and mental health before engaging in research
• Research data must not be traceable to the survivor
• Practitioners and researchers must have specialised training in working with survivors of SV

researchers should have specialised training in the dynamics of SV and be provided with information about risks and safety procedures in carrying out the research. Researchers should receive training on how to recognise their own limitations and capabilities to assist other survivors. They should also be trained to hold the information they obtain in confidence and to not to share it with anyone else besides the project team. Building trust between researcher and participant is also a crucial step. Without trust and a sense of rapport, the participant may not be as willing to share information, especially about such a sensitive topic (Table 7.1).

7.7   Future Directions

We are developing innovative solutions for documenting SV cases to better understand the nature of SV and how to more effectively offer survivor-centred post-rape care services and bring more perpetrators to justice. This work is vital. Even though states are obligated to adopt legislative measures to ensure remedies to victims of SV including restitution, compensation, rehabilitation, satisfaction and guarantees of non-repetition [44, 45], these obligations are not being fulfilled. This has resulted in impunity for perpetrators, the silencing of victims and continued cycles of violence [46]. Our research is focused on strengthening national judicial mechanisms to investigate, prosecute and redress victims of serious crimes. As a first step, cases need to be better documented to build evidence about the factors that contribute to the occurrence of SV, the lack of reporting and case attrition to better advocate for policies and legislation that increase survivors' access to justice.

Along these lines, the Wangu Kanja Foundation has developed mobile application and web portal MobApp, a comprehensive, systematic and independent documentation system to identify the impacts of sexual violence on the survivor's health and well-being and identify barriers to accessing post-rape care services and justice (see examples in Fig. 7.3). MobApp is being used by the Sexual Violence Survivors' Network in Kenya to document cases in all 47 counties. We are researching effective methods of training the survivors to use MobApp to collect reliable and accurate data. Further, we are analysing the data to help officials understand and recognise the scale of SV in Kenya. Comprehensive case documentation can enable authorities, the public and the electorate to understand the full scope of SV and identify new investigation avenues, such as using low-cost techniques for identifying serial perpetrators. Findings from this data will hopefully lead to the creation of one-stop centres, a model for post-rape service provision that has been successful in

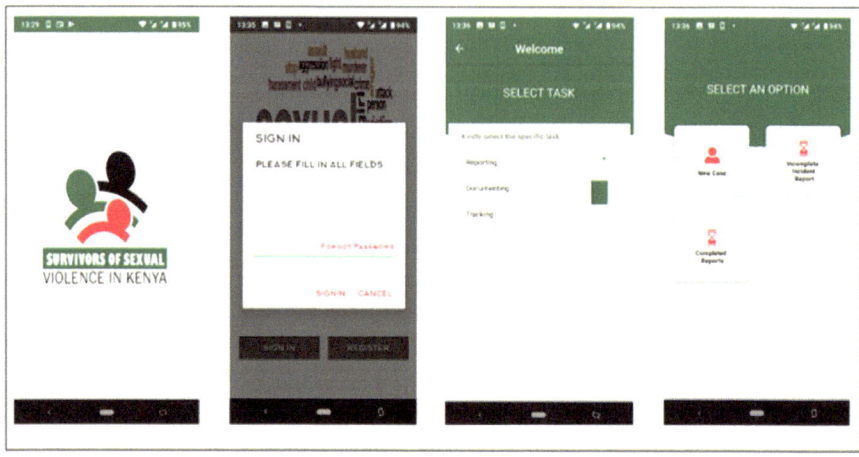

Fig. 7.3 MobApp screenshots courtesy of Wangu Kanja Foundation

multiple countries across the world. By having a centralized location for survivors to access medical and legal services, the hope is that reporting of cases and prosecution of offenders will increase.

References

1. Tulchinsky T, Varavikova E. The New Public Health, Third Edition. Elsevier, San Diego: Academic Press; 2014.
2. Garcia-Moreno C, Jansen HAFM, Ellsberg M, Heise L, Watts C. WHO multi-country study on women's health and domestic violence against women: initial results on prevalence, health outcomes, and women's responses. Geneva: World Health Organization; 2005.
3. World Health Organization/London School of Hygiene and Tropical Medicine. Preventing intimate partner and sexual violence against women: taking action and generating evidence. Geneva: World Health Organization; 2010.
4. UNDP. Gender inequality index. New York: United Nations Development Programme; 2019.
5. Kalra G, Bhugra D. Sexual violence against women: understanding cross-cultural intersections. Indian J Psychiatry. 2013;55(3):244–50.
6. Commission NGaE. National monitoring and evaluation framework towards the prevention of and response to sexual and gender based violence in Kenya. Nairobi: NGEC; 2014.
7. Spross J. The clinical nurse specialist as collaborator. In: Hamric AB, Spross J, editors. The clinical nurse specialist in theory and practice. Philadelphia: WB Saunders; 1989.
8. Frandman J, Hall B, Hayman R, Narayanan P, Newman K, Tandon R. Promoting fair and equitable research partnerships to respond to global challenges. 2018.
9. D'Ignazio C, Klein L. Data feminism. Cambridge: The MIT Press; 2020.
10. KNBS. 2019 Kenya population and housing census. In: Statistics KNBo, editor. Population by county and sub-county, vol. 1. Nairobi: Kenya National Bureau of Statistics; 2019.
11. Njiru R. Political battles on women's bodies: post-election conflicts and violence against women in internally displaced persons camps in Kenya. Soc Without Borders. 2014;9(1):48–68.
12. Presley CA. Kikuyu women, the Mau Mau Rebellion, and social change in Kenya/Cora Ann Presley. Oxford: Westview Press; 1992.

13. Thomas K, Masinjila M, Bere E. Political transition and sexual and gender-based violence in South Africa, Kenya, and Zimbabwe: a comparative analysis. Gend Dev. 2013;21(3):519–32.
14. Blakeley R. State terrorism and neoliberalism: the North in the South/Ruth Blakeley. London: Routledge; 2009.
15. Kenya. Ministry of H, Kenya National Bureau of S, National ACC, Kenya Medical Research I, National Council for P, Development, et al. Kenya demographic and health survey, 2014–2015.
16. International A. Crying for justice: victims' perspectives on justice for the post-election violence in Kenya. London; 2014.
17. Truman JL, Morgan RE, United States. Bureau of Justice Statistics. Nonfatal domestic violence, 2003-2012 [text]. Washington, DC: U.S. Department of Justice, Office of Justice Programs, Bureau of Justice Statistics; 2014.
18. Elkin M. Domestic abuse in England and Wales overview: November 2019. In: Statistics OfN, editor. London: Office for National Statistics; 2019.
19. Decker MR, Latimore AD, Yasutake S, Haviland M, Ahmed S, Blum RW, et al. Gender-based violence against adolescent and young adult women in low- and middle-income countries. J Adolesc Health. 2015;56(2):188–96.
20. UNICEF, Prevention DoV, Control NCfIPa, Prevention UCfDCa, Statistics KNBo. Violence against children in Kenya: findings from a 2010 national survey. Summary report on the prevalence of sexual, physical, and emotional violence, context of sexual violence, and health and behavioural consequences of violence experienced in childhood Nairobi, Kenya UNICEF; 2012.
21. Bridgewater G. Physical and sexual violence against children in Kenya within a cultural context: the Journal of the Health Visitors' Association. Community Pract. 2016;89(2):30–4.
22. Temmerman M, Ogbe E, Manguro G, Khandwalla I, Thiongo M, Mandaliya KN, et al. The gender-based violence and recovery centre at Coast Provincial General Hospital, Mombasa, Kenya: an integrated care model for survivors of sexual violence. PLoS Med. 2019;16(8):e1002886.
23. Moore AM, Awusabo-Asare K, Madise N, John-Langba J, Kumi-Kyereme A. Coerced first sex among adolescent girls in sub-Saharan Africa: prevalence and context. Afr J Reprod Health. 2007;11(3):62–82.
24. Stöckl H, March L, Pallitto C, Garcia-Moreno C. Intimate partner violence among adolescents and young women: prevalence and associated factors in nine countries: a cross-sectional study. BMC Public Health. 2014;14(1):751.
25. Krug EG, Mercy JA, Dahlberg LL, Zwi AB. The world report on violence and health. Lancet. 2002;360(9339):1083–8.
26. Draucker C. Life-course typology of adults who experienced sexual violence. J Interpers Violence. 2010;25(7):1155–83.
27. WHO. Global and regional estimates of violence against women: prevalence and health effects of intimate partner violence and non-partner sexual violence. Geneva: WHO; 2013.
28. Baiocchi M, Friedberg R, Rosenman E, Amuyunzu-Nyamongo M, Oguda G, Otieno D, et al. Prevalence and risk factors for sexual assault among class 6 female students in unplanned settlements of Nairobi, Kenya: baseline analysis from the IMPower & Sources of Strength cluster randomized controlled trial. PLoS One. 2019;14(6):e0213359.
29. Williams LM. Understanding child abuse and violence against women—a life course perspective. J Interpers Violence. 2003;18(4):441–51.
30. Assembly WH. Strengthening the role of the health system in addressing violence, in particular against women and girls, and against children. Geneva: WHO; 2014.
31. Reporting, N. C. f. L. The Sexual Offences Act, Kenya Law Reports, 2009.
32. Wangamati CK, Combs Thorsen V, Gele AA, Sundby J. Postrape care services to minors in Kenya: are the services healing or hurting survivors? Int J Women's Health. 2016;8:249–59.
33. Commission NGaE. Gender-based violence in Kenya: the economic burden on survivors. Nairobo: National Gender and Equality Commission; 2016.
34. Foundation WK. Sexual violence analysis summary report. Nairobi, Kenya; 2017.

35. Ajema C, Mukoma W, Kotut R, Mulwa R. Documenting medico-legal evidence in Kenya: potential strategies for improvement. BMC Proc. 2013;9(Suppl 4):A2.
36. Naimer K, Brown W, Mishori R. MediCapt in the Democratic Republic of the Congo: the design, development, and deployment of mobile technology to document forensic evidence of sexual violence. Genocide Stud Prev. 2017;11(1):25–35.
37. Odhiambo A. "They were men in uniform" sexual violence against women and girls in Kenya's 2017 Elections USA: Human Rights Watch; 2017.
38. Odero M, Hatcher AM, Bryant C, Onono M, Romito P, Bukusi EA, et al. Responses to and resources for intimate partner violence: qualitative findings from women, men, and service providers in rural Kenya. J Interpers Violence. 2014;29(5):783–805.
39. Frankel A, Kanja W, Wood SN, Hameeduddin Z, Decker MR. Research and policy brief: the Wangu Kanja Foundation 2018 data review: supporting SGBV survivors via SMS and Traditional Direct Service. Baltimore.
40. MOPHS M. National guidelines on management of sexual violence in Kenya. 3rd ed. Ministry of Health; 2014.
41. Wangamati CK. Post rape care provision to minors in Kenya: an assessment of health providers' knowledge, attitudes, and practices. J Interpers Violence. 2020;35(5/6):1415–42.
42. Banda F. Researching violence against women: a practical guide for researchers and activists. J Afr Law. 2005;50(2):202–3.
43. WHO. Ethical and safety recommendations for intervention research on violence against women. Building on lessons from the WHO publication putting women first: ethical and safety recommendations for research on domestic violence against women. Geneva: WHO; 2016.
44. UN General Assembly, Declaration on the Elimination of Violence against Women, 20 December 1993.
45. UNGA. Basic principles and guidelines on the right to a remedy and reparation for victims of gross violations of International Human Rights Law and Serious Violations of International Humanitarian Law; 2006.
46. ACHPR. The guidelines on combating sexual violence and its consequences in Africa (the guidelines). ACHPR: The Gambia; 2017.

Part III

Spotlight on Intimate Partner Violence

Intimate Partner Violence in Pregnancy and the Post-partum Period: A Research and Practice Overview

Kathleen Baird

8.1 Introduction

Intimate partner violence (IPV) is an extremely complex and serious social issue that does not lend itself to a one or a simple definition. To help with setting the context for this chapter, the following definition from the World Health Organization (WHO) will be used. The WHO defines IPV as '*violence by an intimate partner which is manifested by physical, sexual abusive acts as well as controlling behaviours*' [1]. Within this chapter, IPV is defined as 'acts of violence against women before, during and after pregnancy perpetrated by a current or previous partner'.

8.2 Pregnancy and IPV

IPV is the most frequent type of violence against women, it occurs across all contexts and all socioeconomic and cultural groups. IPV can have a range of damaging and devastating impacts on women, their families and the wider community. Understanding patterns, correlates and consequences of IPV around the time of pregnancy has important theoretical and clinical implications. International research suggests IPV during pregnancy is common and that the violence can often begin during pregnancy, if violence already exists in the relationship the violence can increase in severity and frequency and continue into the post-partum period [2–4]. Pregnant women experience IPV in the same way as those who are not pregnant. However, the consequences of the violence may include behaviours and consequences that are specific to pregnancy. Pregnant women are often categorised as a high-risk group, as they are particularly

K. Baird (✉)
School of Nursing and Midwifery, Faculty of Health & Centre for Midwifery, Child and Family Health, University of Technology Sydney, Sydney, NSW, Australia
e-mail: Kathleen.Baird@uts.edu.au

© Springer Nature Switzerland AG 2021
C. Bradbury-Jones, L. Isham (eds.), *Understanding Gender-Based Violence*,
https://doi.org/10.1007/978-3-030-65006-3_8

vulnerable to IPV due to an increase in their social, emotional and economic needs during this time [5] or the opposing paradigm may occur that a pregnancy itself could embody a greater sense of autonomy and self-awareness [6]. Some studies have found traditional gender attitudes toward gender roles to be linked to IPV, attitudes and beliefs around domestic chores and women's availability to men in a physical and emotional sense can lead to an increase in violence when a woman's physical and emotional availability during pregnancy may limit their ability to perform the expected traditional roles [2, 7], such beliefs can be intensified during pregnancy, when the male may have a sense of loss of control due to the pregnancy. For example, it is acknowledged that coercive control is a principal and distinguishing feature of IPV, therefore some men may view the pregnancy as threatening to the status quo of the relationship, especially if the pregnancy was unplanned and therefore seek to exert further control over the relationship [7]. Existing IPV prior to pregnancy is associated with experiencing IPV during pregnancy [3, 7, 8], suggesting that IPV prior to pregnancy is an important indicator and risk marker for continued abuse during pregnancy and into the post-partum period.

8.3   Global Prevalence of IPV During Pregnancy

Due to differences in definition and/or variances in research data collection and reporting methods, global prevalence rates vary when assessing IPV and pregnancy. The WHO multi-country study on women's health and domestic violence against women, based on population-based surveys, found the prevalence rates of physical IPV in pregnancy ranged from 1% in Japan to 28% in Peru Province with the majority of sites ranging between 4 and 12% [9]. Further analysis, from the Demographic and Health Surveys and the International Violence against Women Survey, found prevalence rates for IPV during pregnancy to be from 2% in Australia, Denmark, Cambodia and Philippines to 13.5% in Uganda, with the majority ranging between 4 and 9% [10]. A meta-analysis of IPV during pregnancy which included 92 studies from 23 different countries found the average reported prevalence rates of emotional abuse to be 28.4%, 13.8% for physical abuse and 8% for sexual abuse [3]. The highest prevalence rates have been found in Egypt with 32%, followed by India (28%), Saudi Arabia (21%) and Mexico (11%) [11]. Clinical studies from Africa report high prevalence rates of IPV in pregnancy ranging from 23 to 40% for physical, 3 to 27% for sexual and 25 to 49% for emotional violence during pregnancy [12]. However, there continues to be a gap in knowledge about the prevalence and correlates of sexual and psychological IPV during pregnancy, although sexual and psychological IPV around the time of pregnancy are proven to have detrimental consequences for women and their children [1, 5].

Between 60 and 96% of women who are abused during pregnancy were experiencing violence prior to their pregnancy [5], suggesting that violence during pregnancy is in fact a continuation of pre-existing violence for the majority of women.

Taillieu and Brownridge [5] suggest knowing the prevalence, frequency and severity of pregnancy violence is important because it demonstrates the extent to which pregnancy can be considered a particularly vulnerable time.

Reflective Exercise

Please take five minutes to research the current rates of IPV in your country. Once you have obtained this information, consider how they compare with some of the rates from other countries around the world. If your reporting rates are higher or lower, think about some of the reasons why this may be the case.

8.4   IPV and Maternal Health and Well-Being

The perception for many is that pregnancy is a time to nurture and protect both the woman and her unborn child. Media and advertising portray pregnancy as a time when the woman is revered, protected and nurtured and for many couples, pregnancy and the anticipation of a baby is a time of expectation, love and affection. However, regrettably this is not so for all women, for millions of women of reproductive age worldwide, pregnancy is a time of increased risk for experiencing IPV [2, 3, 13, 14]. Indeed, IPV is the leading cause of death for women during pregnancy and is known to increase in frequency and severity during this period of heightened vulnerability [1, 4]. The birth of a baby is a life-changing event; it changes the dynamics within a family relationship and if a relationship is already under stress, then a pregnancy planned or unplanned has the protentional to add further stress to an already fragile relationship [5]. Even when a pregnancy is planned, it still has the possibility to cause jealousy within an intimate relationship. The man's perception that the unborn baby may come between him and his partner whilst obstructing her ability to care for him can be a catalyst for violence [6, 7]. Bacchus et al. suggest that outdated attitudes toward gender roles such as a belief that men control and dominate the home, women should always be emotionally and physically available to men are linked to the execution of IPV in pregnancy [6]. A past history of violence and abuse is one of the strongest predictors of pregnancy violence [7].

Direct consequences of IPV during pregnancy include the potential to develop a high-risk pregnancy and pregnancy-related complications, including spontaneous abortion [15], preterm labour and low birth weight [1, 4, 16], unwanted pregnancy, emotional distress, depression, anxiety, post-traumatic stress disorder and low self-esteem [17]. Indirect contributing factors leading to adverse pregnancy outcomes include but are not limited to: delayed pregnancy care, use of drugs both prescribed and illegal, regular alcohol and nicotine use, recurrent miscarriage, physical impairment from injuries and mental health manifestations including depression, post-traumatic stress disorder and anxiety [1, 7, 18, 19]. The use of alcohol, illegal drugs and nicotine are often used as a means of coping with the violence. Women experiencing physical assaults are at an increased risk of placental abruption, antepartum haemorrhage and foetal and maternal death [4].

A systematic review and meta-analysis conducted by Donovan and colleagues in 2016 found that women who experienced violence during their pregnancy are also at an increased risk of negative birth outcomes maybe affected by the poorer overall health of the mother, such as consuming insufficient nutritious food, substance misuse and smoking [20]. In the post-partum period, living with IPV can lead to disturbances in maternal–child bonding [21] and early cessation of exclusive breastfeeding [13, 22]. Having a newborn baby does not remove the risk for ongoing violence in the home, a new mother will still have to utilise most of her time and energy coping with the determinantal effects of living with IPV as well as trying to adjust to the demands of motherhood. As a consequence, she may find it difficult to bond with her child especially if her mothering skills are constantly being criticised by her partner eroding her esteem as a mother.

8.5   IPV and Maternal Mental Health

A small number of studies have demonstrated that IPV during and after pregnancy is associated with maternal mental health complexities such as anxiety disorders, depression, post-traumatic stress disorder, low self-esteem, negative self-image, less life satisfaction, functional impairment and fear of intimacy [13, 17, 23]. Indeed, perinatal mental health disorders are one of the commonest health complaints associated with pregnancy and the post-partum period [7, 17], and predictably, women who are subjected to IPV are known to experience mental health problems [7]. In addition to depression, women who experience IPV during pregnancy also report a variety of other manifestations of psychopathology, including increased distress levels, and they are more likely to report feelings such as being misunderstood, feeling anxious, fearful and isolated [24]. Post-traumatic stress disorder (PSTD) is also a common consequence of IPV with rates ranging between 19 and 84% [25, 26]. A systematic review and meta-analysis by Howard et al. [17] suggested that women who experienced IPV during their pregnancy had a threefold increase in the odds of experiencing high levels of depression in the postnatal period. Some women exposed to IPV during pregnancy will experience post-partum depression which can often affect the mother– baby relationship [22]. This is supported by a study by McMahon, Huang, Boxer and Postmus [27] who revealed women who experienced physical and emotional abuse during pregnancy had increased rates of depression at 1 year post-partum. Flach and colleagues[28], utilising the Avon Longitudinal Study of Parents and Children (ALSPAC) large cohort study, investigated whether antenatal domestic violence was associated with long-term adverse behavioural outcomes in children at 42 months of age born to women exposed to IPV during pregnancy compared to women who were not exposed to IPV in pregnancy. Results from the study concluded that antenatal domestic violence is associated with high levels of both maternal antenatal and postnatal depressive symptoms and postnatal violence. Both of which are related to future behavioural problems in a child at 42 months. Outcomes from the study confirm the association of antenatal violence and the adverse impact on childhood behaviour. However, it also emphasises the mediating effect of maternal depressive symptoms and ongoing violence in the family after birth. Indicating how difficult it can be to separate which factor is most important, the violence or maternal depression as both can have an extreme effect on a child's development [28].

Suicide is a leading cause of perinatal maternal deaths in industrialised countries [28]. Harrowing and prolonged stress from living with IPV are believed to be major features that result in maternal depression and suicide attempts [8]. Some research intimates that compared with non-pregnant populations, women in the antenatal and postnatal period are at lower risk of suicide. Suggesting that maternal concern for their unborn child may be a protective factor against suicide in the antenatal period [29]. However, other research has found suicidal ideation to be elevated in unplanned pregnancies as well as during depressive episodes [29, 30]. Limited research has examined the association between different types of IPV and suicidal ideation finding women reporting both physical and psychological violence to be at higher risk for suicidal ideation than those women reporting psychological violence only [30].

Maternal suicide is the utmost tragic outcome to manifest in the post-partum period and continues to be a contributor to maternal mortality worldwide [31]. For some women, suicide may be considered as the only escape from the violence; therefore, addressing maternal mental health during the perinatal period is critical. Antenatal visits are an opportune time to assess women for depressive symptoms and related comorbidities. Midwives, and all other healthcare providers, are in a unique position to identify and coordinate treatment for common mental health disorders such as depression, suicidal ideation and exposure to IPV. Yet evidence suggests that overall all healthcare providers' screen rates are relatively low [19]. A number of reasons have been suggested as barriers to screening for mental health and suicide including a lack of knowledge, lack of effective interventions to address, provider self-efficacy, fear of offending women, all highlighting the need to improve education around mental health and the link of mental and IPV during pregnancy [19].

8.6   Pregnancy-Associated Homicide

The most extreme consequence for pregnant women living with IPV is homicide. Available data clearly demonstrates that pregnancy-associated homicide is an important contributor to maternal mortality [32]. Currently IPV during pregnancy is one of the leading causes of maternal death [5]. Within developed countries, the US has the highest reporting rates of IPV-related homicides; however, it is unclear whether the variation rates from country to country can be attributed to better case identification or indeed to actual risk. A recent study from the USA established that of the 119 pregnancy-associated deaths for the years 2016 and 2017 in the state of Louisiana, 13.4% were homicides. For every 100,000 women who were pregnant or in the post-partum period, there were 12.9 homicide deaths, which outnumbered deaths from any single obstetric cause. It also highlighted that overall, the risk of homicide death was twice as high for women and girls during pregnancy and the post-partum period, compared to women and girls who were not pregnant [33]. In the UK between 2009 and 2013, the MBBRACE-UK (Mothers and Babies: Reducing Risk Through Audits and Confidential Enquires across the UK) report (2015) highlighted 13 women were murdered during pregnancy or up to 6 weeks after pregnancy and a further 23 were murdered between 6 weeks and 1 year following birth equating to a total of 36 women. This represented a homicide rate of 0.55 per 100,000, of this number 31 were murdered by a current or former partner. For at least one-third of the murdered women, there were clear signs that the women had been subjected to IPV, yet there was a failure to obtain a history of IPV at any point during their maternity care. Some of the women presented repeatedly to services with unusual and repeated patterns of injuries but no one took a longitudinal lens to the individual case and as a consequence the opportunity to identify a pattern of ongoing abuse was missed. Crucially, most of the women murdered had intersections of other complexities, many belonged to vulnerable and social disadvantaged groups. It is important to acknowledge that not all women experience IPV in similar circumstances. Many black and minority women face issues of racism, culture, language and concern for their immigration status, make the task of accessing services or asking for help from a health professional difficult. The findings from 2015 MBRRACE-UK report confirmed the homicide rate for women from black and/or other ethnic groups to be two and half times higher than white women [34]. The report also highlighted the missed opportunities for IPV screening for all women even when there were high-risk indicators for IPV [34]. Some of the women had presented on several occasions with unusual and/or repeated pattern of injury, and on some occasions, it was noted that the women's partner was verbally aggressive and/or controlling in exchanges with maternity staff [34].

Box 8.1 Case History from the MBRRACE Saving Lives, Improving Mothers' Care 2015 Report

A woman booked for National health Service (NHS) care in her third trimester having previously had private care. No examination of her social circumstances was undertaken and there was no evidence in her case history notes that she has undergone routine enquiry for IPV. She gave birth shortly after booking and during her postnatal stay her partner was verbally aggressive to staff on several occasions. She was murdered by her partner a few weeks later. The subsequent enquiry revealed several attendances at the Emergency Department during her pregnancy with unusual injuries, none of which raised reports/safeguarding referrals by the staff who treated her [34].

8.7   Risk Factors Associated with IPV During Pregnancy and the Post-partum Period

Multiple international studies have found certain socio-demographics characteristics of women associated with an increased risk of experiencing IPV in pregnancy [35], for example younger age and pregnancy intention [5]. Others risk factors such as marital status and social economic status and level of education remain inconsistent, and further research is required to authenticate their association [7]. Regardless of the risk factors highlighted, the strongest predictors of pregnancy violence are, a history of pre-pregnancy violence [7], suggesting that pregnancy violence for many women is a continuation of pre-existing violence. There is some evidence that the pattern of violence for some women may change during pregnancy, for example Martin and colleagues reported that for some women, IPV during pregnancy leads to an increase in psychological and sexual abuse [36].

Several studies have specified that the risk of violence is much higher for younger mothers during pregnancy [21, 37, 38]. Saltzman et al. [37] found that women less than 20 years of age had a 4.3% increased risk of experiencing violence during pregnancy, when compared to women of more than 30 years of age. However, most of the studies use health facility-based samples rather than population-based samples and many are limited in their generalisability [7, 38]. Hospital-based studies differ from population-based studies because the study base is defined secondarily to the identification of cases. Cases are selected regardless of the population from which they arise (e.g. all cases from a given hospital receiving patients from different settings). An effort is then made to identify the study base corresponding to the selected cases. This often translates into important difficulties in the definition of the population from which the controls are to be selected (the source population for cases). According to Taillieu and Brownridge [5] whilst the relationship between age and an increased risk of pregnancy violence is significant in bivariate analyses, the association becomes non-significant once age is controlled in multivariate analysis. However, Martin et al. [36] advises caution when interpreting the association between the increased risk of IPV during pregnancy and age, as different studies use a different definition of 'young age' ranging from 20 years and younger to 30 years of age.

An association exists between pregnancy intention and the risk for IPV during pregnancy [5, 39]. It has been hypothesised that heightened levels of fear and control, as well as sexual violence within abusive relationships, can result in women's inability to prevent pregnancy or to be able to negotiate contraceptive. Several studies have identified an association between unintended pregnancy and domestic IPV [3, 40, 41]. According to Goodwin and colleagues, women with unintended pregnancies in the United States are approximately 2.5 times more likely to have been physically abused than women with intended pregnancies [39]. Using population data from 15 sites in 10 countries, Pallitto et al. [40] explored the association of IPV and unintended pregnancy and abortion in primarily low- and middle-income countries. Results indicate that women with a history of IPV had significantly higher odds of unintended pregnancy in 8 of the 14 sites and of an abortion in 12 of 15 sites. Pallitto and colleagues propose a 50% reduction in IPV would result in potentially reducing unintended pregnancy from 2 to 18% and abortion by 4.5 to 40% [40]. Abortion due to its sensitivity will be under-reported, particularly in countries where it is illegal, nevertheless the inclusion of case control studies involving women provides important evidence of its association [42]. Whether a woman continues with an unintended pregnancy to term or if the pregnancy is terminated through an induced abortion, both outcomes will have huge implications for the mother, particularly when a pregnancy is terminated in settings where abortion is unsafe. Regardless of the strides made in women's healthcare, abortion continues to be one of the leading causes of maternal mortality worldwide [42, 43]. In view of the clear association between IPV, an unplanned pregnancy and termination of pregnancy, healthcare professionals should consider the possibility that any woman seeking a termination of pregnancy may be experiencing IPV. Regardless of undergoing a termination of pregnancy, a woman is vulnerable to ongoing violence within the relationship and therefore may be prevented from accessing future contraception and unable to avoid another pregnancy. Therefore, in view of the relationship between IPV and termination of pregnancy, sexual and reproductive services and the professionals who work in this area represent an appropriate setting in which to test interventions designed to reduce IPV.

8.8   IPV and Neonatal Birth Outcomes

An important consideration is the realisation that IPV during pregnancy does not only carry a risk to the woman but also imposes fatal and non-fatal adverse health outcomes for the growing foetus due to direct trauma as well as the physiological effects of stress on foetal growth and development [16, 44]. The experience of IPV during pregnancy is associated with many negative consequences, miscarriage, preterm labour and birth, (PTB) low birth (LBW) weight and small for gestational age (SGA) [16]. Low birth weight and preterm births are leading causes of neonatal morbidity and mortality. Shah and Shah [16] conducted a systematic review of 30 studies reporting on the rates of LBW, PTB and babies born SGA. Their review identified that women who were exposed to domestic violence during pregnancy had a significant increased risk of LBW and PTB and babies born SGA. During pregnancy, injuries frequently focus on the centre of the woman's body, the abdomen, breasts and genitalia [45], such injuries can cause perinatal death due to placental abruption and maternal uterine rupture [46].

A systematic review and meta-analysis conducted by Donovan et al. [20] revealed that IPV was significantly associated with preterm birth and low birth weight. Women experiencing IPV were at a twofold increase in odds of giving birth to an LBW baby compared with those who did not. Thirty studies reported on the association between IPV and PTB. Again, the analysis showed a twofold increase in the odds of a woman giving birth to a preterm infant when she was experiencing IPV compared with women who were not exposed to IPV. A smaller number of studies examined the association between IPV and SGA. Nevertheless, the seven studies assessed revealed SGA outcomes were significantly increased among women who experienced IPV during pregnancy. Donovan and colleague's meta-analysis of 50 studies in both high- and low-income countries indicate that women who experience IPV during pregnancy are clearly at an increased risk of having an adverse birth outcome compared with women who do not experience IPV during pregnancy [20]. Additionally, ongoing physical and sexual assault can affect birth outcomes via the maternal behavioural or physiological response to stress. Although the research is very limited with the majority of studies carried out on animals, it is considered the stress a women experiences may lead to the release of vasoconstrictors or cortisol, which can cross the placenta resulting in intrauterine growth restriction and increase the risk of premature labour [1, 4, 47]. A deeper understanding of the links between IPV, maternal stress and reduced utero-placental perfusion, leading to poor neonatal outcomes, may provide an important pathway to understanding disparities in neonatal outcomes. Significantly, IPV during pregnancy can significantly affect maternal–child bonding, foetal brain development and breastfeeding practices [48].

8.9   The Impact of IPV on Young Children

It is estimated that one in four children under the age of 4 years is living in a home where IPV and family violence exists [49]. Being exposed to violence can have a wide range of detrimental impacts on a child's development and their mental and physical well-being [49, 50]. Evidence suggests that exposure to IPV during infancy has the potential to disrupt the infant's emotional and cognitive development [51]. According to Jaffe, Wolfe and Campbell [38], young children who are exposed to family violence over a long period of time may develop trauma symptoms, resulting in psychological and physical responses that, if left untreated, can have long-lasting effects on their development, behaviour and well-being. Humphreys et al. argue that IPV should be conceptualised as an assault on the mother–child relationship [52].

An Australian study by Garland and colleagues involving 1507 first-time mothers found 29% of the mothers reported experiencing violence from a male partner in the first 4 years following birth. Accounting for socio-economic and maternal depressive factors, children of the mothers who reported experiencing violence were much more likely to have behavioural and emotional problems at the age of four [49]. Such outcomes confirm the consequences for children growing up in a home where IPV is present even if the children themselves are not physically hurt. The shorter duration that children are exposed to violence allows for recovery, and children in the same study who were exposed to violence at 1 year of age but not at 4 years of age had fewer reported behavioural problems [49]. A study from the United States observed the effects of the continued exposure to IPV in utero up to the age of 10 years and found it was predicative of children's behaviour. Higher levels of cortisol secretion were found in children who had been exposed to IPV in utero and this was an attributing factor in their overall behaviour [53]. A review from the UK, which particularly focused on the impact of domestic violence on mothering and the effects of living with paternal abuse, established that heightened fear and anxiety, sleep problems and difficulty concentrating were all identified as effects for both mother and children [54]. Children who are exposed to the violence over a sustained period of time may also experience trauma symptoms, including PTSD, resulting in psychosocial and sometimes physical responses that, if left untreated, can have long-lasting effects on children's development, behaviour and wellbeing [38]. These include:

- Depression
- Low self-esteem
- Anxiety
- Poor coping mechanisms
- Suicidal thoughts
- Eating disorders
- Self-harm
- Substance abuse
- Physical symptoms such as chronic pain [38]

8.10 Screening for IPV During Pregnancy

Healthcare systems can play a key role in identifying and providing support for women who would not usually access other support services [55]. Although midwives play a key role in a woman's pregnancy and childbirth journey, a woman often continues to engage with many other healthcare professionals during this time, especially when there are ongoing social and medical complications. For that reason, all healthcare professionals play a critical role in the identification of IPV during pregnancy. Indeed, IPV in pregnancy may be the only time a woman can freely engage with healthcare professionals without raising suspicion. However, many healthcare professionals may not see screening as part of their role, many feel unprepared and there is a fear of offending the woman, however the evidence does not support this assumption. It is known that women subjected to violence identify healthcare professionals as a person they would trust with a disclosure about a current or history of family and partner violence [8, 56].

Screening during pregnancy is important as numerous studies have established that IPV escalates during pregnancy and the postnatal period. Consequently, many countries now advocate for screening for IPV and family violence during pregnancy. The antenatal period specifically can provide a window of opportunity and a safe environment where women can safely and confidentially disclose about their experiences of violence and expect to receive a safe and supportive response [42]. Whilst the debate continues as to whether there is enough evidence available justifying screening for all pregnant women, screening nonetheless is now mandated by most major health organisations as indicated by the WHO clinical and policy guidelines [42]. O'Doherty et al. [57] systematic review and meta-analysis involving 11 eligible trials comprising of 13,027 women identified that screening did improve the identification of IPV, especially in the antenatal services.

Midwives have frequent contact with women during their pregnancy and therefore this places them in an ideal position to provide women with advice, support and help [58–60]. However, caution should be exercised before midwives or indeed any health professional feel they should undertake a search and rescue mission in attempt to 'save' women [61]. This belief and action only serve to strengthen the belief that women who experience IPV are feeble and in need of saving. It is the development of a reciprocal and trusting relationship that has been recognised as part of the foundation for enquiry by midwives and other health professionals. Women have identified the importance of the client–health professional relationship when disclosing a history of previous or current abuse. The WHO recommends that all healthcare professionals should be trained to be able to respond effectively [42]. However, there continues to be barriers to screening by healthcare professionals, some do not see it as their role, and they do feel they have the knowledge skills, or time to support a woman who may disclose that she is experiencing IPV [62, 63]. Such findings reconfirm the importance of relationship-based care and the universal provision of continuity of midwifery care throughout the perinatal period by a known midwife. A known midwife enhances the likelihood of effective routine enquiry across time and provides opportunities to link women with support services and to bolster their social support network [2, 8, 64–67].

The main purpose of screening for IPV is to identify women who have experienced or are experiencing IPV and to be able to offer support, yet despite the introduction of routine mandatory screening in many clinical sites, the reported disclosure rates of IPV during pregnancy do not reflect the scale of the problem. Even with direct asking not all women will elect to divulge a history of violence and abuse, and, of those that do, not all will want immediate help or a referral to a woman's support agency. Low disclosure rates may also be a reflection of the woman's wish not to report the violence, or how she views herself as a person, her feelings of shame or that she may not be believed; however, the primary reason for a woman's decision not to divulge about the violence is thought to be the fear of retribution or escalating violence if her partner finds out she has told anyone [42]. It is important for healthcare providers to realise and understand that whilst screening provides an opportunity to identify the immediate safety needs of the woman and her family, there are also other benefits to screening, not least the opportunity for awareness raising about the various support networks available which in itself can be very beneficial to the woman and her family. The majority of pregnant women access maternity care and therefore this provides a unique and important window of opportunity to provide support and a pathway to safety [42, 59, 64].

Midwives and other health professionals should appreciate that if screening/routine enquiry is conducted in a sensitive and professional approach, carried out by a caring and knowledgeable professional, it appears to cause no harm to women [56, 65, 66]. There continues to be many barriers to the effectiveness of routine antenatal screening with the most common being lack of education, training and support for midwives and obstetricians. Consequently, many lack the knowledge about the complexities of IPV and family violence and therefore feel poorly equipped to deal with a woman's disclosure of IPV. This in some part may explain why in some areas the uptake of universal screening assessments has been poor [8].

8.11 Guidelines for Asking About IPV Using Women-Centred Principles

Prior to screening, all healthcare professional should establish a strong rapport with the woman through sensitive and respectful discussion. The ability to assess the physical and emotional safety of the woman is essential. The WHO recommends using the mnemonic LIVES when health professionals are screening for IPV.

Listen	Listen to the woman closely, with empathy and without judging
Inquire about needs and concerns	Assess and respond to her various needs and concerns—emotional, physical, social and practical (e.g. childcare)
Validate	Show her that you understand and believe her. Assure her that she is not to blame
Enhance safety	Discuss a plan with her to protect her from further harm if violence occurs again
Support	Support her by helping her connect to information, services and social support

It is important that women who are experiencing IPV, feel safe to disclose. To do this, the following steps should be followed (*Information taken from: WHO Health care for women subjected to IPV. A clinical handbook (2014)*).

Listen: It is important to provide the woman with an opportunity to say what she wants to say in a safe and private place. Health professionals should ask women about a history of IPV in a confident manner, without predetermined judgement. Be aware of her feelings, hearing both what she says and what she does not say.

Inquire about her needs and concerns: Some women may feel stigmatised and fear that they will not be believed. Acknowledge that the woman may decide to withhold some information until a relationship is formed. Remember for some women there is a genuine fear of the perpetrator finding out and this may lead to her withholding information.

Validate: Let the woman know that you are listening attentively and believe her without judgment or conditions. Some of the responses to consider include:

- 'It's not your fault'; 'You are not to blame'; 'It's okay to talk'; 'Help is available' [only say this if it is true]; 'No one deserves to be hit by their partner in a relationship'; 'Everybody deserves to feel safe at home'.

Enhance safety: Many women who have been subjected to violence have fears about their safety. Assessing and planning for safety is an ongoing process—it is not just a one-time conversation. There are questions you should ask to assess if it is safe for a woman to return to her home. For example, it is important to find out if there is an immediate and likely risk of serious injury. Even women who are not facing immediate serious risk could benefit from having a safety plan. Whatever referral or safety plans are made they should always aim to meet the needs of the individual woman and her family.

Support: It is important that women are connected with community resources for her safety and social support. Do not expect the woman to make decisions immediately. Some women will need to take their time and do what they think is right for them [67].

In addition to utilising the LIVES mnemonic, all healthcare professionals should also consider documentation risk assessment, safety planning and duty of care.

Documentation: Accurate and contemporaneous record keeping of an IPV disclosure is imperative. Recording of a disclosure about IPV or family violence should follow the same practice guidelines as any other aspect of clinical practice. Local polices and guidelines should be adhered too. Clearly a positive disclosure about IPV should not be documented in a woman's handheld notes, or any documentation that the partner or another family member may read. Information pertaining to a disclosure should be handled with care and sensitivity and stored safely. It is imperative that a disclosure should only be shared with those professionals that need know. At all times the safety and well-being of the woman and her children should be paramount to any information sharing or decision-making. However, a healthcare professional/midwife may decide to share the woman's information without her consent if they feel a referral to another agency will protect the woman and her children to prevent a serious crime/harm. At all times healthcare professionals must adhere to their professional codes of conduct and standards and place the well-being and safety of the woman and her children centre and foremost of their decision-making and duty of care.

Risk assessment, safety planning and duty of care: An important point of consideration for all healthcare professionals regardless of the field they work in is the immediate and long-term safety obligations for both the woman and her children. Midwives and other healthcare professionals should make themselves aware of their organisation's protocol for promoting the safeguarding of children and who they should contact if they have any concerns about the safety and well-being of children. Risk assessments should ensure the safety, well-being and emotional needs of a woman and her children. Women from different communities may have different needs due to language difficulties and isolation. Crucially, women should never be encouraged to leave a violent relationship without a full risk assessment being performed and a safety plan put in place. A safety plan should place the needs of the woman and her children at the centre, meet her individual needs and be developed in partnership with local specialised domestic violence services. Working with other agencies is crucial and an essential to achieve the optimal result for the woman and her family.

8.12 Conclusion

In summary, IPV is implicated in poorer maternity and perinatal outcomes, and the consequences may expand long after a woman's pregnancy and birth. Although the prevalence rates across the globe may vary, the detrimental effects on a woman's health and her pregnancy are conclusive. Both fatal and non-fatal effects of IPV during pregnancy have been found to significantly impair women's health, her well-being and her ability to parent effectively, which is associated with infant and childhood development and adjustment issues. All healthcare professionals providing maternity care need to be aware of the risk factors of IPV during pregnancy and be able to identify women who may be at risk for delayed access to maternity care.

The prevalence of IPV and the severity of its impacts during pregnancy and early motherhood continues to suggest that there is an opportunity for early intervention, including referrals to support services, to be made by midwives and other healthcare professionals working in perinatal, maternal and child health services. The vast majority of women are not offended by caring health professionals asking them about a history of IPV; indeed, for many women this may be their only opportunity to disclose about a history of violence. Pregnancy is an optimal window of opportunity, a time when women may be seeking support to escape from the violence.

References

1. World Health Organization. Intimate partner violence during pregnancy information sheet WHO/RHR/11.35, Department of Reproductive Health and Research, World Health Organization, Switzerland. https://www.who.int/reproductivehealth/publications/violence/rhr_11_35/en/. Accessed 10 Apr 2020.
2. Campo M. Domestic and family violence in pregnancy and early parenthood. Overview and emerging interventions. Australian Institute of Family Studies, Child Family Community Australia. 2015. https://aifs.gov.au/cfca/publications/domestic-and-family-violence-pregnancy-and-early-parenthood. Accessed 5 Mar 2020.
3. James L, Brody D, Hamilton Z. Risk factors for domestic violence during pregnancy: a meta-analytic review. Violence Vict. 2013;28(3):359–80. https://doi.org/10.1891/0886-6708.VV-D-12.00034.
4. World Health Organization, Department of Reproductive Health and Research, London School of Hygiene and Tropical Medicine, South African Medical Research Council. Global and regional estimates of violence against women: prevalence and health effects of intimate partner violence and non-partner sexual violence. Geneva: Department of Reproductive Health and Research, World Health Organization; 2013. https://www.who.int/reproductivehealth/publications/violence/9789241564625/en/. Accessed 2 Mar 2020.
5. Taillieu TL, Brownridge DA. Violence against pregnant women: prevalence, patterns, risk factors, theories, and directions for future research. Aggress Violent Behav. 2010;15:14–5.
6. Bacchus L, Mezey G, Bewley C. A qualitative exploration of the nature of domestic violence in pregnancy. Violence Against Women. 2006;12(6):588–604.
7. Brownridge DA, Taillieu TL, Tyler KA, Tiwari A, Chan KL, Santos SC. Pregnancy and intimate partner violence: risk factors, severity, and health effects. Violence Against Women. 2011;17(7):858–81.
8. Baird K. Women's lived experiences of domestic violence during pregnancy. Pract Midwife. 2015;18(3):27–31.

9. García-Moreno C, Jansen HA, Ellsberg M, Heise L, Watts C. WHO multi-country study on women's health and domestic violence against women: initial results on prevalence, health outcomes and women's responses. Geneva: World Health Organization; 2005. https://www.who.int/reproductivehealth/publications/violence/24159358X/en/. Accessed 22 Mar 2020.

10. Devries KM, Kishor S, Johnson H, Stöckl H, Bacchus L, Garcia-Moreno C, et al. Intimate partner violence during pregnancy: prevalence data from 19 countries. Reprod Health Matters. 2010;18(36):1–13.

11. Campbell J, Garcia-Moreno C, Sharps P. Abuse during pregnancy in industrialized and developing countries. Violence Against Women. 2004;10(7):770–89.

12. Shamu S, Abrahams N, Temmerman M, Musekiwa A, Zarowsky C. A systematic review of African studies on intimate partner violence against pregnant women: prevalence and risk factors. PLoS One. 2011;6(3):e17591.

13. Islam J, Broidy L, Baird K, Mazerolle P. Exploring the associations between intimate partner violence and delayed entry to prenatal care: Evidence from a cross-sectional study in Bangladesh. Midwifery. 2017;47:43–55. https://doi.org/10.1016/jmidw.2017.02.002. Accessed 20 Feb 2020.

14. Garcia-Moreno C, Watts C. Violence against women: an urgent public health priority. Bull World Health Organ. 2011;89(1):2. https://doi.org/10.2471/BLT.10.085217.

15. Morland LA, Leskin GA, Block CR, Campbell JC, Friedman MJ. Intimate partner violence and miscarriage examination of the role of physical and psychological abuse and posttraumatic stress disorder. J Interpers Violence. 2008;23(5):652–69. https://doi.org/10.1177/0886260507313533. Accessed 12 Feb 2020.

16. Shah P, Shah J. Knowledge Synthesis Group in Determinants of Preterm/LBW Births. Maternal exposure to domestic violence and pregnancy and birth outcomes: a systematic review and meta-analyses. J Women's Health. 2010;19:2017–31.

17. Howard LM, Oram S, Galley H, Trevillion K, Feder G. Domestic violence and perinatal mental disorders: a systematic review and meta-analysis. PLoS Med. 2013;10(5):e10001452. https://doi.org/10.1371/journal.pmed.1001452.

18. Cha S, Masho SW. Intimate partner violence and utilization of prenatal care in the United States. J Interpers Violence. 2014;29(5):911–27.

19. Taft A, O'Doherty L, Hegarty K, Ramsay J, Davidson L, Feder G. Screening women for intimate partner violence in health care settings. Cochrane Database Syst Rev. 2013;(4):CD007007. https://doi.org/10.1002/14651858.CD007007.pub2. Accessed 22 Feb 2020.

20. Donovan BM, Spracklen CN, Schweizer ML, Rychman KK, Saftlas AF. Intimate partner violence during pregnancy and the risk for adverse infant outcomes: a systematic review and meta-analysis. Br J Obstet Gynaecol. 2016;123(8):1289–99. https://doi.org/10.1111/1471-0528.

21. Janssen PA, Holt VL, Sugg NK, Emanuel I, Critchlow CM, Henderson AD. Intimate partner violence and adverse pregnancy outcomes: a population-based study. Am J Obstet Gynecol. 2003;188(5):1341–7.

22. Kendall-Tackett KA. Violence against women and the perinatal period: the impact of lifetime violence and abuse on pregnancy, postpartum, and breastfeeding. Trauma Violence Abuse. 2007;8(3):344–53.

23. Alhusen JL, Ray E, Sharps P, Bullock L. Intimate partner violence during pregnancy: maternal and neonatal outcomes. J Women's Health. 2015;24(1):100–6. https://doi.org/10.1089/jwh.2014.4872.

24. Casanueva CE, Martin SL. Intimate partner violence during pregnancy and mothers' child abuse potential. J Interpers Violence. 2007;22:603–22.

25. Woods SJ, Hall RJ, Campbell JC, Angott DM. Physical health and posttraumatic stress disorder symptoms in women experiencing intimate partner violence. J Midwifery Health. 2008;53:543–6.

26. Hellmuth JC, Jaquier V, Swan SC, Sullivan TP. Elucidating posttraumatic stress symptom profiles and their correlates among women experiencing bidirectional intimate partner violence. J Clin Psychol, 2014; 70(10):1008–1102. 10.1002/jclp.22100.
27. Mahon S, Huang CC, Boxer P, Postmus JL. The impact of emotional and physical violence during pregnancy on maternal and child health at one-year post-partum. Child Youth Serv Rev. 2011;33:2103–11. https://doi.org/10.1016/j.childyouth.2011.06.001.
28. Flach C, Leese M, Heron J, Evans J, Feder G, Sharp D, Howard LM. Antenatal domestic violence, maternal mental health and subsequent child behaviour: a cohort study. Br J Obstet Gynaecol. 2011;118:1383–91. https://doi.org/10.1111/j.1471-0528.2011.03040.x.
29. Lindahl V, Pearson JL, Colpe L. Prevalence of suicidality during pregnancy and the postpartum. Arch Womens Ment Health. 2005;8:77–87.
30. Gavin AR, Tabb KM, Melville JL, Guo Y, Katon W. Prevalence and correlates of suicidal ideation during pregnancy. Arch Womens Ment Health. 2011;14:239–46.
31. World Health Organization. Global status report on violence prevention. Geneva: World Health Organization; 2014. https://www.who.int/violence_injury_prevention/violence/status_report/2014/en/. Accessed 1 Apr 2020.
32. Cliffe C, Miele M, Reid S. Homicide in pregnant and postpartum women worldwide: a review of the literature. J Public Health Policy. 2019;40:180–216. https://doi.org/10.1057/s41271-018-150-z.
33. Wallace ME, Crear-Perry J, Mehta PK, Theall KP. Homicide during pregnancy and the postpartum period in Louisiana, 2016-2017. JAMA Pediatr. 2020;174(4):387–8. https://doi.org/10.1001/jamapediatrics.2019.5853.
34. Knight M, Bunch K, Tuffnell D, Shakespeare J, Kotnis R, Kenyon S, Kurinczuk JJ, editors. On behalf of MBRRACE-UK. Saving lives, improving mothers' care—lessons learned to inform maternity care from the UK and Ireland Confidential Enquiries into Maternal Deaths and Morbidity 2015-17. Oxford: National Perinatal Epidemiology Unit, University of Oxford; 2019.
35. Martin S, Arcara J, McLean DP, Davis L. Violence during pregnancy and the postpartum period. VAWNet.org. National Online Resource Center on Violence Against Women. 2012. https://vawnet.org/material/violence-during-pregnancy-and-postpartum-period.
36. Martin SL, Harris-Britt A, Li Y, Moracco KE, Kupper LL, Campbell JC. Changes in intimate partner violence during pregnancy. J Fam Violence. 2004;19(4):201–10.
37. Saltzman LE, Johnson CH, Gilbert BC, Goodwin MM. Physical abuse around the time of pregnancy: an examination of prevalence and risk factors in 16 states. Matern Child Health J. 2003;7(1):31–43.
38. Jaffe PG, Wolfe D, Campbell M. Growing up with domestic violence: assessment, intervention, and prevention strategies for children and adolescents. Cambridge: Hogrefe Publishing; 2012.
39. Goodwin MM, Gazmararian JA, Johnson CH, Gilbert BC, Saltzman LE, PRAMS Working Group. Pregnancy intendedness and physical abuse around the time of pregnancy: findings from the pregnancy risk assessment monitoring system, 1996–1997. Matern Child Health J. 2000;4(2):85–92.
40. Pallitto CC, García-Moreno C, Jansen HA, Heise L, Ellsberg M, Watts C. Intimate partner violence, abortion, and unintended pregnancy: results from the WHO multi-country study on women's health and domestic violence. Int J Gynecol Obstet. 2013;120(1):3–9. https://doi.org/10.1016/j.ijgo.2012.07.003.
41. Mercedes M, Lafaurie V. Intimate partner violence against women during pregnancy: a critical reading from a gender perspective. Rev Colomb Enfermería. 2015;10:64–77.
42. World Health Organization. Responding to intimate partner violence and sexual violence against women: WHO clinical and policy guidelines. Geneva: World Health Organization; 2013.
43. World Health Organization. The world health report: 2005: make every mother and child count. Geneva: World Health Organization; 2005. http://whqlibdoc.who.int/whr/2005/9241562900.pdf.

44. Chai J, Fink G, Kaaya S, Danaei G, Fawzi W, Ezzati M, Lienerta J, Smith Fawzid MC. Association between intimate partner violence and poor child growth: results from 42 demographic and health surveys. Bull World Health Organ. 2016;94(5):331–9. https://doi.org/10.2471/BLT.15.152462.
45. Hedin LW, Janson PO. Domestic violence during pregnancy. The prevalence of physical injuries, substance abuse, abortion, and miscarriages. Acta Obstet Gynecol Scand. 2000;79:625–30.
46. Bailey B. Partner violence during pregnancy: prevalence, effects, screening, and management. Int J Women's Health. 2010;2:183–97. https://doi.org/10.2147/ijwh.s8632.
47. Hill A, Pallitto C, McCleary-Sills J, Garcia-Moreno C. A systematic review and meta-analysis of intimate partner violence during pregnancy and selected birth outcomes. Int J Gynecol Obstet. 2016;133(2):69–276. https://doi.org/10.1016/jijgo.2015.10.023.
48. Trabold N, Waldrop DP, Nochajski TH, Cerulli C. An exploratory analysis of intimate partner violence and postpartum depression in an impoverished urban population. Soc Work Health Care. 2013;52(4):332–50.
49. Gartland D, Woolhouse H, Mensah FK, Hegarty K, Hiscock H, Brown SJ. The case for early intervention to reduce the impact of intimate partner abuse on child outcomes: results of an Australian cohort of first-time mothers. Birth. 2014;41(4):374–83.
50. Humphreys C. Children and family violence: finding the right responses. Insight. 2014;9:40–2.
51. Mueller I, Tronick E. Early life exposure to violence: developmental consequences on brain and behaviour. Behav Neurosci. 2019;13:156. https://doi.org/10.3389/fnbeh.2019.00156. Accessed 25 Mar 2020.
52. Humphreys C, Thiara RK, Sharp C, Jones J. Supporting the relationship between mothers and children in the aftermath of domestic violence. In: Stanley N, Humphreys C, editors. Domestic violence and protecting children: new thinking and approaches. London: Jessica Kingsley Publishers; 2015. p. 130–47.
53. Martinex-Torteya C, Bogat GA, Levendosky AA, von Eye A. The influence of prenatal intimate partner violence exposure on hypothalamic—pituitary-adrenal axis reactivity and childhood internalizing and externalizing symptoms. Dev Psychopathol. 2016;28(1):55–72. https://doi.org/10.1017/D09545794150000280.
54. Stanley N. Children experiencing domestic violence: a research review. Dartington, 2011. England: Research in Practice. https://www.barnsley.gov.uk/media/4345/domesticviolence-signpostsresearchinpractice-july2012.pdf. Accessed 23 Feb 2020.
55. Spangaro J. What is the role of health systems in responding to domestic violence? An evidence review. Aust Health Rev. 2017;41:639–45. https://doi.org/10.1071/AH16155.
56. Baird K, Salmon D, White P. A five-year follow-up study of the Bristol pregnancy domestic violence program to promote routine enquiry. Midwifery. 2013;29:1003–10.
57. O'Doherty L, Hegarty K, Ramsay J, Davidson LL, Feder G, Taft AR. Screening women for intimate partner violence in healthcare settings. Cochrane Database Syst Rev. 2015;(7):CD007007.
58. Baird K, Eustace J, Creedy DK, Saito A. An exploration of Australian midwives' knowledge of intimate partner violence against women during pregnancy. Women Birth. 2015;28(3):215–20. https://doi.org/10.1016/j.wombi.2015.01.009.
59. Baird K, Saito A, Eustace J, Creedy DK. Longitudinal evaluation of a training program to promote routine antenatal enquiry for domestic violence by midwives. Women Birth. 2018;31(5):398–406. https://doi.org/10.1016/j.wombi.2018.01.004.
60. Baird K, Creedy DK. Midwives can help detect domestic violence—here's how. The Conversation. 2015. https://theconversation.com/midwives-can-help-detect-domestic-violence-heres-how-37918. Accessed 26 Apr 2020.
61. Dobash RE, Dobash RP. Rethinking violence and social change. London: Routledge; 1998.
62. Feder G, Ramsay J, Dunne D, Rose M, Arsene C, Norma R, Tacket A. How far does screening women for domestic (partner) violence in different health-care settings meet criteria for screening programme? Systematic reviews of nine UK National Screening Committee criteria. Health Technol Assess. 2009;13(16):1–113, 137–347.

63. Hegarty K, Spangaro J, Koziol-McLain J, Walsh J, Lee A, Kyei-Onanjiri M, et al. Sustainability of identification and response to domestic violence in antenatal care: the SUSTAIN study. Sydney: ANROWS; 2019.

64. Eustace J, Baird K, Creedy D, Saito A. Midwives' experiences of routine enquiry for intimate partner violence in pregnancy. Women Birth. 2016;29:503–10. https://www.anrows.org.au/project/the-sustain-study/. Accessed 10 Feb 2020.

65. Spangaro J, Koziol-McLain J, Rutherford A, Zwi AB. "Made me feel connected": a qualitative comparative analysis of intimate partner violence routine screening pathways to impact. Violence Against Women. 2020;26(3–4):334–58. https://doi.org/10.1177/1077801219830250.

66. Zink T, Levin L, Putman F, Beckstrom A. Accuracy of five domestic violence screening questions with nongraphic language. Clin Pediatr (Phila). 2007;46(2):127–34.

67. World Health Organization. Health care for women subjected to intimate partner violence or sexual violence. A clinical handbook. RHR/14.26. Geneva: World Health Organization; 2014.

Supporting the Safety and Welfare of Children Affected by Domestic Violence and Abuse: A Practice Case Study

9

Ben Donagh

9.1 Introduction

Gender-based violence includes a host of harmful behaviours that are directed at women and girls; these can include but are not limited to domestic violence and abuse (DVA), so-called honour-based violence, forced prostitution, female genital mutilation (FGM) and sexual abuse [1]. This chapter focuses specifically on DVA as one form of gender-based violence and critically analyses its impacts on children and young people. DVA is present in the lives of many children and young people, with it being estimated that as many as 275 million children worldwide experience DVA in their home [2]. Aside from the economic cost, experiencing DVA during childhood has a significant impact on the physical, emotional and social development of children and young people [2–4]. To highlight the impact, this chapter is based on a single case study of the Cooper family and their experiences of DVA. This family is hypothetically constructed for the purpose of this chapter, formed from a montage of examples drawn from practice.

9.2 Meet the Cooper Family

Currently employed as the manager of two specialist children's services within a charity, I have over nine years practice experience supporting children and young people to cope and recover from the harm caused by different forms of gender-based violence. From supporting young girls who have experienced child sexual exploitation and rape when giving evidence in a courtroom to helping young people to create emergency safety plans whilst they continue to experience DVA, I could share many journeys of young people I have supported. The case study used for this chapter is

B. Donagh (✉)
Victim Support and University of Birmingham, Birmingham, UK
e-mail: BXD946@student.bham.ac.uk

© Springer Nature Switzerland AG 2021
C. Bradbury-Jones, L. Isham (eds.), *Understanding Gender-Based Violence*,
https://doi.org/10.1007/978-3-030-65006-3_9

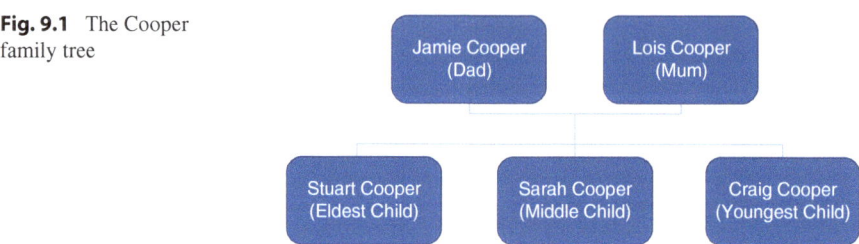

based on the experiences of a family, from an urban location within the United Kingdom (UK), who accessed support after experiencing DVA. Their names and any other identifying information have been changed to protect their confidentiality.

At the age of 16 years, Lois met 22-year-old Jamie through mutual friends. Their relationship developed rapidly, with Lois becoming pregnant after four months. Aged 17 years, Lois and Jamie had their first child, Stuart, and later Sarah and Craig.

Figure 9.1 shows the relationships between the Cooper family members. What has been missed out of this description of their relationship so far is the abusive behaviours Lois and the children experienced from Jamie for many years. Throughout their relationship, Jamie subjected Lois to a myriad of physical, emotional, sexual and financial abuse. He was extremely controlling and would often set Lois unachievable tasks. For example, Jamie would check the mileage on their car before he left for work and again when he returned. He knew it was a six-mile round trip to the children's schools and if there had been more than 12 miles added to the car, he would become extremely abusive, questioning Lois as to where she had been and who with. If Lois was not able to provide an answer he deemed 'acceptable' she would receive multiple injuries often resulting in her needing medical assistance.

Lois would often express the guilt she felt that her children were not able to have a 'normal childhood'. Jamie's abusive behaviours meant the children were not allowed to have friends over after school for fear of them finding out what was happening. They were not allowed to play with toys past 5 pm, as this was Jamie's time to relax, and if any toys were seen past this time the abuse would escalate. Jamie's behaviours resulted in Lois visiting the Accident and Emergency Department on multiple occasions. The police were called on two occasions and this resulted in the Police removing Jamie from the property; however, he would return the following day, apologetic, and move back in.

Whilst Lois knew this behaviour from Jamie was not right, she had come to the conclusion that this behaviour was her 'normal' and Jamie had convinced her she was to blame. Lois also believed abuse within relationships was something most women experienced. Like her children, Lois had experienced DVA as a child with her stepfather being physically and verbally abusive towards her mother. Many families like the Coopers experience an *intergenerational cycle of abuse*. Read Box 9.1.

Children and young people experience abuse within the home in a variety of ways. The Cooper siblings saw a range of abusive behaviours on a regular basis, including seeing their father physically assault their mother. Stuart would take his younger brother and sister to a bedroom to protect them from harm and would also

Box 9.1 The Intergenerational Cycle of Abuse

The intergenerational cycle of abuse or 'intergenerational theory' proposes that children who experience DVA within their childhood go on to be part of abusive relationships as adults [5]. Using this theory, gender has been found as a significant factor, with males who experience DVA in their childhood identified as more likely to perpetrate abuse as an adult and females more likely to experience abuse as victims [6–8]. Gendered patterns can be highlighted through generations of violence against women and girls being perpetrated by men.

Although some boys who experience DVA as children do go on to perpetrate violence as adults, this is not an inevitable or even common pattern. As a practitioner working with children and families, you can play an important role challenging expectations (held by young people and adults) that boys exposed to violence will inevitably become violent men.

Jaffee et al. [9] completed a UK-based study, whereby findings indicated substantial continuity of abuse from one generation to the next. However, there are criticisms of the intergenerational transmission theory and there are a number of rigorous studies that have found that the cycle of abuse is not evident in most families [10, 11]. Some feminists argue that experiencing DVA as a child can increase the likelihood of accepting patriarchial gender norms and this may in turn lead to violence in the next generation [12]. Intergenerational theory is limited, however, with how it explains the impact of violent behaviours on an individual level. Despite these differences of opinion and research findings, it is a commonly held view that children and young people who have a parent who has experienced DVA are at an elevated risk of experiencing or instigating abusive behaviour in adulthood [9].

try to get between his parents hoping this would stop the abuse. On a number of occasions Stuart was physically injured himself. Even when the children were in a different room they would still hear shouting, screams from their mother and objects being smashed and broken. When incidents happened during school hours, the children would come home and experience the aftermath of broken objects on the floor, visible injuries and tension between their parents. The Cooper siblings would often find the experience of a negative atmosphere following a DVA incident the most worrying.

It is a common misconception that children and young people will not be affected by DVA if it happens when they are in a different room or not in the home at all. This is a myth and it is important not to underestimate the impact that unseen abuse can have. When a child or young person overhears abuse taking place, they can often imagine the incident to be much worse than it actually was. It is also important not to underestimate the impact tension and silence can have on children and young people living with DVA. There are many other myths associated with DVA, especially around what abuse looks like, which type of person it happens to and why

Box 9.2 The Use of Language

The ways in which children and young people experience DVA will often go much further than direct observation. For example, being directly involved themselves, overhearing the incidents and experiencing the aftermath [4, 15, 16]. The term 'witnessed' is arguably one of the most utilised within DVA research; however, it fails to capture the varying ways that children and young people experience the abuse.

The language used when supporting children and young people who have experienced DVA can be the difference between whether or not they engage with your support and any future professionals they meet. Practitioners should remain open to challenge from other professionals, and young people themselves, to ensure they are approachable and their support remains accessible.

people '*choose*' to stay in an abusive relationship. Just because the abuse does not mirror the stereotypical media portrayal of DVA does not mean it has any less of an impact. There have been a number of studies that explore DVA myths and the effects these myths can have [13, 14]; having an understanding of this will enhance the approach of front-line practitioners.

Jamie subjected his family to abuse for just over six years, until Lois and the children were able to flee to a place of safety. A fellow parent from the children's school happened to work within a local DVA refuge service and supported the family to leave the abuse safely. This chapter refers to the Cooper siblings as having 'experienced' DVA rather that other terms often used such as 'witnessed' or 'exposed'. The use of language should not be underestimated when discussing the impact of DVA on children and young people (see Box 9.2).

9.3 The Cooper Siblings

Studies have shown the detrimental impact DVA can have on children and young people describing it as a significant risk factor, jeopardising their physical, emotional and social development [2–4]. Compared to those who have not, children and young people who have experienced DVA can have significantly more internalised (depression and anxiety) and externalised (aggression and antisocial) behavioural problems, often persisting after the abuse ends [4, 17–19]. Research is overwhelmingly clear that young people exposed to DVA have much higher rates of trauma symptoms than those not exposed [20].

Experiencing DVA throughout their childhood had a significantly detrimental impact on the Cooper siblings, each affected in different ways. Box 9.3 shows the potential gender differences in relation to the impact DVA can have on children and young people.

Box 9.3 Gender Differences

The impact of experiencing DVA has been found to differ depending on the gender of the young person. Research indicates that boys exhibit more externalised behaviours such as anger and hostility after experiencing DVA, whereas girls exhibit more internalised behaviours such as depression and low self-esteem [4, 21, 22]. In my experience as a practitioner, this is not always the case and it is important not to generalise these viewpoints. There are many young boys who become withdrawn and lack confidence after experiencing DVA as well as many young girls who become aggressive and abusive. Ultimately, whilst research and theories can be useful to influence and guide service structures and approaches, the only way to truly understand how DVA has affected a young person is by focussing on them as individuals; DVA will impact every young person in a unique way.

Stuart Cooper is the eldest sibling. His experience of DVA resulted in him experiencing high levels of anger with an inability to control it. Lois would receive weekly calls from school reporting that Stuart had been verbally aggressive with his teachers, destroyed school property and was caught fighting with other students. Stuart's aggressive behaviours were also present at home; when his dad left, Stuart became very controlling of Lois and his sister, Sarah. He would demand to know where Lois was at all times and would discipline his sister if she had not completed chores around the home as 'this was her role as a woman'. If Lois did not do what he demanded, Stuart would often become both verbally and physically abusive. One incident involved Stuart holding a knife against Lois' throat when she would not do as he said, threatening to take her life. When Lois would try to calm Stuart down and regain control, Stuart would often say 'dad got away with it, women need to know who is in charge'. It was apparent Stuart had a distorted view of gender following his experiences of DVA. Lois would refer to Stuart as a 'mini-me' of his father. Research has found some children and young people can somewhat take over the role of the abusive parent and become abusive to their non-abusive parent and siblings. Some attribute this to Social Learning Theory (as in Box 9.4) where gender can play a significant role.

Sarah Cooper is the middle sibling. Lois would often describe her as the most affected. Once an outgoing, confident young woman, experiencing DVA left Sarah quiet and withdrawn. She struggled to sleep at night as she worried about what might happen to her mother and would experience flashbacks of the trauma. This often left her tired at school and her educational attainment suffered. Sarah would spend her school day worrying about her mother and what might be happening; her ability to concentrate deteriorated significantly as a result of the abuse she experienced. Like home, school also became an unhappy and unsafe place for Sarah. She began to experience bullying from a group of peers. One of them lived on the same street as the Coopers and had seen the police take away Sarah's father. Following this, Sarah was mocked on a daily basis for having a parent who 'needed locking

Box 9.4 Social Learning Theory

Some children and young people who experience DVA may believe this is an acceptable way of resolving conflict or achieving what they want [23, 24]. This is a prime example of Bandura's notion of social learning [25]. If violence and abuse is modelled to young people when developing their own beliefs, they may be likely to adopt these behaviours in later relationships [26, 27]. This may be within their own intimate relationships, or directed at their non-abusive parent, or involve taking over the role of the abusive parent. A young person's perception of right and wrong can be influenced by the abuse that they experience, resulting in them viewing violence and abuse as acceptable within relationships [24].

Further to this, some may also identify with the abused parent [4]. Baldry identified how some young people learn that violence is a normal way to be treated [23]. This has also been described as 'learned helplessness'. This perspective takes a gendered viewpoint, predicting that women and girls who experience DVA may become passive and feel there is nothing they can do to end abuse within their relationships [28]. It is important to recognise that the word 'helplessness' needs to be used with caution when discussing DVA; as highlighted by Walker, those in abusive relationships should not be considered helpless, but resilient for staying alive [29].

Whilst gender differences are often highlighted within social learning theory, it is not as simple as boys identifying with their abusive fathers and girls with their abused mothers. Gender attributes (masculinity/femininity) are learned rather than biological. A young person's understanding of gender and gender norms will change throughout their childhood. They learn about and understand masculine and feminine behaviours within a variety of environments, whether that be their experiences within the home, or their social experiences, peer relationships and education setting [30].

up'. This, combined with the DVA Sarah experienced, resulted in her having very low confidence and self-esteem; Sarah would often appear to be in a very low mood.

Craig Cooper, the youngest of the Cooper siblings was often described as 'totally fine'. Lois attributed this to his age, believing he was too young when the DVA was taking place to understand what happened. At parents evening his school would tell Lois how hard-working Craig was and how they expected him to go far in life. Craig put a lot of effort into his school work and would be the first to complete his homework after school. He would always do his best to help around the house, make sure his toys were tidy and ask Lois whether there was anything else he could help with. Craig always wanted to please his parents and friends. When the DVA was taking place, Craig went through a phase of bed-wetting; however, Lois felt this was more related to his age rather than the abuse. There is a common misconception that younger children are not affected by DVA as they are too young to understand. The impact of abuse can be misinterpreted as typical behaviours

Box 9.5 Not Affected or Overlooked?

The most common way of determining whether or not a young person has been affected by the DVA they experienced is by the behaviours they display. Some may not exhibit the expected internalised or externalised behaviours. For some, their behaviours after experiencing DVA can appear to be no different to how they have always been. This could be for a wide range of different reasons; everyone is affected differently.

Children and young people develop a range of coping strategies to help protect themselves from the harm caused. For some, this strategy can be to overcompensate with their approach to school or their behaviour at home. Some may seek positive attention and reinforcement from adults within their lives. These young people may receive praise and positive feedback, but most importantly to them, they are not being punished or experiencing further abuse. The adults in their lives may see this as a positive and therefore underestimate the impact DVA has had on them; these young people are most at risk of being overlooked.

There is also a common misconception amongst parents, and some professionals, that some children and young people are too young to understand what has happened and will therefore not be affected by DVA in the family home. As a result, they are often not referred into support services or highlighted to statutory services [31]. The question here is are these children, and those who are doing well at school, not affected or being overlooked?

The reality is a lower age limit around the impact of DVA on children does not exist. Experiencing DVA can impact children and young people before they are born. Consequences associated with DVA during pregnancy include premature labour, low birth weights and foetal trauma [32]. Whilst a large proportion of research explores the impact of DVA on children aged 6 and above, those that do look at preschool-aged children highlight how they too can be adversely affected [33].

associated with childhood development. Box 9.5 considers some indicative behaviours and how these might be misinterpreted.

9.4   Access to Support

Despite two police call outs and multiple hospital visits for Lois, the children were not referred to a specialist DVA support service until they were no longer living with the abuse. Originally established within maternity and health visiting settings, 'routine enquiry' is the process of professionals asking their patients or service users about DVA regardless of whether there are any presenting indicators. Lois had been offered support herself on both occasions following reporting DVA to the Police. She has also been asked about her DVA experiences when attending A&E. However, support for the children had not been discussed. Arguably one of the biggest battles for children and young people experiencing DVA is being recognised by professionals as victims who need access to specialist support.

Being recognised as victims by professionals can hold symbolic importance for children in the course of their recovery. It can also result in practical benefits, such as access to specialist support. Experiencing DVA can have significant implications on the physical, emotional and social development of children and young people. Specialist support can help them to not only understand what they have experienced but also begin to recover from the harm caused. This support can take many forms, from one-to-one therapeutic sessions with a specialist practitioner, creating safety plans and developing coping strategies, to connecting with peers who have had similar experiences through accredited group work programmes. Some young people may need bespoke advocacy with their school or college, or advice and information around their rights within the Victim's Code of Practice. Specialist support is delivered by trained practitioners who understand DVA and the impact it can have on children and young people. The support they provide will always depend on the individual needs of the young person accessing support.

Many specialist DVA support services have a Service Level Agreement (SLA) with their local police force whereby they receive Automatic Data Transfer (ADT) referrals. This is where DVA support services receive incident and victim data for every DVA incident recorded on police systems. In addition to very low reporting rates, there is also a lack of victim-status for children and young people experiencing DVA, meaning their details are not shared with support services. There is a reliance upon agencies to make targeted referrals for children and young people if they identify a need for support. The proposed Domestic Abuse Bill in the UK (see details in Box 9.6) marks the potential for a significant change around the recognition of children and young people experiencing DVA.

Children and young people who have experienced DVA want to feel safe and be given the opportunity to talk to someone about what happened [36]. In the UK, whether they are given this opportunity depends on what support is available in the area they live. There is a consistent shortfall in services for young people who experience DVA, with support being described as a 'postcode lottery' [36–39].

The Cooper family lived within a county where their police and crime commissioner had commissioned a specialist service for children and young people experiencing DVA. Initially, only two siblings were referred into their local specialist service by their school; Stuart and Sarah. Craig, the youngest sibling, was not referred for support as it was felt this was not needed. School staff had noticed changes in the children's behaviours, despite being unaware they were experiencing DVA. This lack of knowledge may be due to school staff not receiving sufficient training around DVA and its impact on children and young people, and also due to a lack of communication from the police.

Improvements have been made around communications between schools and statutory services regarding DVA with the introduction of Operation Encompass in 2011 (see Box 9.7); however, the police force where the Cooper family lived had not signed up to it at the time they were experiencing DVA.

Box 9.6 The Domestic Abuse Bill

Legislation around DVA differs around the world with various significant milestone being reached internationally. 1994 saw the first Southeast Asian nation, Malaysia, pass their first Domestic Violence Act. By 2005, most Southeast Asian nations enacted laws against this form of gender-based violence [34].

In December 2019, the UK Government committed to passing a Domestic Abuse Bill, designed to ensure victims felt confident to come forward, assured that support will be available for them and their children. At the time of writing this chapter, the Domestic Abuse Bill was still waiting to be passed through Parliament and had been delayed as a result of Britain leaving the European Union and the COVID-19 pandemic.

The initial proposal of a Domestic Abuse Bill created excitement and expectations that it will result in children and young people who experience DVA being recognised as victims in their own right. Whilst the current bill does not appear to fully achieve this, once passed, it does hope to improve the current circumstances for some young people. In principle, the bill in its latest form claims to introduce a new duty on local authorities in England to provide support to victims and their children with safe accommodation [35]. Whilst this does not fully address the issue of children not being recognised as victims, it marks the next step towards this being a possibility.

Box 9.7 Operation Encompass

Operation Encompass was established as a charitable organisation in 2011 and has since enabled effective communication between police forces and local schools, leading to positive outcomes for children and young people experiencing DVA. On a daily basis, Operation Encompass connects the police to key members of staff within schools to allow early information sharing when a child has been in a home the night before and the police had been called to a DVA incident.

This rapid communication enables the schools to better safeguard the children against the adverse impact of DVA and ensure their well-being is checked following recent incidents of abuse in the home. More information around operation encompass can be found at: https://www.operationencompass.org/.

Such changes are consistently being made in policy and practice, aiming to improve multi-agency working around DVA. The success of this, however, will always rely on the skills and understanding of individual practitioners. An audit of social workers found less than half (45%) had attended DVA training and taken it forward in their work [36]. With DVA being a large proportion of their caseloads, improved understanding around the dynamics of abuse is vital for successful multi-agency work.

Whilst only two of the Cooper siblings were initially referred to the service, all three received support. This was provided on an individual basis, giving each the opportunity to talk through their experiences and develop a range of strategies designed to help them cope and recover from the harm caused. Whilst their support followed a tailored plan created around their individual needs, all received support around safety planning, confidence and self-esteem building and help to develop their own coping strategies. The Cooper siblings engaged well, utilising the opportunity to process their experiences and begin to move forward. Unfortunately, it is not like this for all children and young people who have experienced DVA. Not only are there a lack of specialist services, but an additional barrier can come from their non-abusive parent not identifying their relationship as abusive. Support is most successful when the parent is able to recognise the abuse, and both they and their children are willing to engage with specialist support services.

The same specialist DVA service that supported the Coopers also receive a substantial number of referrals for young people who have experienced DVA and are now subject to child protection or child in need (i.e. satutory safeguarding) plans. A common scenario from these referrals are the non-abusive parent does not feel there is a need for support however accepts it through fear of this reflecting negatively to their social worker. Some social workers have been known to also add significant pressure to non-abusing parents to accept support in the belief that this will reduce the 'risk' of children and young people experiencing further violence and abuse. These parents have often endured periods of someone using power and control against them, which arguably is happening again with their social worker. Even when the benefit of accessing specialist support appears clear, it will only be successful when accessed with true consent and at a time that is right for the non-abusing parent, who will often require enhanced and different support after leaving an abusive partner. Specialist support is designed to empower those experiencing DVA and not to be enforced upon them. A more supportive approach, spending time exploring the abusive nature of their relationship and the potential benefits from accessing support, can make a difference to whether they truly engage with support.

Once support came to an end for the Cooper siblings, it was evident Stuart needed more intensive support, specifically around his aggressive behaviours and distorted view of women. Unfortunately, there were no local services that offered this. This support does exist and there is an example in Staffordshire, UK. New Era, the specialist DVA service, delivers support to children and young people who have experienced DVA and developed their own unhealthy and abusive behaviours. Had the Cooper family lived within Staffordshire, Stuart would have been able to receive the needed support, reiterating the postcode lottery of DVA support services.

9.5   Conclusions

The Cooper family's experiences highlight the impact DVA can have on children and young people. It also raises wider issues about what constitutes best practice for health and social work professionals when working with affected children. The detrimental impact DVA can have on children and young people is undeniable, and the current approach to supporting them is not always appropriate, or even available. It is hoped children and young people will start to be recognised as victims however even without this, our approach as practitioners can make a difference. Whether you are a student, social worker, school teacher, nurse, police officer or domestic abuse practitioner, if you are engaging with a family experiencing DVA do not forget about the children. If there is a specialist service within their area, with their consent, a referral for the children can ensure they are given the opportunity to process their experiences and begin to cope and recover from the harm caused. Whilst this chapter has been able to highlight some of the wider issues around children and young people experiencing DVA, it has been based upon the circumstances of one family. It is important to recognise that all young people will experience and be affected by the abuse in different ways. Where possible, speaking directly with these young people and asking them individually about their circumstances is best practice; this is the only way to be sure support will meet their needs.

Reflective Questions

1. In what ways may we see gender differences between young people who have experienced DVA?
2. What is your understanding of Social Learning Theory within a DVA context? Can you think of any case examples of this?
3. How can an understanding of gender norms and inequalities help to challenge the idea that abuse is inevitable for future generations?
4. What are the potential strengths and challenges of multi-agency approaches to supporting families affected by DVA?
5. Spend some time thinking about any unconscious bias you may have and explore some of the myths associated with DVA to enhance your approach as a practitioner.

References

1. Heise L, Ellsberg M, Gottmoeller M. A global overview of gender-based violence. Int J Gynecol Obstet. 2002;78(1):5–14.
2. UNICEF. Behind closed doors: the impact of domestic violence on children. 2006. http://www.ncjrs.gov/App/abstractdb/AbstractDBDetails.aspx?id=251032. Accessed 15 Apr 2020.
3. Gewirtz A, Edleson J. Young children's exposure to intimate partner violence: towards a developmental risk and resilience framework for research and intervention. J Fam Violence. 2007;22(1):151–63.
4. Holt S, Buckley H, Whelan S. The impact of exposure to domestic violence on children and young people: a review of the literature. Child Abuse Negl. 2008;32(1):797–810.
5. Michael Lloyd Research & Office of the Police and Crime Commissioner for Merseyside. Rapid evidence overview: life course impacts of domestic violence on children and young people. 2014. https://tinyurl.com/yawbfzxa.
6. Brown B, Bzostek S. Violence in the lives of children. Child Trends. 2003;15(1):1–13.
7. Smith C, Ireland T, Park A, Elwyn L, Thornberry T. Intergenerational continuities and discontinuities in intimate partner violence: a two-generational prospective study. J Interpers Violence. 2011;26(18):3702–52.

8. Whitfield C, Anda R, Dube S, Felitti V. Violent childhood experiences and the risk of intimate partner violence as adults. J Interpers Violence. 2003;18(12):166–85.

9. Jaffee A, Bowes L, Ouellet-Morin I, Fisher H, Moffitt T, Merrick M, Arseneault L. Safe, stable, nurturing relationships break the intergenerational cycle of abuse: a prospective nationally representative cohort of children in the United Kingdom. J Adolesc Health. 2013;53(4):4–10.

10. Berlin L, Appleyard K, Dodge K. Intergenerational continuity in child maltreatment: mediating mechanisms and implications for prevention. Child Dev. 2011;82(1):162–76.

11. Renner L, Slack K. Intimate partner violence and child maltreatment: understanding intra- and intergenerational connections. Child Abuse Negl. 2006;30(6):599–617.

12. Namy S, Carlson C, O'Hara K, Nakuit J, Bukuluki J, Namakula S, Nanyunja B, Wainberg M, Naker D, Michau L. Towards a feminist understanding of intersecting violence against women and children in the family. Soc Sci Med. 2017;184(1):40–8.

13. Policastro C, Payne B. The blameworthy victim: domestic violence myths and the criminalization of victimhood. J Aggress Maltreat Trauma. 2013;22(1):329–47.

14. Yamawaki N, Ochoa-Shipp M, Pulsipher C, Harlos A, Swinder S. Perceptions of domestic violence: the effect of domestic violence myths, victim's relationship with her abuser, and the decision to return to her abuser. J Interpers Violence. 2012;27(16):3915–212.

15. CAADA. In plain sight: the evidence from children domestic abuse. 2014. https://safelives.org.uk/sites/default/files/resources/Final%20policy%20report%20In%20plain%20sight%20-%20effective%20help%20for%20children%20exposed%20to%20domestic%20abuse.pdf.

16. Øverlien C. Children exposed to domestic violence: conclusions from the literature and challenges ahead. J Soc Work. 2010;10(1):80–97.

17. Social Services Improvement Agency. What works in promoting good outcomes for children in need who experience domestic violence? 2007. http://www.ssiacymru.org.uk/home.php?page_id=7141. Accessed 29 May 2020.

18. Barnish M. Domestic violence: a literature review. London: HM Inspectorate of Probation; 2004.

19. Mullender A, Hague G, Imam U, Kelly L, Malos E, Regan L. Children's perspectives on domestic violence. London: Sage; 2002.

20. Humphreys C, Houghton C, Ellis J. Literature review: better outcomes for children and young people experiencing domestic abuse—directions for good practice. 2008. https://dera.ioe.ac.uk/9525/1/0064117.pdf. Accessed 12 May 2020.

21. Bogat A, DeJonghe E, Levendosky A, Davidson W, Von Eye A. Trauma symptoms among infants exposed to intimate partner violence. Child Abuse Negl. 2006;30(1):109–25.

22. McIntosh J. Children living with domestic violence: research foundations for early intervention. J Fam Stud. 2014;9(2):219–34.

23. Baldry A. Bullying in schools and exposure to domestic violence. Child Abuse Negl. 2003;27(1):713–32.

24. Bauer N, Herrenkohl T, Lozano P, Rivara F, Hill K, Hawkins D. Childhood bullying involvement and exposure to intimate partner violence. Child Abuse Negl. 2006;118(2):235–42.

25. Bandura A. Aggression: a social learning analysis. London: Prentice Hall; 1973.

26. Carlson J, Voith L, Brown J, Holmes M. Viewing children's exposure to intimate partner violence through a developmental, socio-ecological, and survivor lens: the current state of the field, challenges, and future directions. Violence Against Women. 2019;25(1):6–28.

27. Jaffe P, Baker L, Cunningham A. Protecting children from domestic violence: strategies for community intervention. New York: Guildford Press; 2004.

28. Mazibuko N, Umejesi I. Domestic violence as a 'class thing': perspectives from a South African township. J Gender Behav. 2015;13(1):6584–93.

29. Walker L. The battered woman syndrome. 3rd ed. New York: Springer; 2009.

30. Callaghan J, Alexander J, Sixsmith J, Fellin LC. Children's experiences of domestic violence and abuse: siblings' accounts of relational coping. Clin Child Psychol Psychiatry. 2017;22(4):649–68.

31. Howarth E, Moore T, Stanley N, MacMillan H, Feder G, Shaw A. Towards an ecological understanding of readiness to engage with interventions for children exposed to domestic vio-

lence and abuse: systematic review and qualitative synthesis of perspectives of children, parents and practitioners. Health Soc Care Commun. 2017;27(1):271–92.

32. Jasinski J. Pregnancy and domestic violence. Trauma Violence Abuse. 2004;5(1):47–64.
33. Levendosky A, Huth-Bocks A, Shapiro D, Semel M. The impact of domestic violence on the maternal-child relationship and preschool-age children's functioning. J Fam Psychol. 2003;17(3):275–87.
34. UNIFEM. Domestic violence legislation and its implementation. Thailand: United Nations Development Fund for Women (UNIFEM); 2009.
35. GOV.UK. Domestic abuse bill 2020: overarching factsheet. 2020. https://www.gov.uk/government/publications/domestic-abuse-bill-2020-factsheets/domestic-abuse-bill-2020-overarching-factsheet. Accessed 14 May 2020.
36. Humphreys C, Mullender A. Children and domestic violence. 2015. https://www.nottinghamshire.gov.uk/media/120178/children-and-domestic-violence.pdf. Accessed 12 May 2020.
37. Radford L, Aitken R, Miller P, Ellis J, Roberts J, Firkic A. Meeting the needs of children living with domestic violence in London. City. 2011. https://www.nspcc.org.uk/globalassets/documents/research-reports/meeting-needs-children-living-domestic-violence-london-report.pdf. Accessed 18 May 2019.
38. SafeLives. SafeLives' 2017 survey of domestic abuse practitioners in England and Wales. 2018. https://safelives.org.uk/sites/default/files/resources/SafeLives%202017%20survey%20of%20domestic%20abuse%20practitioners-web_0.pdf.
39. Stanley N. Children experiencing domestic violence: a research review. 2011. http://www.menoresyviolenciadegenero.es/documentos/estudios-sobre-menores-expuestos-a-violencia-de-genero/Children-Experiencing-Domestic-Violence-A-Research-Review.pdf. Accessed 29 May 2020.

Older Women as the Invisible Victims of Intimate Partner Violence: Findings from Two European Research Projects

10

Bridget Penhale

10.1 Introduction

Intimate partner violence (IPV) against older women is a frequently misunderstood and overlooked issue within society, by the general public, older people themselves and professionals from health and human sciences. This often results in inappropriate and unhelpful criminal justice and social care responses. The issue appears to get lost between the topics of intimate partner violence, domestic violence and elder abuse—both in research and in the provision of services [1]. In the past, and to an extent in some places even now, domestic violence services and research have not had a particular focus on the needs of older women or age-related issues, or indeed those of women with disabilities (physical, mental or combined and relating to more complex conditions) [2]. In a number of countries, including the UK, this situation has been changing in recent years, and specific programmes for older survivors are increasingly being offered by domestic violence services, particularly through the provision of outreach programmes rather than a reliance on refuge or shelter provision, which many older women are unlikely to access or, indeed, wish to access. However, it has been apparent that in general, elder abuse and adult safeguarding services within an adult social care or social services context have a predominant focus on vulnerability and issues relating to care and/or welfare, so are usually not sensitive to domestic violence occurring in later life. Also, they tend to ignore the gender-specific dimensions of violence occurring within partnerships or former relationships. An age-specific and gender-specific approach to this type of family violence appears for the most to be part mutually exclusive [3]. To this extent, the experiences and needs of older women have consistently rendered them to a status of invisible victims, a situation that is much in need of redress.

B. Penhale (✉)
University of East Anglia, Norwich, UK
e-mail: B.Penhale@uea.ac.uk

© Springer Nature Switzerland AG 2021
C. Bradbury-Jones, L. Isham (eds.), *Understanding Gender-Based Violence*,
https://doi.org/10.1007/978-3-030-65006-3_10

This gap in relation to service provision has also been reflected in both domestic violence and elder abuse research in Europe. From an initial consideration of older female victims of IPV, a rather blurred picture of a relatively rarely reported phenomenon is apparent. For most European countries, national victimisation and crime surveys do not provide information on prevalence rates for this specific target group and phenomenon, with a focus on younger adult women when considering domestic violence and abuse. Of the few victimisation surveys that include older women (that is, older than reproductive age), these clearly show that IPV is a problem for older women far less frequently than for younger women (for Europe, see e.g. [4, 5]; for the US, see e.g. [6, 7]). Prevalence studies undertaken on the abuse of older men and women by family and household members arrive at similar conclusions [8–10]. The UK prevalence study of elder abuse and neglect, which included establishing the incidence of elder abuse over the past year, found that approximately 3.8% of older women reported experiencing some form of mistreatment within the previous year; in approximately half of these cases, the abuse was inflicted by a spouse or partner and would therefore be considered to be intimate partner violence [11].

Service providers relating to domestic violence often report very small numbers of older victims using their services. In contrast, however, some professionals report severe cases of IPV against older women and emphasise that IPV does not stop at age 60. Professionals also report that barriers to help-seeking and reporting violence appear to be particularly high for older victims and therefore the majority of cases remain undetected.

Research projects specifically addressing the issue of IPV against older women [12–19] and reports related to service provision for older victims [20–22] have mainly been undertaken in the USA, Canada and Australia, with some important contributions also coming from Israel [23, 24]. Within EU countries, initial actions to describe the phenomenon and to identify both service and research gaps appeared quite early within the Daphne programme (see below for futher details). The Daphne funded research project 'Recognition, prevention and treatment of abuse of older women' provided some initial insights, although sampling methods and size and the standardised approach limited exploration of this in depth [25]. This project together with a subsequent Daphne project 'Violence against older women' noted a striking absence of data on the issue of IPV experienced by older women, as well as a lack of services for them [26]. Two further Daphne projects 'Breaking the taboo' [27] and 'Care for Carers' [28] focused on violence against older women occurring within care-giving relationships and therefore had a predominant focus on the relevance of care-giving to the development of violence. Apart from this, only a few studies have been undertaken in the UK—these have mostly been small-scale and based on either a small number of interviews with victims [29–32] or on expert knowledge [33, 34].

Although in general terms (and in comparison with other types of family violence) there has been a lack of research on domestic violence in later life, over the past two decades it has become increasingly acknowledged that: 'no one, young or old, is immune to interpersonal violence' [35, p. 297]. Indeed, consideration of the relevant research that has taken place has established that many older women have been subjected to partner violence throughout their lives and still experience the impacts of this abuse in their old age [16]. Around 500,000 older people are believed to be abused at any one time in the UK [36], with most victims of elder abuse being older women with a chronic illness or disability, according to statistics provided by the government information service [37]. Most of the abuse that is recorded is in the domestic setting, within communities.

When women become 'older', their gender seems to be forgotten or becomes hidden. This means that older women's experiences of gender-based violence are often not recognised or responded to appropriately by such services. The Counting Dead Women project shows that of those women killed, most of the women aged over 60 were killed by a male family member, either a spouse or a son/grandson [38]. Older women experiencing domestic and sexual violence may be afraid and ashamed to seek help or may not know how to access support and are less likely to report crimes or to leave the perpetrator. And due to their relative invisibility, older women are likely to face particular obstacles to disclosure and help-seeking, which have not been adequately acknowledged and are not sufficiently understood or provided for.

Against the backdrop of the global ageing population, it is fundamental that the particular experiences, needs and rights of older women are adequately understood and that health care professionals respond appropriately. Whilst it is understood that the principal setting in which elder abuse and neglect happen is the domestic setting (within the community), and despite some work being undertaken, particularly in a North American context, it is still the case that comparatively little is known about the abuse of older women by their partners or former partners. Gaps in the research include understanding their behaviour in relation to help-seeking by older women or interventions that might assist recovery from abuse and moving forward following such experiences. This is the specific area of interest for this chapter, particularly in relation to two separate, but linked projects that were undertaken, funded by the European Commission within the frame of the EU Justice Department's Daphne programme. This was a specific funding mechanism developed to explore, violence against women and children. Its focus was on action based and innovative projects rather than being oriented towards research. The two specific projects that are the subject of this chapter aimed in the first case to obtain a better understanding of the specific challenges faced by older women, particularly in relation to help-seeking and in the second, follow-up project, to look at improving interventions with the development of training and guidance.

The first project, Intimate Partner Violence against Older Women (IPVoW), was developed to obtain a better understanding of the phenomenon and our knowledge about it. The second project, Mind the Gap!, was a follow-on initiative and innovative project, which aimed to increase knowledge about law enforcement interventions, and also had a focus on knowledge transfer for practitioners in social support services and the police and criminal justice agencies. It aslo aimed to develop, awareness-raising material for more general use. For more information on both projects and to access reports and project materials, see: http://www.ipvow.org. If more UK-specific information is required, please contact the chapter author.

10.2 The Intimate Partner Violence Against Older Women (IPVoW) Project

As stated, this project was supported and funded by the European Commission within the Daphne III programme. It was coordinated by the German Police University (Deutsche Hochschule der Polizei) and consisted of research teams from six European countries (Austria, Germany, Hungary, Poland, Portugal and the UK), which simultaneously explored the topic of violence against women aged more than 60[1] and at the hands of current and former intimate partners.

The fundamental aim of the project was to obtain first-hand knowledge from institutional and organisational perspectives and to understand how professionals and victims themselves described the phenomenon and associated help-seeking behaviours of older women affected by such violence and abuse. National reports (available in the respective national languages and in English) were developed to detail the results of the surveys in all six participating countries. An English summary report of the overall results of the study (and international comparison between the countries) was also produced. The research programme consisted of the phases as shown in Box 10.1.

Box 10.1 Overview of the IPVoW Project
- Compilation and evaluation of data and statistics in each country, together with a review of existing research.
- A survey at national level undertaken with the different agencies and institutions that might be involved in this type of work.
- Interviews with professionals who had knowledge about cases (30–35 per country).
- Interviews with women with experiences of intimate partner violence in old age (approx. 10 per country[2]).
- Development of recommendations for national and international contexts, discussed and developed at an international seminar.

[1] The age of 60 years was agreed as the chronological cut-off point for both projects, as demographic and retirement age variables were not consistent across participating countries, so a decision was taken to work to the youngest denominator in use.

[2] The original aim was to have 10 interviews per country. Due to constraints and circumstances beyond the control of the research team this was not possible to achieve in two countries (which achieved 7 and 9 interviews respectively).

10.3   Key Findings of the IPVoW Project

10.3.1 Data About Intimate Partner Violence Against Older Women

In most of the six countries, we found an overall lack of data on IPV against older women, particularly at the national level. Data are usually not sufficiently disaggregated by gender, age, the relationship between victim and perpetrator and/or the type of offence. However, some (mostly regional) data from services showed that the proportion of older women amongst all female clients reporting domestic violence to services was generally low, but higher in non-residential community-based services than in those providing shelters and refuges. In the UK, in the results from the British Crime Survey module on reported experiences of domestic violence, there was a lack of data concerning women older than 59 years as the module of questions was not available to women older than this cohort.[3] Overall, the extent of case knowledge amongst law enforcement agency participants who took part in the survey or in interviews was low.

10.3.2 Perceptions of Intimate Partner Violence and Older Women

From the interviews that were held in all partner countries, according to both professionals' and victims' reports, women and men involved in violent intimate relationships in later life come from all social and educational backgrounds. Violence was viewed as predominantly perpetrated by cohabiting partners within the context of long-standing relationships. A traditional gender role distribution – with high degrees of economic dependency of the older women and a substantial number of whom had not worked outside of the home – was often reported. All of the women who were interviewed across the different participating countries ($n = 56$) discussed some form of partner abuse within their relationship, some indicating that they had experienced multiple forms of abuse; the majority of women had experienced several types of abuse at the same time (for example physical and psychological/emotional forms of abuse). However, many of the women participants were reluctant to use terms such as 'domestic violence' or 'partner violence' and did not consider these terms, or the concept of violence to refer to their situations. In addition, many of the women appeared to minimise the severity and significance of the abuse they had been subjected to, with some women apparently perceiving such behaviour as normal, particularly within the context of their relationship(s). Most of the women reported that they had experienced violence from the beginning or early stages of

---

[3] This situation remained the case until the age limit for participation in the module was raised to 79 years in 2018.

their relationships and throughout the complete course of the marriage/relationship. Unequal power relations, gender-specific roles and patriarchal societal structures were mentioned by professionals and the older women as causes of IPV against older women (the terms used by the women may not have been exactly these, but broadly referred to such issues). Alcohol consumption/alcoholism, abuse of medication and jealousy were seen as specific triggers for violence that occurred.

In several cases, the violence began or worsened in later life, with a number of factors leading or contributing to a late onset or aggravation of violence. Such factors included: increasing dependency (relating to care, household matters); issues relating to property and household income; mental health disorders such as dementia or relating to substance misuse; retirement of partner (loss of self-esteem and increase in amount of time spent together) and changes in sexual function. Unfulfilled or thwarted expectations, or with additional (perhaps too much) time spent together in retirement, also contributed to the onset or increased levels of violence in a number of relationships.

10.3.3 Older Women's Experiences of IPV

In most of the cases that were described to the researchers, unidirectional violence by the male partner against the woman was reported. These cases were marked by pronounced shame by the women, increased levels of social isolation, psychological disorders, low self-esteem and a perception of reduced options for change. Health problems appeared to play a major role in cases of IPV against older women; these situations increased vulnerability, particularly to the effects of violence, reduced coping opportunities and reduced options for seeking help. Although such health problems related to the women, health problems on the part of husbands/partners were also reported to play a part (for example a partner with a cognitive problem such as dementia becoming violent during the course of the illness).

In our study, from the institutional survey and other reports, it became apparent that often other people in either social proximity or the social network of the older women could also be considered as perpetrators. This included sons (in relatively high numbers, the next most frequent to husbands/partners), neighbours, acquaintances, children of new partners, tenants and staff members of care services. For many older women victims of IPV, experiences of (male) violence appeared to be a biographical constant seemingly across their lives. For some women this included the possibility of the extent of the violence increasing in later life, perhaps because of the women's reduced capacity to deal with the abuse and also because the consequences of such violence were experienced more severely.

Many of the women reported that they had experienced rigid upbringings by their parents and had experiences of violence in their childhood and as young adults. For this generation of women, particularly from the cohort of older than 75 years, many had been brought up to accept traditional gender roles and were taught to perceive marriage as a life-long commitment and one which meant acceptance of the partner as dominant, and which did not allow for divorce or separation.

10.3.4 Leaving or Staying in the Violent Relationship

Although there were many reported reasons for the women not to leave their violent partners, the wish to change their situations and live free from violence was still very strong. Indeed, a number of women who were interviewed had separated from their partners, despite experiencing difficulties in doing so. For example, within the UK sample of 10 women who were interviewed, 8 had successfully left their partners. Identified advantages of leaving included being able to live without fear (of ongoing or future violence), having improved relationships with their children and other family members and the possibility of improved 'peace of mind'. Difficulties that were experienced either during or after leaving the violent relationship included increases in levels of violence that happened, or changes in the type of violence encountered, with former partners finding other ways to exert control over the women; financial consequences of leaving, or loss of the family home (for those women who moved out on separating from their partners), and raised levels of loneliness for those who had also moved to a different area. For the two women who were still in their relationships at the time of interview, relevant factors influencing the decision to stay with the partner included being able to stay in the family home, small but significant changes that happened in the situations (so that they felt safer) and acknowledging a need for financial security (which would not have been the case had they separated from the partner). This was counter-balanced, however, by the reported continuation of unhappy relationships in overall terms for both women.

10.3.5 Intersectional and Contextual Factors

Our study showed that the intersection of age-, gender- and generation-specific factors played a key role on a number of different levels; additionally, some specific problems were reported by women with migration backgrounds, who were ageing in adopted countries rather than native contexts. Although there were not many immigrant women in the study overall, the problems experienced by this subsample, particularly in relation to help-seeking, appeared to be substantial. Amongst the reported continuing and even persistent effects of long-term abuse were severe physical health and psychological problems, including exacerbation of illnesses unrelated to the violence, as well as low self-esteem and increased financial dependency in later life. This could make it more difficult for older women to end the relationship than for younger women who have been in their relationships for a comparatively shorter time and who probably have the ability to attain financial independence and rebuild their lives and self-esteem, albeit over a period of time. For older women who experience IPV, however, time is not generally on their side.

The historical and current societal contexts in the different participating countries also shaped women's experiences of IPV. Examples of country-specific differences were the differential importance of religion, of alcohol abuse, particular experiences of dictatorship and war, specific country/cultural values, attitudes and gender roles, the current economic situation and country-specific urban–rural gaps. For all the partner countries, it became clear that in most cases IPV against older women is deeply rooted in inequality, power and intersectional issues in the relations between men and women. In addition, age-related vulnerability to increased risk of harm, marginality and in some cases dependency served to worsen the situation for many older women. Furthermore, it was also apparent from the interviews that IPV against older women could also be caused by a partner/former partner who had mental health problems, either of a long-standing nature or that the man had developed in later life. It is therefore very important to differentiate between individual cases and situations and to explore the precipitating factors in the circumstances presented within cases as these will likely be quite different between individuals undergoing what might appear, externally, to be quite similar situations and even experiences.

10.3.6 Help-Seeking and Provision of Support

For the professionals who took part in interviews, working with older women victims of IPV often meant facing bigger challenges than working with younger women in apparently quite similar situations. From the IPVoW study, and specifically from the interviews held with older women across the different partner countries, when older women victims of IPV seek support, there were a number of relevant key factors. These included finding out information about their rights and finding someone with whom they could build a trusting relationship and share their feelings and experiences and explore possible options for change. Older women appear to separate from their violent partners or press charges against them somewhat less often (exact figures for this are unknown, but a brief comparison of relevant reporting rates across the police and public prosecution services in the different partner countries within the subsequent Mind the Gap! study suggested such a trend). This can be for a variety of different reasons but includes at times a lack of available and suitable alternative accommodation—for example our partners in Hungary noted this impediment to separation for older survivors. Additionally, older women do not know about or make use of services as often as younger women who experience these types of violence [39, 40]. In one of the interviews held in the UK, the woman said that she had been persuaded to make contact with the local Women's Aid group (in the area in which she was living at that time) after her daughter had been in touch to receive assistance for herself and had then told her mother that she thought that such contact could also be of assistance to her; this daughter had instigated contact with Women's Aid and accompanied her mother to her first meeting.

In the IPVoW study, specialist professionals/workers in this area reported that they quite often saw a particular demand for support of older women, which, according to their accounts, was not sufficiently well met at that time. Some respondents suggested that this could be due to resource issues within their agencies, one example of this being unable to undertake long-term work with any of the women in contact with the agency but acknowledging that older women might be more likely to be in need of longer periods of support and assistance. The study provided evidence, however, that older women do seek help through a variety of different ways. This could be through (initial) contact with relatives, neighbours, organisations working in the field of domestic violence, the police and other law enforcement agencies and from doctors and other health services and social services and social support agencies[4] (for example Non-Governmental Organisation (NGO) or third-sector organisations working either with older people in a more general sense or with domestic violence).

One of the key findings from the series of interviews held with professionals as well as with the older women was that partner violence does not appear to decrease or stop as women become older and enter 'later life'. However, it is of note that in some cases, the type(s) of violence that women were subjected to did change in later life. Situations were described in which perpetrators who were no longer capable of physical violence (for example due to the development of health problems or physical frailty) chose to use alternative methods of abuse—for instance through increased forms of psychological and emotional abuse. In the UK context, women felt that it was fear that had often caused them the greatest difficulties when it came to leaving their violent relationship, considering leaving the situation or accessing help for the violence that they had experienced. This comprised fear of other people's reactions, fear that the violence would get worse if they tried to leave or sought help and/or fear that they would not be able to support themselves financially if they left the situation. These were all significant barriers to leaving and even to seeking help in more general terms. The findings indicated that a proportion of older women could be at an increased level of situational vulnerability because of the dependence on their partners for financial security and/or their healthcare needs—and that in some circumstances a double dependency might occur, which could further heighten risk for individuals. Both the professionals and the older women who were interviewed reported that there was limited information available to older female victims of IPV relating to available help and support for older women who have experienced (or are experiencing) IPV.

If older women are exposed to violence by their partners, amongst the greatest needs reported in the study by older women and professionals working on this issue were in the areas of health, finance and housing-related issues. Housing was indicated as one of the main problems older women have to deal with, and as one of the strongest limitations within the interventions that support agencies could be successfully involved in. From the survey findings, most of the respondents from the different institutions were critical about the lack of resources to provide appropriate support to older women, including adequate accommodation and, additionally, the lack of close cooperation with other organisations that was apparent in a number of situations. A central theme derived from the interviews with both professionals and the older women themselves highlighted a clear need for more awareness across several

---

[4] As formal, state provided social services were not available across all the countries in the study, the term social support agencies was adopted to denote both state and NGO or third sector organisation involvement in this field.

contexts—amongst the general public, but also amongst older women—about 1) IPV and other forms of elder abuse and 2) what organisations can provide assistance and support to affected older women.

10.4 The Mind the Gap! Project

The work that had commenced in the IPVoW project was continued in the context of a second Daphne project and again involved seven different partner agencies from six EU countries; these were the same as those previously involved in the IPVoW study, providing useful continuity within this strand of work. This follow-up project aimed to transfer the knowledge gained in the previous IPVoW study into practice, specifically within the settings of law enforcement and social support agencies and, particularly, to gain additional knowledge and understanding of the ways in which law enforcement agencies deal with cases of IPV against older women. The project aimed to obtain further insight into possible effective and adequate interventions, and support by law enforcement and social support agencies, to raise awareness about older women as victims of IPV. The underpinning aim of which was, to encourage agencies to tackle the problem and to improve outreach to this subgroup of victims by raising awareness about this issue. There was also an additional objective to strengthen the capacity of law enforcement and social support agencies so that they could respond to and intervene more successfully in such cases, through participatory and co-production activities with professionals and organisations in this field of work. One of the awareness raising activities that was especially undertaken with social support agencies was the development of awareness-raising promotional materials for older women; more detail and information on this will be provided in a later section.

10.4.1 Analysis of Police and/or Public Prosecutor Files

In order to gain a better understanding about what happens when police, public prosecution and courts intervene in situations of IPV against older women and to gain knowledge about possible good practice, an analysis of selected police, public prosecutor or court files involving cases of IPV against older women was carried out in all six participating countries and using an agreed analytical framework. In some countries, access could be gained to public prosecutors' files, in other countries, we analysed police or court files. In the UK, analysis of 150 police case files across seven different police forces in England and Wales was undertaken; the same number of cases was also accessed and subject to analysis in Germany. In smaller countries, or those where law enforcement responses to domestic violence/IPV were less well developed, 75 such cases were analysed. Preliminary discussions of the results from all the partner countries determined that some of the issues connected with police/judicial intervention in cases of IPV against older women appeared to be relevant in all or most of the countries, and some clear similarities between the types of cases were seen. Similarities between cases included the following factors: in the majority of cases, victim–perpetrator relationships were generally long-lasting and of many years duration, partners were usually cohabitating (or partly separated but living under one roof), but also a number of short-term relationships were reported, although these tended to be of more than five years duration [41].

In many countries there was, however, a sizeable proportion of younger perpetrators, with perpetrators being middle-aged rather than older, as seen in the following Table 10.1, containing the mean ages of the perpetrators. Within the comparative analysis, the mean ages of suspects and victims were relatively close together; however, the age range was broader for perpetrators. In the total sample, 12.5% of victims were more than 9 years older than the suspected abuser. In Poland, this ratio was the lowest (2.9%) and in Hungary the ratio was much higher (21%). The age gap between those intimate partners who were not living together at the time of the reported incident and ex-intimate partners appeared particularly large (at more than 50%).

To provide some further comparison, in the UK, it was found that in the analysed cases, just over three-quarters (76%) of the victims were aged between 60 and 69 years old (with over half the sample, 56%, between 60 and 64). A further 18% of reported victims were between 70 and 79 years. However, just under half (49%) of the sample of perpetrators were between 60 and 64 years, whereas 16% were aged between 50 and 59 years and a further 7% were in the 41–49 range. Almost three-quarters of the sample (72%), therefore, were aged between 41 and 64 years. Additionally, a considerable percentage of perpetrators were reported as intoxicated at the time of the violent incident (or incidents), as seen in the following Table 10.2, which compares levels of intoxication (at the time of the incident) for perpetrators and victims.

In the field of domestic violence generally, it is often reported that intoxication increases the risk of violent behaviour happening. Within our samples of case files, partner countries differed significantly from each other concerning this aspect. In Poland, almost every perpetrator was reported as intoxicated during the incident, but none of the victims were recorded as intoxicated through alcohol or drug use at

Table 10.1 Mean ages of perpetrators, by country

	Austria	Germany	Hungary	Poland	Portugal	UK	Total
Mean age	67.9	68.1	65.5	63.8	67.7	65.4	66.3
Min–max age	46–90	40–90	28–90	52–82	47–86	41–90	28–90

Table 10.2 Reported rates of intoxication (alcohol and/or drug use) at the time of the incident

	Austria	Germany	Hungary	Poland	Portugal	UK	Total (Mean)
Perpetrator intoxicated	42.7	31.5	31.7	95.7	23.7	44.7	43.8
Victim intoxicated	7.3	8.7	11	0	0	22.7	10.3

that time. In the UK, there was a relatively high percentage of rates of intoxication amongst both perpetrators and victims. The lowest level of recorded IPV incidents by intoxicated persons occurred in Portugal. Within the samples, information was only coded if it was clearly recorded in the case file. If information about drug or alcohol use was vague, incomplete or contradictory, this was coded as unclear. In the case files from both the Hungarian and German samples, most of the information was unclear. However, files from Poland, UK and Portugal contained the most detailed information about the intoxication of victim; whereas the Polish and UK files were the most detailed concerning perpetrators. Across the sample, quite different drug/alcohol consumption patterns relating to IPV against older women were apparent. Additionally, it is of note that many perpetrators committed acts of IPV without the use of any kind of drugs or alcohol, as with other types of domestic, or familial violence.

Of the risk factors that were identified for perpetrators across a number of domains, the following Table 10.3 provides a comparison between the partner countries.

As seen in Table 10.3, despite some variation between countries, overall the main risk factor for perpetrators concerning intimate partner violence was substance use. All the perpetrators in the Polish sample of cases had reported problems with substance use and another 50% had some kind of health problem (physical, or mental health related, or both). As seen in Table 10.4, below, in relation to the victims, the main risk factors appeared to be health problems and being in a caring situation (either providing care for the perpetrator or being cared for due to their own health problem(s)).

In those countries where further proceedings could be tracked, a very high percentage of cases did not proceed—which mirrors findings for IPV cases in general. Whilst across the total sample (all countries) the police initially instigated criminal proceedings in almost three-quarters (73%) of the situations, full prosecution did not always proceed, for a variety of reasons and in only 13% of cases ($n = 91$) was the prosecution successful and resulted in conviction of the perpetrator. It appears

Table 10.3 Comparison of perpetrator risk factors, by country, across several domains

	Austria	Germany	Hungary	Poland	Portugal	UK
Caring situation	12.2	17.1	0	4.3	15.8	32
Health problem	22	37.1	15.9	50	21.2	19.3
Substance abuse	34.1	14.9	15.9	100	46.1	12.7
Economic dependency	1.2	0	8.5	10	6.6	3.3

Table 10.4 Comparison of victim risk factors, by country, across several domains

	Austria	Germany	Hungary	Poland	Portugal	UK
Caring situation	13.5	16	0	4.3	13.2	31.4
Health problem	23.2	21.3	18.3	48.5	18.4	31.3
Substance abuse	0	2.1	7.3	1.4	0	5.3
Economic dependency	7.3	4.3	6.1	1.4	31.6	4

that one of the prime reasons that prosecution did not proceed was due to a reluctance on the part of the victim. Throughout the full sample, a third of the victims (33.8%) was fully supportive of criminal prosecution of the perpetrator. It is of some interest that the highest proportion of victims who fully supported prosecution was found in Hungary (66.3%) and in Poland (55%), although in these countries the extent of organised and legal actions in relation to IPV have the shortest history (and in Hungary, domestic violence is not wholly recognised or recorded as a crime). However, in Poland, only files relating to court proceedings were analysed, which could mean that only the most severe cases were contained in the sample—or the fact that these cases were subject to full prosecution could be due to the victims being more supportive of prosecution. In Hungary, police case files were analysed (as in the UK sample), but in the former situation, the majority of reports to and requests for intervention by the police were made by victims. In addition to this, the highest proportion of recorded major injuries related to victims in Hungary (40.2%, with a further 24.4% of records containing reports of moderate injuries). This might explain the higher proportion of Hungarian victims being supportive of prosecution. The lowest number of supportive victims was found in the UK and German samples—in the UK sample, 42% of victims were recorded as either mainly or totally reluctant towards prosecution (as opposed to 34% who were mainly or fully supportive), although it must be borne in mind that the UK sample included initial investigation files, rather than (exclusively) prosecution or court files.

Older women victims often made reports and involved the police when they were in need of safety and had a clear wish to stop the violence, but this quite often happened in the context of uncertainty or lack of knowledge about where to obtain help from. However, many of the women did not really wish there to be any criminal prosecution of their partner or ex-partner, or were rather ambivalent in this respect, perhaps withdrawing a complaint after initial agreement that the police should proceed with investigations and so forth. In this respect, although the majority of reports to the police were made by the older women themselves (somewhat contrary to the expectations of the research team), such reports appear to relate more to a 'cry for help' rather than any desire for punishment of the partner or former partner.

Questions about how to ensure inter-agency cooperation are important in all cases of IPV, but perhaps become more crucial when victims and/or perpetrators are in some way dependent, are chronically ill or frail. The important role of the police in recognizing healthcare and/or social needs and initiating procedures to obtain a substantiated medical diagnosis and associated necessary support was clear in such cases, particularly as in the case files this did not always appear to have happened. There was also an evident need for an agency to assume case (or care) management functions for complex cases and to ensure collaborative and transdisciplinary working. UK structures with police officers who specialised in dealing with domestic violence and/or safeguarding vulnerable adults seemed more likely to ensure that such issues concerning dependency and frailty were tackled, and this might be a useful model for other countries to develop and use.

Several countries appeared to lack any protocols for inter-agency cooperation or information sharing, and in others domestic violence, perhaps especially towards older women, did not appear to be perceived as a crime at all. However, even in the UK, it was apparent that it was still a challenge to bridge the gap between procedures, specialists and concepts of domestic violence and adult safeguarding (or elder abuse) within police forces and also other agencies. Due to a number of issues, including for example the consequences of a long period of austerity and associated resource restrictions, it is likely that this situation (of challenges) still pertains now. Problems encountered in the participating countries were also related to insufficient or inadequate risk assessment procedures; this seemed to be due, at least in part, to the fact that such assessments did not fully consider age-related issues and were not particularly adapted to or focused on the intersectional issues that exist in relation to older women's experiences of violence in later life, whether this concerned IPV or some other form of elder abuse.

Final results of the case file analysis are available in the national languages (English, German, Hungarian, Polish and Portuguese), together with summaries in English on the homepage of the internet site developed for the IPVoW study (see: http://www.ipvow.org). A further summarising report was produced that also brought together national results of the law enforcement analyses from across the six countries.

10.5   Capacity Building for Law Enforcement: Development of a Manual and Training

On the basis of findings from IPVoW, the file analysis and participatory discussions with experts from justice agencies, in each country a manual was developed for capacity building for police and other law enforcement agencies working in the field of domestic violence, in order to develop awareness of and increase responsiveness to the needs of older women victims. A framework for training police and other law enforcement agencies was also developed in a co-productive manner with relevant justice agency representatives. The guidance manuals and training template were designed to contain information about the characteristics of cases of IPV against older women and some of the typical problems in dealing with these cases. Possible measures to improve the handling of such cases, together with possible partners for collaboration, and information sources and resources relevant to each country were also included. In most countries, the training that was developed was also tested out.

In the UK, the training framework was developed and agreed with the (then) National Policing Improvement Agency (NPIA) and then passed to the College of Policing on its inception, for incorporation into their curriculum on Protecting Vulnerable People. The framework was in the form of learning objectives and scenario-based case compilations derived from the analysis of case records, which illustrate different discussion and learning points. Overall, this was framed within a modular format for the NPIA to use and potentially to develop further; unfortunately, at that time it was not possible to fully test the framework due to organisational reasons within the College of Policing and in any case, implementation was determined to be an internal matter for the police.

National differences found across the partner countries within the project meant that different approaches to guidance and training documentation were established to be necessary. Whilst in some of the partner countries the development of new curricular concepts and manuals was needed, in others the modification of existing curricula and manuals concerning domestic violence was possible and undertaken. In some places, several of the participating partners preferred to develop training and guidance (manuals) for both law enforcement agencies and social support agencies together. In both Austria and Portugal, multi-agency training sessions were devised, through co-production, working with the principal organisations involved in work in this area. Such sessions involved professionals with specialist backgrounds in both IPV and working wth older people. Examples of training materials and manuals developed across the countries are also available from the project website both in national languages and in English.

10.6   Awareness Raising to Improve Social Support Agency Outreach to Older Victims

Within the scope of the project, awareness raising materials (posters, postcards, flyers and information leaflets or brochures) were developed for professionals, the general public and particularly for older female victims of IPV. In the UK, this initiative centred on the development of posters. Well-developed participatory and consultative processes were undertaken in each country, involving experts, practitioners and older women themselves, including some who had experienced IPV in later life, to gain valuable information about the design and content of such material and what would be both acceptable and most likely to be beneficial. Following such methods of consultation and feedback, different needs were identified across the partner countries and therefore six different posters were developed, although the design centred on a common theme. On all posters a free space appearing in the bottom section was created to enable support organisations to add their own specific contact details before use in a local area or in a particular context. On completion of the project, a USB stick containing a copy of the UK poster templates was disseminated to the participating agencies and organisations (and similar approaches adopted for the resources developed in other partner countries). This followed consultation about the preferred type of dissemination requested by partner organisations—although virtually all opted for this method. Following further dissemination of the project findings via presentations at relevant conferences and meetings, links to a downloadable copy of the UK poster templates and other project resources that had been developed were made available for use. In addition, a link to a downloadable copy of the UK poster templates was circulated in a Women's Aid (England) member's bulletin during 2018. Copies of the relevant material in one of the other languages used within the project (German, Hungarian, Polish or Portuguese) were also made available to download through the project website, available at www.ipvow.org as stated earlier.

10.7 Capacity Building of Social Support Agencies: Development of Guidance

Following the findings from IPVoW and the file analysis information across all countries, materials were also developed for social support agencies which might have contact with older women affected by IPV, for example women's shelters/refuges, intervention centres, crisis intervention units and a variety of care services. In Austria, following the participatory methods and consultative approaches, a special brochure for older women was created, whilst in the other countries, separate guidance for practitioners and organisations was produced. In the UK, in addition to the more general booklet-type document provided for organisations (both statutory and voluntary or third sector organisations), a smaller sized, more portable version of the guidance for practitioners was produced so that this would be more readily accessible for use. This separation of the material into two distinct elements also occurred as a result of the co-production methods used within the project and again were made generally available via the project website on completion of the project. This is also the case for the resources developed in other countries; these are provided in national languages, with some English versions also made available.

Reflective Questions

- Identify the main areas of improvement needed at professional and organisational levels in order to improve responses to older victims-survivors of IPV.
- Think about whether these are similar (or different to) established responses that exist in relation to younger adult women who experience IPV.
- Consider if these are similar (or different to) established responses that exist in relation to older people who encounter elder abuse (outside of an intimate of former relationship).
- What appear to be some of the main similarities between older and younger women when disclosing abuse and/or seeking support?
- Identify some of the key differences between older and younger women when disclosing abuse and/or seeking support?

10.8 Concluding Comments

In order to further develop the field and to improve professional practitioner responses to older women in such situations, a number of different approaches need to be used. It is apparent that there is a need to improve awareness and recognition of mistreatment, across the general public, professionals and the older population themselves, perhaps most importantly older women. Work needs to take place to develop knowledge and to understand about abuse and neglect, the interrelated aspects of causal factors and consequences and the interaction of gender and power relations within such situations. Development of theoretical and conceptual frameworks and foundations are also of central importance here [42, 43] and these need to include gender perspectives, as appropriate. Social perspectives on abuse must also be fully incorporated in such frameworks. Above all, it is imperative that the voices of older people, particularly those who have experienced abusive and neglectful situations, are central to such developments and that such voices include those who are the most marginalised and excluded, many of whom are women.

Several of these approaches will need thorough research and development to happen. There is a need for intervention studies to be undertaken to try and discover which techniques work best and in which circumstances. This might include the development of model projects concerning different interventions, with appropriate and rigorous evaluation of the different projects in order to establish necessary areas for future development. Research on effectiveness and impact, not just of interventions including the effect(s) of processes and interventions but also the impact of abuse and neglect on individuals who have experienced or are at risk of abuse and harm, also needs to be undertaken. Further work on the differing models of service provision (for example different types of specialist teams) should also take place, but as it is not yet clear which model might work best, in which situation or type of abuse, and for whom. In-depth research and evaluation of such models would be valuable and would be likely to be beneficial for developmental reasons (to develop the field further, including health and care practice with individuals who experience such violence and abuse).

Equally, a need for sufficient focus on individualised and personalised approaches for people who experience mistreatment and harm is required; as far as possible these types of approaches should be tailored to the needs of particular individuals. Key and central issues here relate to autonomy, choice, empowerment and independence, with further essential elements relating to individuals' capacity and consent. Self-determination, independence and service user control are not necessarily juxtaposed to matters concerning individual safety and protection. Indeed, most safety planning for older people aims to support and empower individuals to keep themselves safe and to change their own situations (if they are willing and able to do so). If we wish to achieve the aim of assisting all older people to live their final years free from abuse, neglect and exploitation, perhaps particularly older women who are the most disenfranchised segment of cohorts of older people, there must be more research, development and evaluation of practice initiatives and transdisciplinary collaboration to further counteract the differing and pervasive forms of mistreatment that exist. Attention to issues relating to gender equality and the specific needs of older women who experience IPV will undoubtedly strongly support this undertaking.

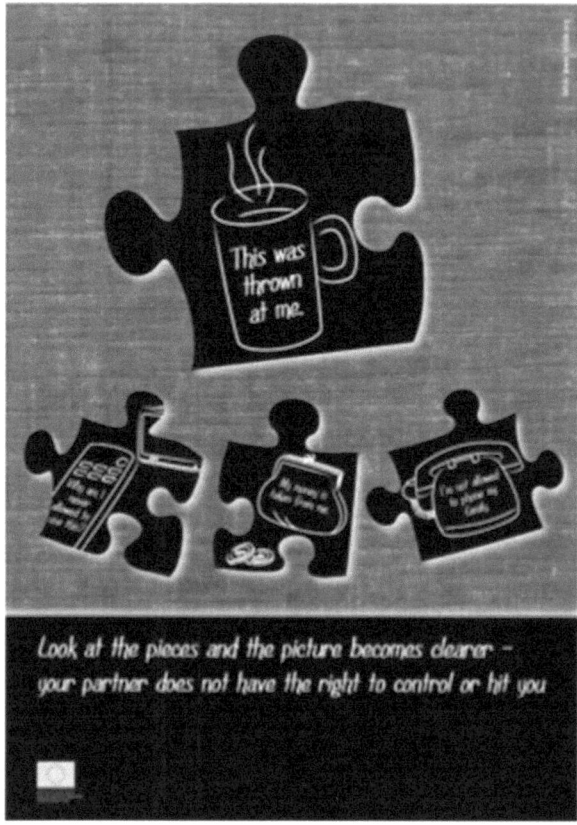

One of the UK posters developed as part of the Mind the Gap! project, available from www.ipvow.org/en/campaign-material

Acknowledgements Acknowledgements are due to all those who took part in these studies: those who participated and freely gave their experiences, expertise and time. This also includes our partners in the other five EU countries; the European Commission DAPHNE Programme (DG Justice) for providing funding and our thanks to Dr. Jenny Porritt (IPVoW) and William Goreham (Mind the Gap!) for acting as researchers on the respective projects.

References

1. Wydall S, Zerk R. Domestic abuse and older people: factors influencing help-seeking. J Adult Protect. 2017;19(5):247–60.
2. Penhale B. Elder abuse, ageing and disability. In: Shah S, Bradbury Jones C, editors. Global perspectives on disability, violence and protection over the life-course. London: Routledge; 2018.
3. Penhale B. Gender issues in elder abuse. In: Phelan A, editor. Advances in elder abuse-research, practice, legislation and policy. London: Springer Books; 2020.
4. Schröttle M. Gewalt gegen Frauen in Paarbeziehungen. Eine sekundäranalytische Auswertung zur Differenzierung von Schweregraden, Mustern, Risikofaktoren und Unterstützung nach erlebter Gewalt. Berlin: Bundesministerium für Familie, Senioren, Frauen und Jugend; 2008.

5. Stöckl H, Watts C, Penhale B. Intimate partner violence against older women in Germany: prevalence and risk factors. J Interpers Violence. 2012;27(13):2545–64.
6. Zink T, Fisher B, Regan S, Pabst S. The prevalence and incidence of intimate partner violence in older women in primary care practices. J Gen Intern Med. 2005;20(10):884–8.
7. Bonomi A, Anderson M, Reid R, Carrell D, Fishman P, Rivara F, Thompson R. Intimate partner violence and older women. Gerontologist. 2007;47(1):34–41.
8. Mouton C, Rodabough R, Rovi S, Hunt J, Talamantes M, Grzyski R, Burge S. Prevalence and 3-year incidence of abuse among post-menopausal women. Am J Public Health. 2004;94(4):605–12.
9. Görgen T, Nagele B. Sexuelle Viktimisieutring im Alter. Z Gerontol Geriatr. 2006;39(5):382–9.
10. Soares J, Barros H, Torres-Gonzalez F, Ioannidi-Kapolou E, Lamura G, Lindert J, de Dios Luna J, Macassa G, Melchiorre M-G, Stankumas M. Abuse and health of elderly in Europe. Kaunas: Lithuanian University of Health Sciences Press; 2010.
11. Luoma M-L, Koivusilta M, Lang G, Enzenhofer E, De Donder L, Verte D, Reingarde J, Tamutiene I, Ferreira-Alves J, Santos A-J, Penhale B. Prevalence study of violence and abuse against older women: results of a multi-country study. Helsinki: National Institute of Health and Welfare (THL); 2011.
12. Beaulaurier RL, Seff LR, Newman FL. Barriers to help-seeking for older women who experience intimate partner violence: a descriptive model. J Women Aging. 2008;20:231–48.
13. Bergeron R. An elder abuse case study: caregiver stress or domestic violence? You decide. J Gerontol Soc Work. 2001;34(4):47–62.
14. Fisher B, Regan S. The extent and frequency of abuse in the lives of older women and their relationship with health outcomes. Gerontologist. 2006;46(2):200–9.
15. Hightower J. Hearing the voices of abused older women. J Gerontol Soc Work. 2006;46(3/4):205–27.
16. Mears J. Survival is not enough: violence against older women in Australia. Violence Against Women. 2003;9:1478–89.
17. Montminy L. Older Women's experiences of psychological violence in their marital relationships. J Gerontol Soc Work. 2005;46(2):3–22.
18. Rennison C, Rand M. Non-lethal intimate partner violence against women: a comparison of three age cohorts. Violence Against Women. 2003;9:1417–28.
19. Teaster P, Roberto K, Dugar R. Intimate partner violence of rural aging women. Fam Relat. 2006;55(5):636–48.
20. Vinton L. A model collaborative project towards making domestic violence centers elder ready. Violence Against Women. 2003;9:1504–13.
21. Brandl B, Hebert M, Rozwadowski J, Spnagler D. Feeling safe, feeling strong: support groups for older abused women. Violence Against Women. 2003;9(12):1490–503.
22. Brownell P. Psycho-educational support groups for older women victims of family mistreatment: a pilot study. J Gerontol Soc Work. 2006;46(3/4):145–60.
23. Winterstein T, Eisikovits Z. The experience of loneliness of battered old women. J Women Aging. 2005;17(4):3–19.
24. Winterstein T, Eisikovits Z. "Aging out" of violence: the multiple faces of intimate partner violence over the life span. Qual Health Res. 2006;19(2):164–80.
25. Barnes-Holmes Y, Barnes-Holmes D, Morichelli R, Scocchera F, Sdogati C, Morjaria A, Furniss F. Mistreatment of older women in the European Community: estimated prevalence and service and legal responses. A review of the situation in three member states. DAPHNE project 2000-125. Final report. http://ec.europa.eu/justice_home/daphnetoolkit/html/projects/dpt_2000_125_w_en.html. Accessed May 2020.
26. Ockleford E, Barnes-Holmes Y, Morichelli R, Morjaria A, Scocchera F, Furniss F, Sdogati C, Barnes-Holmes D. Mistreatment of older women in three European countries: estimated prevalence and service responses. Violence Against Women. 2003;9(12):1453–64.
27. Strümpel C, Gröschl C, Hackl C. Breaking the taboo project. Violence against older women in families: recognizing and acting. Vienna: Austrian Red Cross; 2010.

28. ISTISS. Care for Carers—violence against Alzheimer elderly women. DAPHNE Programme project, 2005. http://ec.europa.eu/justice/grants/results/daphne-toolkit/content/care-carers-violence-against-alzheimer-elderly-women_en. Accessed May 2020.
29. Pritchard J. The needs of older women: Services for the victims of elder abuse and other abuse. Bristol: The Policy Press; 2000.
30. McGarry J, Simpson C, Hinchliff-Smith K. The impact of domestic violence for older women. Health Social Care Commun. 2010;19(1):3–14.
31. Bows H. Sexual violence and older people. London: Routledge; 2019.
32. Bows H. The other side of late-life intimacy? Sexual violence in later life. Aust J Ageing. 2020;39(S1):65–70.
33. Scott M, McKie L, Morton S, Seddon E, Wasoff F. '…and for 39 years I got on with it.' Older women and domestic violence in Scotland. Edinburgh: Health Scotland; 2004.
34. McGarry J, Simpson C. Domestic abuse and older women: exploring the opportunities for service development and care delivery. J Adult Protect. 2011;13(6):294–301.
35. Lundy M, Grossman S. Domestic violence service users: a comparison of older and younger women victims. J Fam Violence. 24:297–309.
36. O'Keeffe M, Hills A, Doyle M, McCreadie C, Scholes S, Constantine R, Tinker A, Manthorpe J, Biggs S, Erens B. UK study of abuse and neglect of older people: prevalence survey report. London: NatCen; 2007.
37. NHS Digital. Safeguarding adults, 2018–2019. https://digital.nhs.uk/data-and-information/publications/statistical/safeguarding-adults/annual-report-2018-19-england. Accessed May 2020.
38. Long J, Harvey H. The femicide census: annual report on UK femicides, 2018. London: Nia/Women's Aid; 2020.
39. Blood I. Older women and domestic violence, help the aged/HACT. www.ageuk.org.uk/documents/en-gb/for-professionals/communities-and-inclusion/id2382_2_older_women_and_domestic_violence_summary_2004_pro.pdf?dtrk=true. Accessed May 2020.
40. Lives S. Safer later Lives: older people and domestic abuse. London: Safe Lives; 2016.
41. Amesberger H, Haller B, Toth O. Mind the gap: improving interventions in intimate partner violence against older women-summary report. Vienna: Institut fur Konfliktforschung (IKF); 2013.
42. Ploeg J, Fear J, Hutchinson B, Macmillan H, Bolan G. A systematic review of interventions for elder abuse. J Elder Abuse Negl. 2009;21:187–210.
43. Podnieks E, Penhale B, Görgen T, Biggs S, Han D. Elder abuse: an international narrative. J Elder Abuse Negl. 2010;22(1):131–63.

Supporting People Affected by Intimate Partner Violence in Emergency and Crisis Situations

11

Simon Sawyer

11.1 Gender-Based Violence and Health

Gender-based violence can be broadly defined as any acts of violence or abuse directed at someone because of their gender and is usually used to define violence against women [1]. Isolated acts of GBV between strangers, such as assaults or verbal abuse, occur regularly in society [2]. These isolated acts can have a number of negative healthcare outcomes, for example trauma from physical assaults or adverse mental health outcomes such as PTSD. Health and social care workers may encounter patients seeking care due to an isolated incident of GBV occurring between strangers; however, individuals are far more likely to experience GBV from known individuals, and in particular from family members [2].

Family violence is the term widely used in Australia to refer to all acts of violence, abuse and neglect within a family unit and occurs when an individual uses physical, sexual, psychological or any other form of abuse to control or otherwise harm another person in their family [2]. As distinct from isolated acts of violence or abuse between strangers, family violence often is often *ongoing* and *escalates* over time, meaning it often causes continued and increasing harm over a longer period of time [3]. While family violence perpetrated against children or elders does occur, the most common manifestation of GBV within the subset of family violence is intimate partner violence (IPV) [3]. Intimate partner violence occurs between two people in an intimate relationship, such as married or de facto partners, dating couples or other informal relationships [2]. Intimate partner violence is known to occur in both heterosexual and same-sex relationships [3]. The gender makeup of the people in the intimate relationship can vary and may include individuals who identify as female, male, transgender or another gender-identity.

S. Sawyer (✉)
Australian Catholic University, Melbourne, VIC, Australia

© Springer Nature Switzerland AG 2021
C. Bradbury-Jones, L. Isham (eds.), *Understanding Gender-Based Violence*,
https://doi.org/10.1007/978-3-030-65006-3_11

When considering the gendered nature of family violence, and in particular IPV, it is known that the majority of the most damaging violence is perpetrated by men against women [2]. The reason why men are more likely to use violence and women are more likely to experience violence in a relationship is complex and there is no single unifying theory as to why all acts of family violence occur. Research which helps us understand the connection between gender and family violence has shown that men often perceive their roles in society and within relationships differently to women. For example men who use violence in their relationships may be more likely to believe in gender roles and norms and advocate for the use of abuse and violence to maintain their own status (and that of their gender), while also seeking to oppress women and the status of their gender. Across most of the world, men hold the balance of power, and the societal systems and structures that are created and maintained are often designed to favour men and their interests, which includes creating a system that allows the use of violence and prevents or creates high barriers for women from seeking help [4]. Conversely we know that men can also experience family violence; however, the drivers for that violence are often quite different. Research has shown that when women use violence against male intimate partners, it is often (but not always) the result of self-defence [5]. Therefore, we can say that males tend to use violence to help control their female partners; while females tend to use violence to achieve freedom from the control of their male partners.

Because of the inequality that gender brings, we see the disproportionate impact of GBV, and in particular family violence, on the health outcomes of women and children. Later in this chapter, we will discuss the known healthcare outcomes associated with IPV, such as physical injuries, adverse reproductive outcomes, stress-mediated symptoms and poor mental health outcomes. Further to this harm, it is important to note that GBV within a family often impacts more than one person, for example studies in Australia have shown that in cases of IPV reported to police, children were present in at up to 48% of cases [6]. Therefore, when you do encounter a person experiencing GBV within a family (and in particular IPV), there may be more than one person who requires care and support.

Family violence brings a huge social, economic and health burden on society [20]. While the response to family violence is complex and requires action from all facets of society, the remainder of this chapter will focus on the role of health and social care workers. Much of the research used to inform this chapter has focused on IPV, and this is where it is expected the majority of health impacts will be seen by non-GBV-specialist health and social care workers. Likewise, research has generally focused on IPV-related presentations and the needs of women who are experiencing violence and abuse. Therefore, women experiencing IPV will often be the main focus of this chapter. However, unless otherwise stated, the information presented in this chapter can be used to inform the response of health and social care workers to GBV for any individual, irrespective of age, sexuality or gender identity. The information presented is intended as a guide to informed GBV practice.

11.2   GBV Emergency Health and Social Care Presentations

As we have discussed, GBV and family violence brings a huge health burden on society. While many countries have begun funding a specialist GBV and family violence workforce who are largely responsible for advocacy and support of people living with GBV, the entire health and social care workforce needs to be prepared to identify GBV early and help people access these support services.

In the context of GBV, defining exactly what would constitute an 'emergency' presentation or who would be considered an 'emergency' health and social care worker is difficult given the broad range of medical conditions associated with GBV. However, it is possible to identify three different categories of presentations that health and social care workers are likely to encounter:

1. Health or social care seeking post a single discrete event (e.g. after an assault or attempt at self-harm).
2. Health or social care seeking for ongoing treatment of a chronic condition which is associated with GBV, even if the patient is unaware that GBV is occurring or is related to their condition (e.g. treatment for PTSD, hypertension or asthma).
3. Health or social care seeking post an acute exacerbation of a chronic condition (e.g. an anxiety attack, chest pain or migraines).

Case Study 1: Jenny

Jenny is a patient living in an abusive relationship who has been struck by her partner across her face after an argument over disciplining one of their children. Jenny has been assaulted by her partner before, but he usually just pushes her and shouts at her.

Jenny may present to a number of different health or social care workers due to this incident. For example Jenny may call for an ambulance or present to a hospital emergency department immediately with traumatic head injuries. However, she may be afraid to seek help immediately (for her or her children's safety), and instead she may present to a physiotherapist a number of days later due to ongoing pain. Likewise, Jenny may be already regularly attending her GP or a pharmacist for repeat prescriptions of medication to control anxiety related to her experiences. Jenny may seek the support of a psychologist or counsellor for ongoing panic attacks or PTSD symptoms brought on by past assaults. Jenny may encounter a social worker at her child's school if, for example, her child is identified as not meeting educational outcomes.

Regardless of which of the previous health and social care workers encounter Jenny (and it may be more than one), each has an opportunity to identify the potential for GBV and provide initial support and care for Jenny. It is especially important that these health and social care workers are properly educated and trained as Jenny may not be aware that her relationship is abusive. Likewise, she may not see how her experiences of GBV are impacting on her children even if they are not being directly assaulted or abused. Jenny may also not fully understand the link between her experiences of GBV and her injuries or symptoms or the behaviours of her children.

It may require the concern and skill of a health or social care workers to assist Jenny to identify her experiences as GBV and seek support. The earlier this happens, the earlier Jenny will be able to make informed choices, which may reduce the amount of violence and abuse Jenny and her children experience and reduce future harm.

In Case 1, Jenny could present for a number different reasons to any number of different health or social care workers. Each situation provides an opportunity for the health or social care worker to identify the potential for GBV and, if the person does disclose violence or abuse to them, the worker can become an 'emergency' health worker who can provide an emergency health response to the patient. In this context, an emergency health response is one which focuses on the immediate medical and social needs of the person as well as addressing any ongoing safety concerns [7].

Therefore, for the remainder of this chapter, any health or social care worker should be considered as a potential emergency worker if they are required to treat or support a patient presenting with an acute or chronic health or social complaint which may be related to GBV. It is perhaps more useful to consider the concept of an 'emergency response' rather than specific emergency responders. In this context, it is not the individual worker or the type of medical condition or social issue being treated, but rather the situation itself that defines the emergency. Later in the chapter, we will look at what actions can be undertaken immediately by health and social care workers in support of people experiencing GBV.

11.3   The Impact of Disasters in GBV

In addition to the day-to-day response of emergency health and social care workers to GBV, disasters and other states of emergency are also known to impact on GBV rates [8]. In one recent systematic review, it was found that most forms of violence increase during and post disasters, including rape and sexual assault, intimate partner violence and child abuse [9]. Types of incidents studied have included bushfires, hurricanes, floods, tsunamis and earthquakes. As this chapter is being written in mid-2020, we are in the midst of the Covid-19 pandemic. While it is still too early to accurately measure the impact of Covid-19 on GBV, preliminary research is indicating that family violence is rising in Australia and indeed worldwide [10].

Research on why a disaster may increase the prevalence of GBV is emerging but gaps in knowledge remain; however, preliminary evidence shows associations between increased homelessness, unemployment and alcohol and drug use [8]. The links between these situations and increases in GBV come from multiple factors. For example unemployment may result in an individual becoming more reliant on their partners for income to provide basic needs for themselves and any children. This may create a power imbalance, where one partner is reliant on the other, or may increase the barriers to leaving abusive partners or seeking help. A similar power imbalance can occur when a person (and potentially their children) become homeless and are forced into controlling relationships to access basic needs such as food or lodgings. Alcohol and other drug abuse can increase as people use these substances to help cope with the stress they are placed under during an emergency. Alcohol and drug effected states can then increase the rates and magnitude of GBV as it reduces inhibition and reduces the person's ability to find non-violent solutions to problems [11].

11.4   The Health and Social Care Response to GBV

Regardless of which health or social care worker an individual experiencing GBV presents to, the initial emergency response should be largely the same, whether you are responding as a physician or nurse, paramedic or physiotherapist, social worker or psychologist. While ongoing specialist care of patients experiencing GBV is essential, the initial response is also vital. This response consists of identification and the provision of initial, front-line care for the patient, usually in the form of catering for immediate medical, safety and social needs through referrals to the right care or advocacy agencies.

This response can be described by the four Rs: Recognise, Respond, Refer and Record [12]. This method, which is detailed in the following section and in Table 11.1, is a simple method for health and social care workers to learn how to respond appropriately. The method is not dissimilar to the extended response that a specialist GBV worker may provide; however, it is often less detailed and focuses on the key, immediate needs of a patient. Many health and social care workers report feeling unprepared to ask patients about GBV [13], and the intention of this method is to help prepare the health and social care workforce with simple and direct actions they can perform for the benefit of the patient. This method is a basic

Table 11.1 The Four Rs of GBV

RECOGNISE	Keep an open mind and look for indications that the people you encounter may be experiencing GBV, and that this may impact on their health and social welfare
RESPOND	When you see indications that a person may be experiencing GBV, do not ignore it or try and explain it away. Talk to your patients about GBV in an open, compassionate and non-judgemental way, and ask them if they feel safe or if they might benefit from further care or support
REFER	If a person does disclose to you that they are experiencing GBV, explore their needs with them and where possible provide them with resources and referrals to further care and support
RECORD	Make sure that you document these encounters properly while ensuring confidentiality. These documents may be needed to help the patient in the future and can be used for research to improve the response of the health and social care sector

approach, which can be modified depending on the context of the scene. Health and social care practitioners with a greater scope of practice may take hours engaging in this process, or it may be less than a minute during time-sensitive presentations that a paramedic or nurse encounters.

Many organisations and professional health and social care bodies now have formal guidelines and protocols for responding to GBV, and we recommend that all health and social care professionals undergo comprehensive training and adhere to relevant occupational and professional guidelines. The following should be considered not as an exact method to respond to GBV, but rather a set of principles which refer to best practice and can be applied appropriately by any health or social care worker in an emergency presentation.

11.5   Working with the Four Rs

11.5.1 Recognise

Health and social care workers respond to a wide variety of health and social care presentations. Often the focus of their action is to identify and manage symptoms or injuries.

As Case 2 demonstrates, while the injuries from GBV are often plain to see, we do not always think about or recognise the *cause* of the injury unless we make the

---

Case Study 2: Regina

Regina is an 80-year-old female who lives in her adult child's home with their eldest child Jake acting as her primary carer. One day, Regina falls at home and an ambulance is called. The paramedics assess Regina and find she has fractured her right hip. The paramedics treat her pain and transport her to the local emergency department (ED) where the doctors and nurses provide further assessment and treatment for her hip.

While the role of the paramedics and ED staff may be to assess Regina for injuries sustained during the fall, they would be remiss if they did not consider the *cause* of the falls. For example why did Regina fall? Was this an isolated incident, or could this be related to family violence? For example, Jake withholding Regina's walking frame to prevent her from leaving the house.

---

effort to go looking for it. We know that people living with GBV are expected to experience ongoing and potentially escalating violence, abuse or neglect, and therefore rather than treat the symptoms only, such as injuries from a fall, we should also consider the cause. By undertaking this process, health and social care workers may discover indications that GBV may be contributing to the patient's overall health, which allows them to then connect people with the right care and support to help reduce the damage caused by GBV.

Routine screening to assess for GBV of all patients who seek health and social care is not currently recommended, and therefore a more common approach is indicator-based screening. A person experiencing GBV may present to a health or social care worker in a number of different ways. Research with IPV has shown there are common injuries and known associated conditions which often present to other services, including EDs and GP clinics, which can guide health and social care workers (See Table 11.2 [14]). While these indications were identified as associated with IPV, many of these would also be likely to be associated with all forms of

Table 11.2 Health consequences and health risk behaviours associated with experiencing IPV [14]

Brain and nervous system	Cardiovascular system	Somatic symptoms
Headaches	Angina	Chronic fatigue
Migraines	Cardiovascular disease	Chronic pain
Memory problems	High blood pressure/	Fibromyalgia
Seizures	hypertension	Temporomandibular disorder
Speech difficulties	High cholesterol	Somatic symptoms
Traumatic brain injury	Stroke	
Gastrointestinal system	**Reproductive system**	**Adverse pregnancy outcomes**
Constipation	Chronic pelvic pain	Abortion
Diarrhoea	Genital injuries	Increased abortion rate
Frequent indigestion	Hysterectomy	Multiple induced abortions
Functional gastrointestinal	Lack of sexual pleasure	Delayed prenatal care
disorder	Sexual dysfunction	Foetal death, foetal loss
Gastric reflux	Painful intercourse	(miscarriage, spontaneous
Gastrointestinal	Painful menses	abortion)
disturbances	Pelvic inflammatory	Interference with contraception
Inflammatory bowel	disease	Low birth weight
syndrome	Poor sexual health	Neonatal death
Irritable bowel disorder	Sexually transmitted	Preterm delivery
Spastic colon	infections	Premature labour
Stomach ulcers	Vaginal bleeding	Premature rupture of
Stomach/gastrointestinal		membranes
problems		Unintended pregnancy
Other health outcomes	**Mental health outcomes**	**Musculoskeletal system**
Asthma	Anger/hostility	Activity limitations
Chronic health conditions	Anxiety	Arthritis
Delayed diagnosis of	Depression	Broken bones
breast, cervical,	Mental health disability	Joint disease
endometrial, and ovarian	Poor mental health	Physical disability
cancer	Posttraumatic stress	Functional impairment
Hearing loss	disorder	Physical injuries
Physical symptoms	Psychological distress	
Poor general health	Sleep disturbance	
Poor physical health	Suicidality	
Immune and endocrine	**Genitourinary system**	**Health risk behaviours**
function	Bladder/kidney	Decreased preventive care use
Chronic pain	infections	Heavy or binge drinking
Inflammation	Genitourinary problems	HIV and other sexually
Metabolic syndrome/		transmitted disease risk factors
diabetes		Not having check-up with
		physician in the past year
		Smoking

GBV. These health consequences do not constitute an exhaustive list, but rather the signs that would be relevant and likely presentations which emergency health and social care workers might witness.

This list is long and encompasses many different situations. Beyond these conditions, some health and social care professions are focusing on indications based on feelings, behaviours, general medical complaints, controlling people and trauma (see Table 11.3).

In addition to the previously listed indicators, there are several risk factors which are relevant to health and social care practitioners and are known to be associated with a higher likelihood of experiencing GBV. The presence of these risk factors do not indicate violence in themselves; however, an awareness of them may increase a worker's index of suspicion. Risk factors include young age, alcohol or other drug abuse (particularly in care givers to children or other dependants), low

Table 11.3 Potential indicators of family violence [12]

Feelings	• The patient appears depressed/withdrawn, anxious/distressed or fearful without an apparent reason
Behaviours	• Suicidality or self-harm • Alcohol or other drug abuse • Repeated/suspicious presentations with no clear diagnosis • Inconsistent or implausible explanations for injuries/symptoms • Scene findings or behaviours of those on scene which indicate an unsafe environment (physically or psychologically), particularly for children, elderly or the disabled
Medical signs	• Unexplained chronic symptoms (e.g., pain; gastrointestinal, or genitourinary symptoms) • Pregnancy related complications or trauma, or delays in care • Evidence of malnutrition or medical neglect, particularly in children, elderly or disabled patients
Controlling people	• The presence of intrusive or controlling people in the consultation (especially a partner or ex-partner) • The patients (or their children/dependants) are unwilling to respond without approval from controlling person • The presence of a controlling person who states things like the patient is 'crazy', 'mad', 'unstable' or other similar terms • The presence of a potential abuser who attempts to minimise, distract or explain away injuries, or who states the patient is not to be believed (particularly with children, elderly or disabled patients) • The presence of withholding communication/mobility devices, access to funds/resources/services, over/under medication (especially for elderly or disabled patients)
Trauma	• A presentation related to an assault or suspicion of assault (e.g. there is the presence of weapons, or signs of violence) • The patient has suspicious bruises or injuries, especially to the neck, face, breasts or genitals. Note that toddlers are likely to have bruises, and therefore this may be a poor predictor in this group • The patient states or indicates someone has threatened to kill or harm them, their children/dependants or their pets • Evidence of sexual assault (actual or attempted)

socio-economic status, separated or divorced marital status and pregnancy [15]. There is some subtlety on why each of these risk factors can increase the likelihood of GBV; however, broadly speaking, young age and low social economic status increase the marginalisation of a person, meaning they are less visible and violence and abuse can occur without being as easily detected. When considering marital status and pregnancy, IPV often first occurs or is escalated during pregnancy, and males can become more violent and controlling when their partner attempts to leave them [7].

When a health or social care worker sees indications of GBV, it is important that they do not ignore the indicators or attempt to minimise or justify behaviours. Individuals living with GBV can be helped, and there are key actions that health and social care workers can undertake to support them, which we will discuss in the next section.

11.5.2 Respond

The presence of indicators of GBV does not necessarily mean a person is currently experiencing GBV, or that they require any further support. This is why some form of screening is necessary. At present, universal screening for GBV is not recommended, as studies have shown there is no benefit to screening every person [16], and in fact it appears that the likelihood that a person discloses GBV is more about the skill of the worker who asks, rather than the screening tool or method. Regardless, due to the evidence that universal screening is not beneficial, indicator-based screening is usually preferred. There is currently no consensus on the best method of screening in every setting, which is why principles of care may be more important. Each organisation should have their own policies on responding to GBV and should provide advice on screening procedures, which should be followed.

Based on the context of the scene, the patient's presentation, and the professional or organisational context, screening usually involves asking a person a number of specific or general questions about GBV. This might take the form of a specific screening tool, such as the Composite Abuse Scale [17] which asks specific questions about violence and abuse. It may also involve a more general approach, such as simply asking the person about their experiences and if they require support. Individual organisations and professions should have advice on preferred methods and you should follow local or professional body advice. Either way, the conversation can be confronting and difficult for an untrained worker, which is why before engaging in screening, it is recommended that comprehensive training is provided.

When you are concerned that GBV may be an issue, you should attempt to create the opportunity to let the person know that you are concerned for their safety and that you want to support them. Research shows that women experiencing family violence want to be asked by health and social care workers, provided it is in a sensitive, empathetic and non-judgemental manner [18]. While the response of health and social care workers may vary between professions and contexts, general principles apply to all, and we will discuss some of these now.

11.5.2.1 Privacy and Confidentiality

Before asking any questions, ensure you are in a private environment. Take care not to let anyone else present know that you suspect GBV (for example a potential offender), and do not talk to a person about GBV in front of anyone else unless you are certain the person is comfortable with this. Some people may prefer to have a support person present when you attend to them. When this is case, you should make every effort to ensure the patient's confidentiality.

Some health and social care workers may find this easier than others, for example a radiologist may routinely be left alone with a patient in a controlled environment, while a paramedic may be more likely to treat a patient with family or other bystanders present and in people's homes or community spaces. You may have to create a diversion to get the patient alone, for example you may ask bystanders to move to another room so you can perform a proper assessment. Admittedly this can be difficult at times, and you are not always going to be able to get the patient alone. This can be particularly true when the abuser is aware that you may wish to ask the patient about GBV and they wish to prevent you.

Sadly, there is sometimes no way to arrange for privacy in some situations, and in these situations the health or social care worker may have to think creatively about alternative options, such as passing on concerns to another practitioner who will have future contact, or arranging for follow up appointments in a more private setting.

11.5.2.2 Reassurance

Individuals experiencing GBV often feel fear about disclosing [18], and letting them know that you will keep what they say confidential, and that they are in a safe place and would not be over heard can help them to feel more comfortable. Remember that many people will deny experiencing GBV or abuse if they do not feel safe, so you should take your time to prepare them and the scene, build rapport and make them feel comfortable.

11.5.2.3 Using Fear and Safety Questions

There is no one right way to ask a patient about GBV. One recommendation is to use *fear and safety* questions, which means questions which focus on how the patient feels [7]. This conversation should be natural and while memorising a screening question may be of use to some, it is often best to adapt a simple questioning framework to the individual situation.

11.5.2.4 Avoid Negative Comments

There are also many things that you should not ask or say. Questions or comments that imply the patient was at fault or that excuse the violence, such as '*what did you do to make them angry?*' or '*I'm sure they love you, this is just the way they show it*' can be very damaging and can actually prevent the person disclosing the violence or seeking help in the future [18]. When in doubt, it is best to simply listen and respond with empathetic statements.

11.5.2.5 Remain Supportive

When talking to patients, consider that it is common for someone to self-blame or make excuses for injuries. This does not mean they do not want you to ask about GBV and you should still offer care and support. It is also ok to ask the same person about GBV again if you see them in subsequent consultations, even if they always decline help. It is likely that the more a patient is offered help and support the more likely they will be to seek help in the future.

11.5.2.6 Children

The general principles to the response to children is largely the same as to adults; however, these situations are often far more complex (especially legally), dynamic, and the child may be at a higher risk than adults. For these reasons, we do not recommend that generalist health and social care workers respond directly to children where they have concerns about GBV. For example how you approach GBV with a 4-year-old child would vary considerably to how you would approach GBV with a 15-year-old adolescent. Health and social care workers should contact their local specialist service, so that properly trained practitioners can undertake this role.

11.5.3 Refer

If you ask a person about GBV and they do disclose to you, after validating what they say, you can move to considering their ongoing needs. It is not always necessary to provide a referral, and sometimes simply bearing witness to another person's story can be incredibly therapeutic. The needs of a person experiencing GBV can be very broad, and there is no one right referral option. It is important that, where possible, health and social care workers consult with and attempt to find the service which meets the individual's needs. Options will vary based on availability in the local area, however as a guide you might consider options such as:

- General advocacy, information and counselling services.
- Legal assistance.
- Safe housing or refuge accommodation.
- Specialist sexual assault services.
- Child protection services.
- Specialist services for culturally and linguistically diverse patients, disabled patients, children or the elderly.
- Specialist services for indigenous peoples.

Referrals can be made by providing details to individual, so that they can contact services in their own time. It is not advised that health and social care workers routinely contact services on the person's behalf or without their consent, unless in cases of mandatory reporting or where the individual requests your assistance. It is also advised that individual health and social care services make printed referral materials available upon request, or display them in consultation and waiting rooms [15].

11.5.4 Record

Recording encounters with individuals experiencing GBV is important and must be done in an appropriate way. The confidentiality of medical records should be the primary concern. Each profession will have different standards of documenting encounters; however, some general advice concerning documenting GBV is provided below. Documentation of encounters should include:

- A description of the observed indicators, including a description of any injuries, indicative symptoms or behaviours and any evidence or statements about who inflicted them. It can be useful to write direct quotes where appropriate.
- Note if there were any children or other witnesses present and if they were involved at all.
- If you discussed GBV with the patient or provided a referral include a note of which referral option was provided.
- Any other relevant findings or statements made by the patient or potential perpetrators.

Remember that your notes should be objective and complete. These notes may be required in the future for legal proceedings, and accurate and thorough notes can help a patient prove their claim. Be mindful as well that such notes can be used by researchers to improve the response of the entire health and social care workforce.

11.6 The Future and Challenges for Health and Social Care Workers to Respond to GBV

The future of the health and social care response lies largely in increased training for practitioners to recognise indications of GBV and to provide supportive care (this is covered extensively in Chap. 2). Already accreditation programs and professional bodies are increasing resources for practitioners, such as educational packages, guidelines and protocols for responding. Coupled with this should be programmes to streamline communication and access between health and social care workers and advocacy groups. For example the ability for health and social care workers to work alongside specialist GBV advocates in collaborative care models would allow for much greater cohesion between health and social care needs and GBV advocacy.

A major limitation to such educational efforts is the availability of support services for people experiencing GBV. While many governments are building their health and social care capacity, there remains a critical workforce shortage of GBV advocates as well as underfunding of essential services, such as safe housing. One emerging challenge for the health and social care workforce will be supporting patients to access the limited care and support available for GBV. With increased risks for dramatic climate events and potential for disaster events, unless the drivers of GBV are addressed across society, it is likely we will also see increases in

GBV. Therefore, greater disaster preparedness from governments and response agencies will ensure that individuals impacted by disasters are able to retreat to safe environments and access timely care and support should they experience GBV.

Finally, the impact of GBV on the health and well-being of the health and social care workforce remains unclear; however, initial evidence indicates that health social care workers may be at greater risk of experiencing some forms of GBV [19]. Likewise, the risk of vicarious trauma to health and social care professionals by asking patients about their experience remains unclear. Greater research, as well as access to care and support for health and social care workers, may assist their response to GBV.

Summary and Key Points
- GBV is known to be associated with a wide variety of chronic and acute medical complaints and therefore health and social care workers are expected to encounter these patients.
- Any health or social care worker might be considered an emergency responder in the context of GBV, and the skills to recognise and respond should be taught to all health and social care workers.
- Disasters, either natural or human-made, are known to lead to increased rates of GBV, and workers present at these events should be mindful of GBV and its impact on the population.
- An appropriate response from health and social care workers to GBV should include the four Rs: Recognise, Response, Refer and Record.
- The future of the emergency health and social care response to GBV is largely based on greater education and training for practitioners to perform these roles and support people to access the right care and support to end the violence and abuse in their lives.

Case Study 3 (Part 1): Anna
You are employed as an emergency health and social care worker in an emergency health centre which was erected in a camp set up for displaced people following a major earthquake two weeks ago. While on duty, you are approached by a 30-year-old female named Anna, who asks you for help with neck pain. She does not request any specific treatment, but asks for some pain medication as she is having trouble sleeping. Anna provides you with a completed pre-appointment form which shows that she is a non-smoker and does not drink alcohol, she has two children at home (a 4-year old and a 3-year old), she is currently unemployed, she takes medication for anxiety and depression and she did not complete high school.

You ask Anna about her neck pain and how it started. She says she is not really sure but it has been getting worse over the last few days and now she can hardly turn her head. You notice some bruising around Anna's neck and ask her about it, she says she is not sure and that it must have happened during the earthquake. You ask Anna about where she is living and what family she has and she says that she is living in a tent in the camp with her two children and husband, they are waiting to get access to emergency accommodation until they can rebuild their house. Anna is very reluctant to discuss her situation further with you, and again asks if you could just help her get some pain relief so she can sleep. You make a plan for her to see the appropriate health-care practitioner, but also you recognise signs of GBV and decide that while she is waiting, you want to ask her if she needs any support.

Before reading on, try and answer the following questions.

Reflective Questions

1. When considering Anna's case, do you see any indications or risk factors for GBV? State which of each you see in Anna's case and provide a rationale for how they are linked to GBV.
2. In the case of Anna, is there any specific form of GBV that you think she may be particularly at risk of experiencing?
3. If you were going to ask Anna about GBV, how would you go about this? Is there anything you would do before asking her? How would you broach the subject?

Case Study 3 (Part 2): Anna

You say to Anna that you are concerned about her neck, and you want to ask her some more questions. You make sure to explain that they are alone and would not be overheard, and that anything she tells you is confidential. Anna nods and so you ask if everything is going ok for her at the moment? She gives a non-committal nod, so you ask her about how her children are coping at the moment? Anna says that it has been hard but they seem to be ok. You ask Anna about her relationship with her husband and if everything is ok at home? At this question, Anna looks away and says everything is fine. She adds that it has been really hard since the earthquake but everyone is struggling and she just wants things to go back to normal. You ask Anna if she is feeling safe or if anyone at home or in the camp is making her afraid and she says it is hard in the camp but everyone is being supportive. You ask if she is feeling safe with her husband and she says that he is a good person and she loves him very much. You ask if her husband has done anything to hurt her or make her feel afraid. Anna says that they have a good relationship, but since the earthquake her husband has been under a lot of stress.

You pause to see if Anna will continue talking and after a few seconds Anna states 'he didn't mean to hurt me, he's just been under a lot of stress'. You tell Anna that you understand what she has said and ask if there was something that happened with her husband related to her neck. She says that they were arguing one night about what they were going to do and they both said some mean things to each other and her husband grabbed her and threw her to the ground. Anna adds that her husband 'might have just had too much to drink' and that his drinking has increased since the earthquake. Anna is quick to add that her husband said he was sorry straight away and has not hurt her again. You thank Anna for telling you this and empathise with her situation. You ask Anna if she is safe to return home, is she afraid of her husband or what he might do to her or her children. Anna states that while they have argued in the past, this is first time he has ever been physically violent, and he apologised straight away and she does not think he will be violent again.

You ask Anna if she needs any help at the moment with her husband, and she says she just wants her pain medication, but maybe someone could speak with her husband to help him with his stress. You say to Anna that there are some GBV advocate services available through the health centre and that she could speak to someone who can help her with her situation with her husband. You ask if it is ok if you make an appointment for her to speak to someone and she says that she is happy to talk to someone. You also ask if it is ok if you explain to the doctor about how her neck injury occurred and Anna gives her permission.

You hand over Anna to the Dr. who will help her with her neck pain, explaining her situation and that you have arranged for her to speak to someone. When recording your patient care notes, you make reference to the bruises you saw on Anna's neck, her responses when you asked about GBV and who you referred her to see. You make sure that your notes are kept confidential.

Concluding Reflective Questions

1. What term would be used to define the particular form of GBV that Anna is experiencing?
2. What are the four Rs of responding to GBV? Provide examples of how the worker in this case performed each of these tasks? Considering your own occupation, how might you have done this differently, is there any aspect you would have changed?
3. How might you engage in self-care if you were working in a similar environment? If you started to feel overwhelmed with hearing about other people's experiences with GBV, or you had trouble with recurring or intrusive thoughts from a particular case, what might you do to ensure your own personal well-being?

References

1. UN General Assembly. Declaration on the elimination of violence against women, a/ RES/48/104. UN General Assembly; 1993.
2. Krug E, Dahlberg J, Mercy J, Zwi A, Lozano R. World report on violence and health. Geneva: World Health Organization; 2002.
3. Garcia-Moreno C, Jansen H, Ellsberg M, Heise L, Watts CH. Prevalence of intimate partner violence: findings from the WHO multi-country study on women's health and domestic violence. Lancet. 2006;368(9543):1260–9.
4. Bagshaw D, Chung D. Gender politics and research: male and female violence in intimate relationships. Women Against Violence. 2000;8:4–23.
5. Swan SC, Gambone LJ, Caldwell JE, Sullivan TP, Snow DL. A review of research on women's use of violence with male intimate partners. Violence Vict. 2008;23(3):301–14.
6. Department of Justice. Victorian family violence database volume 5: eleven year trend analysis (1999–2010). Melbourne: Victorian Government; 2012.
7. World Health Organization. Health care for women subjected to intimate partner violence or sexual violence: a clinical handbook. Geneva: WHO; 2014.
8. Parkinson D, Zara C. The hidden disaster: domestic violence in the aftermath of natural disaster. Aust J Emerg Manag. 2013;28(2):28.
9. Rezaeian M. The association between natural disasters and violence: a systematic review of the literature and a call for more epidemiological studies. J Res Med Sci. 2013;18(12):1103.
10. Pfitzner N, Fitz-Gibbon K, True J. Responding to the 'shadow pandemic': practitioner views on the nature of and responses to violence against women in Victoria, Australia during the COVID-19 restrictions. Melbourne, Australia; 2020.
11. Room R, Babor T, Rehm J. Alcohol and public health. Lancet. 2005;365(9458):519–30.
12. Sawyer S, Coles J, Williams A, Williams B. Paramedics as a new resource for women experiencing intimate partner violence. J Interpers Violence. 2018:0886260518769363.
13. Sprague S, Madden K, Simunovic N, Godin K, Pham NK, Bhandari M, et al. Barriers to screening for intimate partner violence. Women Health. 2012;52(6):587–605.
14. Black MC. Intimate partner violence and adverse health consequences implications for clinicians. Am J Lifestyle Med. 2011;5(5):428–39.
15. World Health Organization. Responding to intimate partner violence and sexual violence against women: WHO clinical and policy guidelines. Geneva: WHO; 2013.
16. Taft A, O'Doherty L, Hegarty K, Ramsay J, Davidson L, Feder G. Screening women for intimate partner violence in healthcare settings. Cochrane Libr. 2013;(4).
17. Ford-Gilboe M, Wathen CN, Varcoe C, MacMillan HL, Scott-Storey K, Mantler T, et al. Development of a brief measure of intimate partner violence experiences: the composite abuse scale (revised)—short form (CASR-SF). BMJ Open. 2016;6(12):e012824.
18. Feder GS, Hutson M, Ramsay J, Taket AR. Women exposed to intimate partner violence: expectations and experiences when they encounter health care professionals: a meta-analysis of qualitative studies. Arch Intern Med. 2006;166(1):22–37.
19. McLindon E, Humphreys C, Hegarty K. "it happens to clinicians too": an Australian prevalence study of intimate partner and family violence against health professionals. BMC Womens Health. 2018;18(1):113.
20. Campbell L. Health consequences of intimate partner violence. Lancet. 2002;359(9314):1331–6.

Part IV

Responses and Innovations

Adopting a Trauma-Informed Approach to Gender-Based Violence Across the Life Course

Mickey Sperlich, Patricia Logan-Greene, and Adair Finucane

> **Box 12.1 Key Terminology Relevant to This Chapter**
>
> *Gender-based violence (GBV)* refers to violence that is directed against a person because of their gender; women are disproportionality affected by GBV due to power inequalities between women and men [1].
>
> *Traumas* include physical injuries and psychologically and/or emotionally deeply distressing experiences.
>
> *Sequelae* refers to after-effects of traumatic exposures and gender-based violence.
>
> *Maladaptive coping* refers to coping mechanisms that may initially provide some relief from the effects of trauma and violence but which carry with them their own negative consequences, including avoidance, withdrawal, aggression, substance use and self-harm.
>
> *Trauma-informed approaches* recognise the widespread impact of trauma and its effects; it includes responsiveness in the form of integration of this knowledge into policies, practices and procedures in order to support recovery efforts and resist re-traumatisation [2].
>
> *Proximal trauma responsivity* refers to interventions and supports that are offered following a recently experienced traumatic event.
>
> *Distal trauma responsivity* refers to interventions and supports that are offered in relation to trauma that took place at some point in the past.
>
> *Nested setting* refers to the concept that people exist within multiple ecological systems, which are nested within each other, simultaneously. The microsystem (family, school, peers, etc) exists within the mesosystem

M. Sperlich (✉) · P. Logan-Greene · A. Finucane
University at Buffalo, Buffalo, NY, USA
e-mail: msperlic@buffalo.edu; pblogang@buffalo.edu; afinucan@buffalo.edu

© Springer Nature Switzerland AG 2021
C. Bradbury-Jones, L. Isham (eds.), *Understanding Gender-Based Violence*,
https://doi.org/10.1007/978-3-030-65006-3_12

(interconnections between microsystems), the mesosystem exists within the exosystem (social services, neighbours, etc), the exosystem exists within the macrosystem (culture at large), and all are influenced by the progression of time (chronosystem) [3].

Developmental epochs are age periods in which critical experiences may affect the trajectory of developmental progress.

12.1 Introduction

Gender-based violence (GBV) is part of a complex picture of cumulative risk that is attended by contextual factors that both facilitate and result from its commission. Exposures and outcomes related to GBV are many, varied and stratified across the lifespan. Life course approaches frequently used for studying long-term effects of chronic disease [4, 5] may be applied to understanding trajectories of development and how these are influenced by early-life exposures and accumulated trauma and adversity. These may be particularly useful for looking at how violence exposure in early life influences personal and social development [6]. Key features of life course models include: (1) recognition of *critical or sensitive periods* in the life course that are highly influential for later development and (2) attention to the *accumulation of risks*, which may either cluster together in patterned ways or link together in 'chains of risk' that accumulate over time and may trigger deleterious outcomes [4]. Finding places where such links may be broken through preventative intervention is a main goal of the life course perspective.

Examining long-term effects of violence can help illuminate such opportunities for GBV and other traumas and adversities. For instance, Greenfield [7] urges that child abuse should properly be conceptualised as a 'life-course social determinant of adult health for both clinical and public health purposes', p. 51. This is consistent with recent framing of childhood adversities as social determinants of mental health [8], although such framing stops short of recognizing the inherent fluid connection of mind and body and the need for addressing social determinants of physical *and* mental health in concert [9]. Although evidence is increasing regarding the ways in which adverse/traumatic childhood experiences and subsequent adult traumas negatively impact lifelong health and functioning [10], and GBV specifically, across stages of development [11], much more work needs to be done to translate what we know from research [12]. With the rise of such evidence, there has been a concomitant rise in calls for trauma-informed approaches in multiple service sectors, including for intimate partner/gender-based violence [13]. For intervention purposes, addressing GBV across the life course necessitates trauma responsivity, not only for improving the lives of affected individuals but also for implementing needed changes at the various socioecological levels of influences that surround the affected individual.

12.2   Adopting a Trauma-Informed Approach

A first step toward being trauma-responsive is to become familiar with the trauma-informed approach and its principles. Awareness of the trauma-informed approach has dramatically increased in recent years, and the concepts have been embraced across a variety of academic and service sector settings [14, 15]. At the core of the approach is a basic recognition that trauma is affecting the lives of many individuals and their families. Essential practices of organizations and systems that adopt a trauma-informed approach include the '4 Rs': *realizing* the widespread impact of trauma and understanding potential paths for recovery, *recognizing* the signs and symptoms of trauma in clients, families, staff and others, *responding* to trauma by fully integrating knowledge about trauma into policies, procedures and practices, and seeking to actively *resist retraumatisation* [2]. Six key principles or values of trauma-informed care have become widely accepted and include (1) *safety* (both physical and psychological), (2) *trustworthiness* and *transparency,* (3) *peer support* and *mutual self-help,* (4) *collaboration* and *mutuality,* (5) *empowerment, voice and choice* and (6) attention to *cultural, historic and gender issues* [2, 16].

Becoming 'trauma-informed' may help equip practitioners who interact with survivors of GBV through increased understanding of their clients' needs, particularly related to the paramount need for safety in the context of the caregiving relationship [15]. But this is merely a first step toward being trauma-*responsive,* which suggests not only being informed but also building capacity to provide trauma-specific interventions that directly address trauma and its effects through a variety of practices, modalities and services, as well as trauma-specific services that offer a continuum of interventions from screening to treatment to recovery supports.

A continuum of responsivity is needed not only for victims of GBV but also for the families, communities and systems that surround victims. Responding will therefore need to take place at multiple levels of the ecological model; this includes the affected individual but also takes into consideration their nested influences, including the immediate setting that most directly impacts development, also called the *microsystem* (family, school, peers, etc), the *mesosystem* (interconnections between microsystems), the *exosystem* (social services, neighbours, etc), the broader *macrosystem* that includes the influences of culture at large and the *chronosystem,* which portrays the movement of these nested influences through time [3]. The ecological framework has been useful for examining sexual assault [17] as well as sexual revictimisation [18].

Responding to GBV across the nested levels of influence with trauma-informed awareness and trauma-focused interventions will likely be much more effective if we can respond proximally to the occurrence of exposures, in acute phases of the trauma, rather than distally to the occurrence when sequelae of the violence will likely be magnified [19]. A simple organizing framework for considering how we might apply a trauma-informed and trauma-responsive approach to GBV across the lifespan emerges, involving interventions that could be applied either

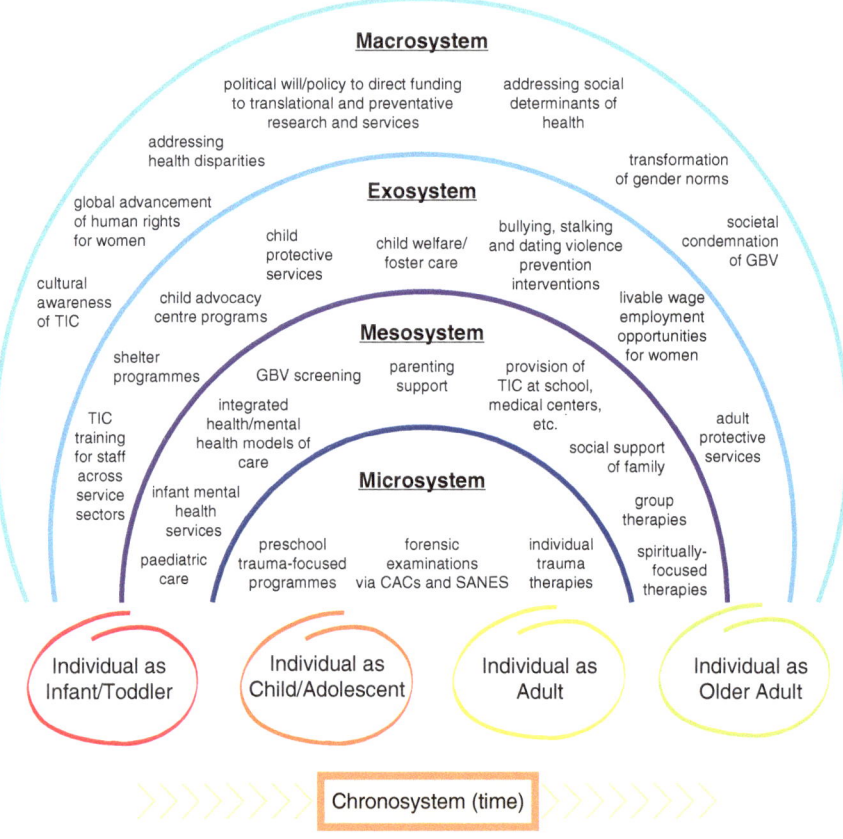

Fig. 12.1 A socioecological model of trauma-responsivity to gender based violence across the life course

proximally or distally to GBV traumatic exposures at each stage of development (see Fig. 12.1). Generally speaking, responding immediately after violence has occurred in a trauma-informed manner might preclude the need for also addressing mental health and other sequelae distal to the violence. Distal responding must include addressing both the immediate effects of trauma and the sequelae in tandem. At both the proximal and distal levels, trauma-responsive interventions must be varied and person-centred in nature in order to consider the heterogeneity of experiences of those affected by GBV, and should involve the nested levels of influence, including caregivers and the broader systems in which they live. Trauma responsivity should also include clinicians and their trauma responses, which will be highly influential for each step in responding to trauma. At each level of the ecological model, we follow the individual across the chronosystem/developmental stages of life (infancy and early childhood, middle childhood and adolescence, adulthood and older adulthood) and consider what form proximal and distal trauma responsiveness might take.

12.3 Infancy and Early Childhood

GBV occurring in early life includes direct maltreatment and witnessing violence. All children may experience both exposures; however, there is evidence that girls are maltreated more often than boys—this is especially true of sexual abuse [20]. In this epoch, infants and children are largely dependent on their parent or caregiver for accessing and receiving interventions. As such, interventions and treatments must consider attachment and child-caregiver functioning in addition to the individual needs of the child related to traumatic exposure [21]. Identifying and intervening early with affected dyads may also serve to disrupt and break intergenerational patterns of maltreatment and psychiatric vulnerability [22].

Proximal Trauma Responsivity in Early Life. Responding to direct maltreatment in early life to address both physical and mental traumatic sequalae includes attention to medical traumas that infants and toddlers sustain, acute psychological stress and early relational trauma; paediatric medical care is an excellent opportunity for these initial steps. Ideally, such care will involve working to minimize any potential traumatic effects of medical care itself, address any evident distress, provide reassurance, hope and emotional support, encourage a child's return to developmentally appropriate activities as possible, encourage family members to provide effective emotional support to the child, provide screening for distress and risk factors and refer to additional services as needed and provide attention to family members to also address their distress in relation to their child [23]. Paediatric care teams can respond in a trauma-informed way by recommending early infant mental health services to affected families to prevent disruptions for all families, and specifically for parents with premature or otherwise medically fragile infants [24].

Child Advocacy Centres (CACs) provide critical wrap-around services for trauma-exposed children and their families. CAC services include being child-friendly in nature, utilizing a multidisciplinary team, conducting investigative/forensic interviews, providing medical examinations, offering mental health services for children as well as non-offending family members, advocating for victims and case review and tracking [25]. However, there is limited evidence related to the efficacy of CAC services for addressing the mental and emotional needs of very young children; one qualitative investigation suggests that CAC personnel have variable perceptions about the effects of trauma in young children, suggesting more training is needed [26].

Another avenue for proximal responding to GBV in early life is through day care centres and preschools. Many of these employ social-emotional learning (SEL) programmes, which teach social and emotional skills in addition to traditional academic curricula to help students develop competencies related to affective self-regulation and interpersonal relating and which aim to increase prosocial behaviours, decrease behavioural problems and emotional distress and improve academic performance [27]. Ideally, SEL programmes should also be taking TIC into consideration in their curricula and application [28]. Although there is little extant literature outlining the direct coordination of SEL and TIC principles, early education programmes might adopt basic recommendations outlined by Perry [29] as guidelines for fostering trauma responsivity. A few trauma-informed programs have been examined with promising results. These include *Head Start Trauma Start,* an adaptation of the existing Head Start preschool programmes in the United States [30] and the Circle Preschool Program [31], which emphasizes a multidisciplinary approach that incorporates trauma-informed play therapy with a goal of promoting self-regulatory capacities in young children, as well providing caregiver therapy. It is a positive sign that there has been a recent proliferation of educational research into TIC practices in schools [32]; however, a recent systematic review of multi-tiered programmes for promoting TIC in schools suggests that this research is none-theless in an early stage of development and that future research needs to involve evaluation efforts to link the development of TIC models in schools to outcomes in a more robust manner [33]. Also needed is increased uptake of TIC principles and policies in early care and education programmes more broadly [34].

Distal Trauma Responsivity in Early Life. Depending on the age at which the infant or toddler is exposed to GBV, some of the proximal interventions already described might in fact be distal responses (e.g. for a preschooler with emotional/behavioural challenges pursuant to exposures sustained during infancy). However, a young child with cumulative trauma may not have been identified in these settings and might not receive support until larger systems become involved, including child welfare and protection systems. Also influential to the presentation of post-traumatic symptoms is whether or not the young child has experienced direct physical violence, has witnessed GBV or has experienced both exposures [35].

Although many children with trauma end up interfacing with child welfare systems, screening is still under-utilised, despite growing interest [36]. However, several projects underway that are attempting to simultaneously embed screening processes as well as TIC-informed principles, trainings, trauma-focused evidence-based interventions and procedures in child welfare systems; a rapid review of these shows by and large these are having promising results [37]. However, such programs are not ubiquitous, and although there is a rise in general awareness of TIC among child-service providers, providers vary widely as to whether or not they have had access to skills and strategies with which to respond to children who have experienced trauma [38]. This is important for early childhood because, unless child service workers and other human service professionals can intervene proximally or distally to trauma and adversity exposure in early life, challenges related to such exposures are likely to compound and be carried into school age and beyond.

12.4 Middle Childhood and Adolescence

Trauma-responsivity among school-aged children and adolescents shares similarities with early life in that individual interventions are needed for both proximal and distal responding, and these systems are also influential on trauma sequelae and needed responses. How these responses differ is that although parents are still highly influential to the well-being and protection of the child, and play an important role in connecting the child to treatments and interventions, the child is no longer exclusively dependent on parent/child dyadic functioning through which all intervention efforts must be filtered. This independence also brings risks of new forms of exposure, including peer bullying (seeking to harm, intimidate or coerce), stalking (unwanted contact or surveillance by individuals or groups that communicates threat or induces fear) and dating violence (physical, sexual or emotional harm from a romantic partner). For children and adolescents, as well as early childhood, both proximal and distal trauma responsivity are needed to address traumatic reactions to such exposures and to prevent future challenges and comorbidities that may follow the adolescent into adulthood.

Proximal Trauma Responsivity in Childhood and Adolescence. Following single-incident trauma exposures, a meta-analytic review suggests that extant interventions likely to help are largely behavioural and cognitive in nature and include psychoeducation, attention to developing coping skills and social support and sometimes include some kind of trauma exposure therapy (debriefing and reconstruction of the traumatic event through creation of a trauma narrative) [39]. Provision of such interventions in response to acute trauma may help disrupt the formation of maladaptive trauma-related appraisals, excessive early avoidance and negative social and interpersonal processes that may ultimately lead to the persistence of post-traumatic symptomatology [40].

As with younger children in relation to preschool interventions, provision of school-based interventions is also an important avenue of trauma responsivity for children. Middle childhood and adolescence introduce potential new GBV traumas as children engage with peers and school settings, including bullying [41], stalking [42] and dating violence [43]. Many evidence-based trauma treatments are utilised in school settings and may work for some instances of bullying, stalking and dating violence; however, programmes specific to these exposures have also been developed [41].

A meta-analytic review [44] identified 31 common elements of effective trauma-based school interventions to treat trauma symptoms broadly; prominent among these were social and coping skills training, relaxation techniques and techniques for engaging creative expressive capacities. For addressing GBV exposures in children specifically, group counselling may be an efficient way for school mental health practitioners to respond to GBV exposures in children that might enhance positive socialisation and encourage mutual peer aid and support [45]. In recognition of the importance of the school setting for recognizing and treating trauma in children, school-wide TIC programs are being implemented and evaluated; one such program, Trauma-Informed Elementary Schools (TIES) [46], is providing resource liaisons to classroom teachers to support their ability to recognise and respond to indicators of trauma in their students. Initial evaluation of effectiveness of the program was encouraging in multiple domains, including positive emotional climate in the classroom, effective behavioural management and teacher productivity [46]. The TIES program is in line with calls to establish multi-tiered programs for trauma treatments in schools that provide professional development for staff, students and families and provide expert consultation as well as clinical supports that utilise evidence-based interventions [47]. Such initiatives are dependent not only on educational staff training and application of TIC interventions but also on macro-level components, including the leveraging of school policies and financing, in order to sustain TIC practices [48].

One novel system-level approach to responding to child exposure to GBV is the Greensboro Child Response Initiative (CRI) [49]. This community-coordinated response involves training police officers in trauma-responsive principles to be CRI advocates embedded within the police department to be dispatched when children are involved in GBV instances as witnesses or victims. The CRI advocate engages with the adult and the child at the scene (with the adult's permission), provides information related to common reactions to trauma, assesses the incident in relation to active or pending Child Protective Services (CPS) involvement and involves any social workers assigned to the child's care. With the social worker, the advocate coordinates processes to promote safety, including safety assessment and engagement in CAC services as needed for forensic investigation and ongoing trauma services. Initial evaluation of the CRI program showed that it was facilitative of faster engagement in service utilisation and was acceptable to both caregivers and law enforcement personnel [49].

Distal Trauma Responsivity in Childhood and Adolescence. Children who are not able to benefit from early intervention proximal to trauma exposure, or who suffer from ongoing and untreated trauma, may develop complex trauma, which is related to diminished regulatory and interpersonal relating capacities and can have lifelong implications for psychiatric problems, substance using, chronic illness and other problems [50]. For distal trauma responsivity, treating complex trauma necessitates attention not only to the trauma but also to these additional sequelae.

A review of the evidence base for various treatments suggests that individual cognitive behavioural therapy (CBT) treatments, both with and without parent involvement and in both individual and group settings, have well-established efficacy [51]. Interventions with probable or possible efficacy include eye movement desensitisation and reprocessing (EMDR), individual integrated psychoeducation/therapy models for complex trauma and provision of group mind–body skills. A common form of evidence-based CBT used with children is trauma-focused CBT (TF-CBT); this model of phased treatment includes psychoeducation for children and parents, support for parents to understand their child's trauma reactions, relaxation, affective and cognitive skills training, trauma narration and processing, joint sessions with therapist, children and caregivers to consolidate learning and enhance future safety and development [52].

Sustained or very serious traumatic exposure often leads to engagement in Child Protective Services and entry into the foster care system; it is estimated that 90% of children in placement have experienced trauma, and, that of those, almost half have experienced four or more types of traumas [53]. Clinicians working with children in the foster care system have the double mandate of recognizing and addressing traumatic antecedents to behaviours and emotions and processing those, as well as addressing and treating compounded behavioural and emotional reactions that have ensued [54]. Individuals in the foster care system experience trauma before, during and after placement; as such, earlier interventions for families involved in the system are needed, as well as increased access to caring adults who might listen to foster care youth, provision of trauma-responsive parenting skills training for foster parents and mechanisms to supply continuity of relationships and opportunities for leadership training for youth in the system [55]. A pilot study of using one such resource, the National Child Traumatic Stress Network's trauma-informed parenting workshop, was conducted with foster, adoptive and kinship caregivers and demonstrated acceptability and increases in knowledge and self-efficacy for parenting a child with a trauma history [56].

Children with prior trauma are more at risk for sex trafficking, as well [57]. More attention is now being directed to addressing human trafficking of children and adolescents and recognizing this as a critical health threat [58]. As such, trauma-informed guidelines and recommendations have been developed for paediatric clinicians [59], nurse practitioners [58] and for systems who provide aftercare for trafficking victims [60, 61].

12.5 Adulthood

GBV in adulthood includes sexual violence, intimate partner violence and sexual harassment in campus and workplace settings. Proximal responsivity to adult-onset incidences of GBV may prevent the development of traumatic stress sequalae including PTSD and other chronic mental health and physical health conditions. Distal trauma responsivity necessitates addressing post-trauma sequalae in addition to addressing these attendant chronic conditions. Parenting in relationship to GBV is a crucial consideration because victimisation impacts parenting practices.

Proximal Trauma Responsivity in Adulthood. As with other epochs, medical staff are often the first line of response because they are treating the physical wounds of violence; therefore, integrated health and behavioural healthcare models are needed to facilitate engagement with preventative services and help increase safety for affected individuals. One excellent example is the sexual assault nurse examiner (SANE) programme, which is associated with improved outcomes related to psychological recovery of victims [62], provision of needed medical care (including emergency contraception, pregnancy testing and addressing sexually transmitted infection risk), collection and documentation of forensic evidence, enhancing efforts to prosecute perpetrators and connecting survivors to resources in the community [63, 64]. Other programmes may be promoted in healthcare settings, including psychological treatments, safety planning and advocacy, including home visitation and peer support programmes and parenting and mother–child interventions [65].

Domestic violence shelters and programmes are another important resource for victims of violence and are generally operating with principles that align to TIC [66]. Providing a physically and psychologically safe environment for victims of GBV and their children is a main purpose of domestic violence shelter services; this provides parents the opportunity to feel better to be able to keep themselves and their children safe [67, 68]. However, as of this writing, there are no published reports of how the provision of these shelter-specific services may specifically improve outcomes for affected children.

Responding to the needs of survivors of GBV during contacts for reproductive healthcare is another avenue of opportunity, and one with promise for breaking intergenerational cycles of violence [22]. A systematic review by Shah and Shah [69] found that women who experienced GBV during pregnancy were at increased risk for having a low birth weight or premature infant and that underreporting of GBV violence is quite likely, despite the opportunity that more frequent healthcare contacts represents. Often, GBV victims also experience a variety of mental health challenges as well, which may be directly related to GBV but which may also have roots in prior trauma. TIC during reproduction is paramount for the provision of care during abortion-seeking [70], during midwifery care [15], obstetric care [71] and doula care [72].

GBV trauma responsivity is also important in educational and workplace settings for adults. Stalking, sexual harassment and sexual assault on university campuses are prevalent, with LGBTQ individuals and disabled people being particularly at risk. Given that often these are new traumas for students [73], proximal TIC responsivity is indicated. Calls for TIC on university campus settings have been described [74], and counselling services for trauma victims are in place across campus settings. Application of TIC principles to campus responding to GBV have also appeared in the literature [75]. However, given that often sexual assault on campuses is underreported, particularly among those of minority race [76], more is needed to encourage a TIC climate across campuses to promote disclosures and to evaluate TIC initiatives longitudinally.

The worldwide #MeToo movement has brought the issue of sexual harassment and GBV in the workplace to the fore and presents an opportunity for redress in the public health arena. GBV in the workplace includes sexual harassment and violence stemming from workplace exposures (from staff or clients), as well as GBV that stems from personal relationships that follows an individual into their work setting. A recent systematic review of GBV exposures originating in the workplace among healthcare, social care and education workers [77] found significant associations between GBV and poor mental health and sickness absence. Sexual harassment and assault in military settings are also highly prevalent and are associated with a variety of mental and physical health outcomes for victims. Calls for application of TIC principles in military settings are increasing as a result [78].

Distal Trauma Responsivity in Adulthood. Many of the TIC approaches and treatments outlined for proximal responding also have utility for responding distal to the occurrence of GBV exposures; however, treatments will need to tailor service delivery toward recognizing and attending to comorbid post-trauma sequalae and taking care to avoid re-traumatising clinical encounters. Considering that health practitioners are often the first line of treatment for many of these comorbid conditions, calls for application of TIC principles and practices in health settings are rising across health and mental health service sectors.

12.6 Older Adulthood

Older adults face a unique set of challenges, especially as impairments become prominent. These may include physical and cognitive declines that make them more vulnerable to GBV and other forms of abuse. Most victims of all forms of maltreatment in this age group are women, and they frequently experience multiple types of abuse or maltreatment [79, 80]. These can include GBV, neglect, financial abuse and physical abuse by caregivers [81]. In this era, prior traumas continue to be a risk factor for more maltreatment, and symptoms related to prior trauma may have delayed onset or reemergence [82]. This age group and responses to their needs are drastically under-researched compared to other epochs.

Proximal Trauma Responsivity. Perhaps more than any other age group, the increasing likelihood of health conditions means that doctor's offices provide a prime opportunity for early detection of GBV and other forms of abuse among older adults. Unfortunately, detection and reporting rates remain low; barriers to reporting include a lack of knowledge and protocols for identification and response, fear about professional repercussions and concern about the lack of available services [83]. Training programs are needed for medical professionals, and TIC principles should be incorporated.

Detecting and responding to all forms of maltreatment is frequently complicated both by the increasing dependence, this population may have on their caregivers as well the relationships; for example if the abuser is the older adult's child [81]. Unlike child protective services, the mirror program for adults (Adult Protective Services) must respect the victim's desire for autonomy, which may include wishing to remain with their abuser or in otherwise unsafe conditions. This can present challenges for ethical and trauma-informed interventions for this vulnerable population [84]. Due to these complexities, all professionals who interface with this population would benefit from TIC training [85]. Unfortunately, there is little literature on this and an ongoing need for development of evidence-based trainings.

Distal Trauma Responsivity. Minimal research has examined the effectiveness of trauma-focused interventions with older adults, and only a few studies have been tested for any form of elder abuse [86]. In one small randomised trial with older (ages 55 and up) women in the community, Bowland and colleagues [82] found that a 'spiritually-focused' group intervention for trauma had promising results. This type of intervention may be a good match for older adults, who tend to be more spiritual than other age brackets. Compared to the control group, participants reported diminished anxious, depressive and somatic symptoms at follow up. Similarly, a psychoeducational group for elder survivors of maltreatment found improvements compared to the control group, although results were not significant for any measure [87]. Clearly, there is a need to develop and test more interventions for traumatic experiences in this population.

The populations of many nations are aging, meaning that an increasing proportion are older adults. This will put a strain on many structures and systems and will make the need for more developed responses to trauma and abuse among elders more pressing. This is due to their vulnerability to abuse as well as effects of prior and accumulating traumas which may re-emerge in later years, both as emotional and psychological difficulties and as chronic illnesses. Unfortunately, older women who are victims of GBV may fall into the cracks between systems designed for elder abuse and those for younger victims of IPV [88]. We need better responses for our elders, ranging from increased recognition and reporting, to effective interventions for victims, to improved trainings for all professionals who interface with this population. Given the needs, the paucity of research at this date is troubling.

12.7 Intergenerational Patterns

It is important to note that there are intergenerational patterns and influences on the transmission of trauma that also affect the life course; a phenomenon that is currently being described as 'transgenerational trauma' [89]. Nascent literature suggests that it is transmitted through both epigenetic and environmental pathways and affects physical health [90] behaviours, [89, 91] attitudes [92], values [93] and socioeconomic statuses [94]. Little in the way of specific interventions for responding to transgenerational trauma have been developed. However, a tool for identifying 'transgenerational scripts' with therapy clients has been developed [95], and parental attachment insecurity in the transmission of transgenerational trauma has been explored [96, 97]. Further identification of epigenetic influences might help us identify at-risk individuals and allow us to target interventions [98]. Better understanding of transgenerational trauma, as well as ways in which victimization and re-victimisation from caregivers [99], and also from the institutions with which an individual interacts, influence development and health [100], will help us develop TIC interventions for GBV that span generations.

12.8 Conclusion

GBV affects individuals across the life course in a variety of ways and involves many relationships and systems across socioecological levels of influence. Because of this heterogeneity of experiences, influences and trajectories, we need heterogeneity of TIC responsivity that includes responding to acute trauma, cumulative and complex trauma, the attendant sequelae, as well as transgenerational trauma across developmental epochs. We also must attend to family members, caregivers, clinicians, the institutions with which individuals interact, the communities in which they live and the larger society, with attention to implementing policies that are also trauma-informed [101].

Much of what we have described as trauma responsivity are nascent and aspirational models and/or initial evaluative efforts of TIC interventions; clearly much more work must be done to translate these models into intervention, and trial, evaluate and scale up such interventions and prevention programming, especially for marginalised groups who have elevated risk. These efforts will also need to take country and context into consideration; in low- and middle-income countries, community culture and traditional gender norms will need transformation, in addition to needed reforms for empowerment for women, engagement of multiple stakeholders, policy formulation and legal protections, as well as service integration and policy and legal protections.

It has been suggested that in this stage of our collective understanding, TIC should be properly viewed as a 'universal precaution' [102]. Our understanding is also evolving toward recognizing that in addition to responding to trauma, we need to identify and promote factors that increase resilience for individuals throughout the life course. In order to build resilience, however, we need to concomitantly reduce the number and severity of stressors and traumas and respond in trauma-informed ways to reduce these effects. Those who receive the disclosures and otherwise work with those affected by GBV are also worthy recipients of TIC, particularly in light of risk for vicarious traumatisation, compassion fatigue and burnout [103]. TIC, in any setting, in any epoch, represents simple good principles, practices and frameworks for responding to any individual. However, for those with trauma history, TIC principles represent a real opportunity to redress past trauma and its effects, prevent re-traumatisation and influence life trajectories in a positive and meaningful way.

Reflective Questions

Where/how is your client population most at risk for GBV?

How might you characterise distal versus proximal trauma in the population you work with?

Are there any interventions mentioned in this chapter already being applied in your work environment?

Are there any interventions mentioned that you think could be helpful in your work environment? What kind of collaboration with professionals from other fields might this require?

Has your organisation considered doing a self-assessment of the degree to which your services are trauma-responsive? Several trauma-informed organisational self-assessment tools have been developed, for example the Trauma-Responsive Understanding Tool (TRUST; information is available at https://trust-survey.com/Learn-About-TRUST-and-TRUST-S).

To what degree does your organisation or clinical practice embody the six key principles/values of trauma-informed care?

- How do you help clients and staff feel physically and psychologically *safe*?
- Are organisational and clinical operations and decisions conducted with *transparency*, with a goal of building (and maintaining) *trust* with clients and staff?

- Does your service delivery provide opportunities for clients and staff to engage in *peer support* and *mutual self-help*?
- Are the concepts of *collaboration* and *mutuality* evident in how power is shared within your organisation and its decision-making?
- How does your practice or organisation seek to recognise the unique strengths, as well as needs of clients and staff and promote *empowerment*, *voice* and *choice*?
- To what extent does your practice or organisation address *cultural, historical* and *gender issues*? How are you striving to address cultural stereotypes and biases, honour traditional cultural healing perspectives and traditions, recognise the pervasive effects of cultural and historic trauma and develop and offer culturally responsive services?

References

1. European Institute for Gender Equality. What is gender based violence? https://eige.europa.eu/gender-based-violence/what-is-gender-based-violence. Accessed 20 Aug 2020.
2. Substance Abuse and Mental Health Services Administration. SAMHSA's concept of trauma and guidance for a trauma-informed approach. HHS Publication No (SMA) 14–4884; 2014.
3. Bronfenbrenner U. The ecology of human development. Cambridge, MA: Harvard University Press; 1979.
4. Ben-Shlomo Y, Kuh D. A life course approach to chronic disease epidemiology: conceptual models, empirical challenges and interdisciplinary perspectives. J Epidemiol Community Health. 2002;31:285–93.
5. Lynch J, Smith GD. A life course approach to chronic disease epidemiology. Annu Rev Public Health. 2005;26:1–35.
6. Macmillan R. Violence and the life course: the consequences of victimization for personal and social development. Annu Rev Sociol. 2001;27(1):1–22.
7. Greenfield EA. Child abuse as a life-course social determinant of adult health. Maturitas. 2010;66(1):51–5.
8. Sederer LI. The social determinants of mental health. Psychiatr Serv. 2016;67:234–5.
9. Sperlich M. Social determinants of maternal mental health and the need for integrated models of care. J Womens Health. 2020;29:1023–4.
10. Felitti VJ, Anda RF, Nordenberg D, Williamson DF, Spitz AM, Edwards V, Marks JS. Relationship of childhood abuse and household dysfunction to many of the leading causes of death in adults: the adverse childhood experiences (ACE) study. Am J Prev Med. 1998;14(4):245–58.
11. Costa BM, Kaestle CE, Walker A, Curtis A, Day A, Toumbourou JW, Miller P. Longitudinal predictors of domestic violence perpetration and victimization: a systematic review. Aggress Violent Behav. 2015;24:261–72.
12. Becker-Blease KA. As the world becomes trauma–informed, work to do. J Trauma Dissociation. 2017;18:131–8.
13. Oral R, Ramirez M, Coohey C, Nakada S, Walz A, Kuntz A, Benoit J, Peek-Asa C. Adverse childhood experiences and trauma informed care: the future of health care. Pediatr Res. 2016;79(1):227–33.
14. Elliott DE, Bjelajac P, Fallot RD, Markoff LS, Reed BG. Trauma-informed or trauma-denied: principles and implementation of trauma-informed services for women. J Community Psychol. 2005;33(4):461–77.

15. Sperlich M, Seng JS, Li Y, Taylor J, Bradbury-Jones C. Integrating trauma-informed care into maternity care practice: conceptual and practical issues. J Midwifery Womens Health. 2017;62(6):661–72.
16. Harris ME, Fallot RD. Using trauma theory to design service systems. San Francisco: Jossey-Bass; 2001.
17. Campbell R, Dworkin E, Cabral G. An ecological model of the impact of sexual assault on women's mental health. Trauma Violence Abuse. 2009;10(3):225–46.
18. Pittenger SL, Huit TZ, Hansen DJ. Applying ecological systems theory to sexual revictimization of youth: a review with implications for research and practice. Aggress Violent Behav. 2016;26:35–45.
19. Bell KM, Naugle AE. Intimate partner violence theoretical considerations: moving towards a contextual framework. Clin Psychol Rev. 2008;28(7):1096–107.
20. Moody G, Cannings-John R, Hood K, Kemp A, Robling M. Establishing the international prevalence of self-reported child maltreatment: a systematic review by maltreatment type and gender. BMC Public Health. 2018;18(1):1–5.
21. Lieberman AF. Traumatic stress and quality of attachment: reality and internalization in disorders of infant mental health. Infant Ment Health J. 2004;25(4):336–51.
22. Sperlich M, Seng J, Rowe H, Fisher J, Cuthbert C, Taylor J. A cycles-breaking framework to disrupt intergenerational patterns of maltreatment and vulnerability during the childbearing year. J Obstet Gynecol Neonatal Nurs. 2017;46(3):378–89.
23. Marsac ML, Kassam-Adams N, Hildenbrand AK, Nicholls E, Winston FK, Leff SS, Fein J. Implementing a trauma-informed approach in pediatric health care networks. JAMA Pediatr. 2016;170(1):70–7.
24. Del Fabbro A, Cain K. Infant mental health and family mental health issues. Newborn Infant Nurs Rev. 2016;16(4):281–4.
25. Jackson SL. A USA national survey of program services provided by child advocacy centers. Child Abuse Negl. 2004;28(4):411–21.
26. Vanderzee KL, Pemberton JR, Conners-Burrow N, Kramer TL. Who is advocating for children under six? Uncovering unmet needs in child advocacy centers. Child Youth Serv Rev. 2016;61:303–10.
27. Durlak JA, Weissberg RP, Dymnicki AB, Taylor RD, Schellinger KB. The impact of enhancing students' social and emotional learning: a meta-analysis of school-based universal interventions. Child Dev. 2011;82(1):405–32.
28. Pawlo E, Lorenzo A, Eichert B, Elias MJ. All SEL should be trauma-informed. Phi Delta Kappan. 2019;101(3):37–41.
29. Perry BD. Examining child maltreatment through a neurodevelopmental lens: clinical applications of the neurosequential model of therapeutics. J Loss Trauma. 2009;14(4):240–55.
30. Holmes C, Levy M, Smith A, Pinne S, Neese P. A model for creating a supportive trauma informed culture for children in preschool settings. J Child Fam Stud. 2015;24(6):1650–9.
31. Ryan K, Lane SJ, Powers D. A multidisciplinary model for treating complex trauma in early childhood. Int J Play Ther. 2017;26(2):111.
32. Thomas MS, Crosby S, Vanderhaar J. Trauma-informed practices in schools across two decades: an interdisciplinary review of research. Rev Res Educ. 2019;43(1):422–52.
33. Berger E. Multi-tiered approaches to trauma-informed care in schools: a systematic review. Sch Ment Health. 2019;1:1–5.
34. Bartlett JD, Smith S. The role of early care and education in addressing early childhood trauma. Am J Community Psychol. 2019;64(3–4):359–72.
35. Showalter K, Yoon S, Maguire-Jack K, Wolf KG, Letson M. Are dual and single exposures differently associated with clinical levels of trauma symptoms? Examining physical abuse and witnessing intimate partner violence among young children. Child Fam Soc Work. 2020;25(2):439–47.
36. Lang JM, Ake G, Barto B, Caringi J, Little C, Baldwin MJ, Sullivan K, Tunno AM, Bodian R, Stewart CJ, Stevens K. Trauma screening in child welfare: lessons learned from five states. J Child Adolesc Trauma. 2017;10(4):405–16.

37. Bunting L, Montgomery L, Mooney S, MacDonald M, Coulter S, Hayes D, Davidson G. Trauma informed child welfare systems—a rapid evidence review. Int J Environ Res Public Health. 2019;16(13):2365.
38. Donisch K, Bray C, Gewirtz A. Child welfare, juvenile justice, mental health, and education providers' conceptualizations of trauma-informed practice. Child Maltreat. 2016;21(2):125–34.
39. Kramer DN, Landolt MA. Characteristics and efficacy of early psychological interventions in children and adolescents after single trauma: a meta-analysis. Eur J Psychotraumatol. 2011;2(1):7858.
40. Kassam-Adams N. Design, delivery, and evaluation of early interventions for children exposed to acute trauma. Eur J Psychotraumatol. 2014;5(1):22757.
41. Menesini E, Salmivalli C. Bullying in schools: the state of knowledge and effective interventions. Psychol Health Med. 2017;22(sup1):240–53.
42. Smith-Darden JP, Reidy DE, Kernsmith PD. Adolescent stalking and risk of violence. J Adolesc. 2016;52:191–200.
43. Smith-Darden JP, Kernsmith PD, Reidy DE, Cortina KS. In search of modifiable risk and protective factors for teen dating violence. J Res Adolesc. 2017;27(2):423–35.
44. du Mello Kenyon G, Schirmer J. Common practice elements of school-based trauma interventions for children and adolescents exhibiting symptoms of post-traumatic stress disorder: a systematic review. J Psychol Couns Sch. 2020;1:1–7.
45. Thompson EH, Trice-Black S. School-based group interventions for children exposed to domestic violence. J Fam Violence. 2012;27(3):233–41.
46. Rishel CW, Tabone JK, Hartnett HP, Szafran KF. Trauma-informed elementary schools: evaluation of school-based early intervention for young children. Child Sch. 2019;41(4):239–48.
47. Phifer LW, Hull R. Helping students heal: observations of trauma-informed practices in the schools. Sch Ment Health. 2016;8(1):201–5.
48. Kataoka SH, Vona P, Acuna A, Jaycox L, Escudero P, Rojas C, Ramirez E, Langley A, Stein BD. Applying a trauma informed school systems approach: examples from school community-academic partnerships. Ethn Dis. 2018;28(Suppl 2):417.
49. Graves KN, Ward M, Crotts DK, Pitts W. The Greensboro child response initiative: a trauma-informed, mental health–law enforcement model for children exposed to violence. J Aggress Maltreat Trauma. 2019;28(5):526–44.
50. Cook A, Spinazzola J, Ford J, Lanktree C, Blaustein M, Cloitre M, DeRosa R, Hubbard R, Kagan R, Liautaud J, Mallah K. Complex trauma in children and adolescents. Psychiatr Ann. 2017;35(5):390–8.
51. Dorsey S, McLaughlin KA, Kerns SE, Harrison JP, Lambert HK, Briggs EC, Revillion Cox J, Amaya-Jackson L. Evidence base update for psychosocial treatments for children and adolescents exposed to traumatic events. J Clin Child Adolesc Psychol. 2017;46(3):303–30.
52. Cohen JA, Deblinger E, Mannarino AP. Trauma-focused cognitive behavioral therapy for children and families. Psychother Res. 2018;28(1):47–57.
53. Stein BD, Zima BT, Elliott MN, Burnam MA, Shahinfar A, Fox NA, Leavitt LA. Violence exposure among school-age children in foster care: relationship to distress symptoms. J Am Acad Child Adolesc Psychiatry. 2001;40(5):588–94.
54. Fratto CM. Trauma-informed care for youth in foster care. Arch Psychiatr Nurs. 2016;30(3):439–46.
55. Riebschleger J, Day A, Damashek A. Foster care youth share stories of trauma before, during, and after placement: youth voices for building trauma-informed systems of care. J Aggress Maltreat Trauma. 2015;24(4):339–60.
56. Sullivan KM, Murray KJ, Ake GS III. Trauma-informed care for children in the child welfare system: an initial evaluation of a trauma-informed parenting workshop. Child Maltreat. 2016;21(2):147–55.
57. Fedina L, Williamson C, Perdue T. Risk factors for domestic child sex trafficking in the United States. J Interpers Violence. 2019;34(13):2653–73.

58. Peck JL, Meadows-Oliver M, Hays SM, Maaks DG. White paper: recognizing child trafficking as a critical emerging health threat. J Pediatr Health Care. 2020:13.
59. Leopardi NM, Hovde AM, Kullmann LV. The intersection of child trafficking and health care: our unique role as pediatric clinicians. Pediatr Clin. 2020;67(2):413–23.
60. Batts RA. Using trauma-informed and victim-centered approaches to provide assistance to survivors of human trafficking. Doctoral dissertation, Valdosta State University.
61. Gaillard-Kenney SF, Kent B, Lewis J, Williams C. Effects of trauma-informed care training on healthcare providers caring for victims of human trafficking. Internet J Allied Health Sci Pract. 2020;18(3):13.
62. Campbell R, Greeson MR, Fehler-Cabral G. With care and compassion: adolescent sexual assault victims' experiences in sexual assault nurse examiner programs. J Forensic Nurs. 2013;9(2):68–75.
63. Campbell R, Patterson D, Lichty LF. The effectiveness of sexual assault nurse examiner (SANE) programs: a review of psychological, medical, legal, and community outcomes. Trauma Violence Abuse. 2005;6(4):313–29.
64. Schmitt T, Cross TP, Alderden M. Qualitative analysis of prosecutors' perspectives on sexual assault nurse examiners and the criminal justice response to sexual assault. J Forensic Nurs. 2017;13(2):62–8.
65. Hegarty K, Tarzia L, Hooker L, Taft A. Interventions to support recovery after domestic and sexual violence in primary care. Int Rev Psychiatry. 2016;28(5):519–32.
66. Wilson JM, Fauci JE, Goodman LA. Bringing trauma-informed practice to domestic violence programs: a qualitative analysis of current approaches. Am J Orthopsychiatry. 2015;85(6):586.
67. Sullivan CM, Virden T. An eight state study on the relationships among domestic violence shelter services and residents' self-efficacy and hopefulness. J Fam Violence. 2017;32(8):741–50.
68. Tutty LM Effective practices in sheltering women leaving violence in intimate relationships: executive summary: prepared for YWCA Canada. Phase II report, 2006. YWCA Canada; 2006.
69. Shah PS, Shah J. Maternal exposure to domestic violence and pregnancy and birth outcomes: a systematic review and meta-analyses. J Womens Health. 2010;19(11):2017–31.
70. Ely GE, Rouland Polmanteer RS, Kotting J. A trauma-informed social work framework for the abortion seeking experience. Soc Work Ment Health. 2018;16(2):172–200.
71. Stevens NR, Holmgreen L, Hobfoll SE, Cvengros JA. Assessing trauma history in pregnant patients: a didactic module and role-play for obstetrics and gynecology residents. MedEdPORTAL. 2020;16:10925.
72. Mosley EA, Lanning RK. Evidence and guidelines for trauma-informed doula care. Midwifery. 2020;83:102643.
73. Galatzer-Levy IR, Burton CL, Bonanno GA. Coping flexibility, potentially traumatic life events, and resilience: a prospective study of college student adjustment. J Soc Clin Psychol. 2012;31(6):542–67.
74. McCauley HL, Casler AW. College sexual assault: a call for trauma-informed prevention. J Adolesc Health. 2015;56(6):584–5.
75. Oehme K, Perko A, Clark J, Ray EC, Arpan L, Bradley L. A trauma-informed approach to building college students' resilience. J Evid Based Soc Work. 2019;16(1):93–107.
76. Wolitzky-Taylor KB, Resnick HS, Amstadter AB, McCauley JL, Ruggiero KJ, Kilpatrick DG. Reporting rape in a national sample of college women. J Am Coll Health. 2011;59(7):582–7.
77. Nyberg A, Kecklund G, Hanson LM, Rajaleid K. Workplace violence and health in human service industries: a systematic review of prospective and longitudinal studies. Occup Environ Med. 2020:15.
78. Herzog JR, Whitworth JD, Scott DL. Trauma informed care with military populations. J Hum Behav Soc Environ. 2020;30(3):265–78.
79. Lundy M, Grossman SF. Elder abuse: spouse/intimate partner abuse and family violence among elders. J Elder Abuse Negl. 2005;16(1):85–102.

80. Ramsey-Klawsnik H, Miller E. Polyvictimization in later life: trauma-informed best practices. J Elder Abuse Negl. 2017;29(5):339–50.
81. Schiamberg LB, Gans D. Elder abuse by adult children: an applied ecological framework for understanding contextual risk factors and the intergenerational character of quality of life. Int J Aging Hum Dev. 2000;50(4):329–59.
82. Bowland S, Edmond T, Fallot RD. Evaluation of a spiritually focused intervention with older trauma survivors. Soc Work. 2012;57(1):73–82.
83. Schmeidel AN, Daly JM, Rosenbaum ME, Schmuch GA, Jogerst GJ. Health care professionals' perspectives on barriers to elder abuse detection and reporting in primary care settings. J Elder Abuse Negl. 2012;24(1):17–36.
84. Band-Winterstein T, Goldblatt H, Alon S. Giving voice to 'age at the edge'—a challenge for social workers intervening with elder abuse and neglect. J Fam Violence. 2014;29(7):797–807.
85. Ernst JS, Maschi T. Trauma-informed care and elder abuse: a synergistic alliance. J Elder Abuse Negl. 2018;30(5):354–67.
86. Ploeg J, Fear J, Hutchison B, MacMillan H, Bolan G. A systematic review of interventions for elder abuse. J Elder Abuse Negl. 2009;21(3):187–210.
87. Brownell P, Heiser D. Psycho-educational support groups for older women victims of family mistreatment: a pilot study. J Gerontol Soc Work. 2006;46(3–4):145–60.
88. Straka SM, Montminy L. Responding to the needs of older women experiencing domestic violence. Violence Against Women. 2006;12(3):251–67.
89. Krippner S, Barrett D. Transgenerational trauma: the role of epigenetics. J Mind Behav. 2019;1:40(1).
90. Crusto CA, De Mendoza VB, Connell CM, Sun YV, Taylor JY. The intergenerational impact of genetic and psychological factors on blood pressure study (InterGEN): design and methods for recruitment and psychological measures. Nurs Res. 2016;65(4):331.
91. Jawaid A, Mansuy IM. Inter-and transgenerational inheritance of behavioral phenotypes. Curr Opin Behav Sci. 2019;25:96–101.
92. Bakó T, Zana K. The vehicle of transgenerational trauma: the transgenerational atmosphere. Am Imago. 2018;75(2):271–85.
93. Akyil Y, Prouty A, Blanchard A, Lyness K. Parents' experiences of intergenerational value transmission in Turkey's changing society: an interpretative phenomenological study. J Fam Psychother. 2014;25(1):42–65.
94. Ryabov I. Intergenerational transmission of socio-economic status: the role of neighborhood effects. J Adolesc. 2020;80:84–97.
95. Gayol GN. Untangling the family tree: using the transgenerational script questionnaire in the psychotherapy of transgenerational trauma. Trans Anal J. 2019;49(4):279–91.
96. Maisel JS. Insecure attachment's role in transgenerational trauma: healing unmet needs to stop the cycle. Doctoral dissertation, Pacifica graduate institute. 2020.
97. Velotti P, Rogier G, Beomonte Zobel S, Chirumbolo A, Zavattini GC. The relation of anxiety and avoidance dimensions of attachment to intimate partner violence: a meta-analysis about perpetrators. Trauma Violence Abuse. 2020:1524838020933864.
98. Howard AE. Transgenerational effects of trauma through epigenetic mechanisms. Doctoral dissertation, Azusa Pacific University. 2020.
99. Drury SS, Mabile E, Brett ZH, Esteves K, Jones E, Shirtcliff EA, Theall KP. The association of telomere length with family violence and disruption. Pediatrics. 2014;134(1):e128–37.
100. Bjørnholt M. The social dynamics of revictimization and intimate partner violence: an embodied, gendered, institutional and life course perspective. Nord J Criminol. 2019;20(1):90–110.
101. Bowen EA, Murshid NS. Trauma-informed social policy: a conceptual framework for policy analysis and advocacy. Am J Public Health. 2016;106(2):223–9.
102. Racine N, Killam T, Madigan S. Trauma-informed care as a universal precaution: beyond the adverse childhood experiences questionnaire. JAMA Pediatr. 2020;174(1):5–6.
103. Brend DM, Krane J, Saunders S. Exposure to trauma in intimate partner violence human service work: a scoping review. Dent Traumatol. 2019;26(1):127–36.

From Surviving to Thriving: A Feminist Empowerment Approach to Supporting Women Affected by Intimate Partner Violence

13

Isobel Heywood and Jacky Mulveen

13.1 Introduction

Whilst men, boys and those who identify as LGBTQ+ can be victims of domestic violence and abuse (DVA) [1], the majority is carried out against women by their—predominantly male—intimate partners [2]. Global estimates indicate that almost a third (30%) of women worldwide who have been in a relationship have experienced some form of physical or sexual violence by an intimate partner in their lifetime [3]. In the UK, DVA refers to 'any incident or pattern of incidents of controlling, coercive or threatening behaviour, violence or abuse between those aged 16 or over who are or have been intimate partners or family members regardless of gender or sexuality' [4]. Abuse can be psychological, physical, sexual, financial or emotional and can involve controlling behaviour, coercive control, harassment, stalking and online or digital abuse such as revenge pornography [5]. Current estimates indicate that from March 2018 to March 2019, 7.5% of women (1.6 million) and 3.8% of men (786,000) in the UK experienced DVA in some form [6], and the UK prevalence of lifetime exposure to DVA in the female population is estimated to be 27.1% [7]. It is important to note here that this data does not allow for important context and information, such as the severity and frequency of abuse, and who experienced abuse within a wider context of power and control. When these factors are considered, the gendered nature of DVA becomes apparent.

The mental and physical impacts of DVA on an individual are 'many and profound' [8]: it causes substantial harm to women's physical, sexual, and reproductive health [9]; can result in chronic health conditions including gastrointestinal issues

I. Heywood (✉)
University of Birmingham Alumni (Masters in Public Health), Birmingham, UK

J. Mulveen
WE:ARE (Women's Empowerment and Recovery Educators), Birmingham, UK
e-mail: jacky@weareuk.org

© Springer Nature Switzerland AG 2021
C. Bradbury-Jones, L. Isham (eds.), *Understanding Gender-Based Violence*,
https://doi.org/10.1007/978-3-030-65006-3_13

and gynaecological problems and is a major cause of poor mental health including depression, PTSD [10] and chronic stress [8]. Recent research found an increased risk of subsequent cardiovascular disease, type 2 diabetes mellitus and all-cause mortality in female survivors of DVA [7]. Moreover, the social and economic cost of DVA was totalled at £66,192 million for 2016–2017 in England and Wales [11], and the global cost of violence against women is thought to amount to approximately 2% of the global gross domestic product (GDP), equivalent to $1.5 trillion [12].

13.2 Background

In 2018, Heywood et al. conducted a qualitative study into the 'thrivership' process; how an individual can move from simply 'surviving' to positively 'thriving' after DVA [13]. Initially developed as a post-graduate dissertation, later published in Women's Health BMC Journal as an empirical paper, it was hoped that studying this topic would allow further exploration of how women recover from long-term DVA, so that others may be enabled to achieve the same sense of thriving. The term 'survivor' is often used within this context. However, heralding 'surviving' abuse as the end goal does not necessarily represent the optimal outcome for healing [14]; 'survivor' crucially fails to explore the long-term nature of recovery from abuse, focusing instead on more immediate freedom [15]. 'Thrivership' offers a resolution to these issues; if someone thrives, they 'prosper' or 'flourish' [16]. Thus, thriving exceeds the absence of problems to signify vigorous, even superlative health and well-being [17]. The study resulted in the development of the Thrivership Model (see Fig. 13.1).

The Thrivership Study involved 37 female participants in qualitative focus groups, all of whom had experienced DVA from a male intimate partner and were recruited via WE:ARE: Women's Empowerment And Recovery Educators; a well-established, independent charitable organisation providing a unique pathway of awareness and empowerment programmes (see Table 13.1), with additional support, for women who have experienced DVA in Birmingham, UK. An evaluation of WE:ARE services took place simultaneously to the Thrivership Study by the same researchers, the findings of which have been partly incorporated into this chapter.

This chapter explores how women can be empowered to move from simply surviving, to positively thriving post-DVA. The core concepts of the 'Thrivership Model'—'Provision of Safety; 'Sharing the Story', and 'A Social Response'—are used as a framework to illustrate the practical ways in which women can be empowered, with examples of WE:ARE's important work in this area. Several reflective exercises have been included to encourage readers to contemplate topics covered in further detail. References are provided, all of which we recommend for further reading on this topic, and participant quotes have been included with assigned numbers to protect participant identity. It is intended that practitioners and students within the health and social care sector who may encounter survivors, consider how they might adopt the model.

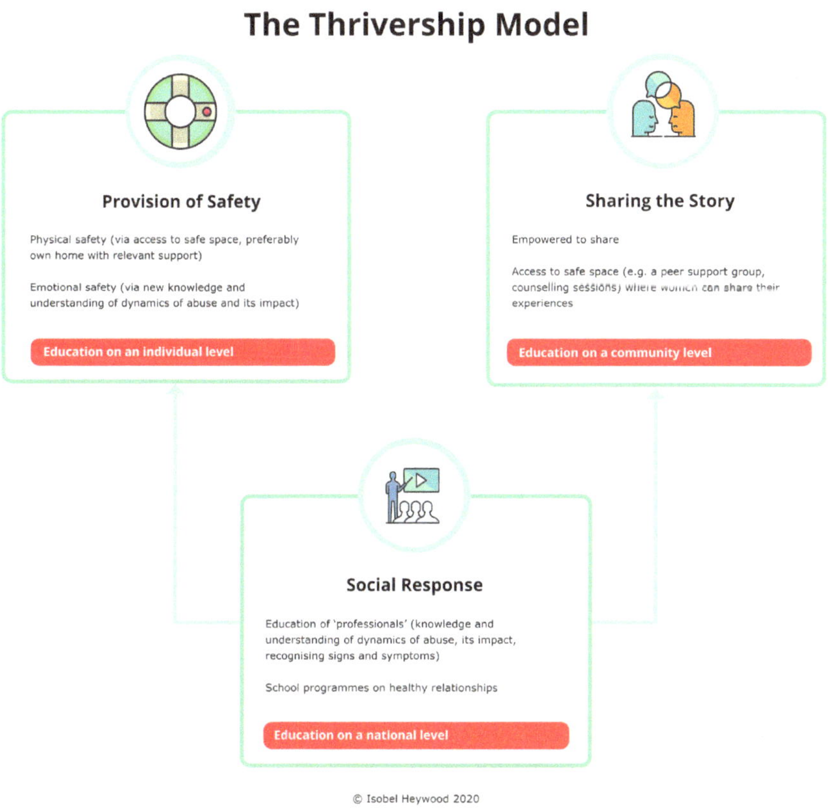

The Thrivership Model

Provision of Safety

Physical safety (via access to safe space, preferably own home with relevant support)

Emotional safety (via new knowledge and understanding of dynamics of abuse and its impact)

Education on an individual level

Sharing the Story

Empowered to share

Access to safe space (e.g. a peer support group, counselling sessions) where women can share their experiences

Education on a community level

Social Response

Education of 'professionals' (knowledge and understanding of dynamics of abuse, its impact, recognising signs and symptoms)

School programmes on healthy relationships

Education on a national level

© Isobel Heywood 2020

Fig. 13.1   The Thrivership Model (Revised version 2020)

13.2.1 Empowering Women to Thrive

The Thrivership Model (Fig. 13.1) by Heywood et al. illustrates the fundamental requirements for thriving post-DVA. The key components are: (1) Provision of Safety, (2) Sharing the Story, (3) Social Response. 'Education' and building awareness around DVA at an individual, community or national level is required for the model to be successfully implemented [13].

13.3   Provision of Safety

"Knowledge is everything"—P32

The Thrivership Study found that 'provision of safety' is needed for women to thrive—physical safety and emotional safety. Physical safety typically came via women having a *'safety bubble'* of their own—preferably their own home. Once

Table 13.1 WE:ARE Programme Pathway

Programme	Author and website	Focus	After-session activity
Freedom Programme	Pat Craven freedomprogramme.co.uk	Explores the abusive tactics, controlling behaviours and belief systems of the personas of the dominator and the effects on women and children's health and well-being [18]	Yoga
You and Me, Mum	Adapted by Women's Aid Northern Ireland Available via: womensaid.org.uk	Aims to empower and support survivors in furthering their understanding of their role as mothers and in addressing the needs of children and young people who have lived with domestic abuse [19]	Art class
Own My Life	Natalie Collins Ownmylifecourse.org.uk	Using a feminist approach to empowerment, educates women about the impact abuse has on an individual, within the context of wider societal patriarchal power structures [20]	Zumba

All programme sessions delivered within group setting. Additional one-to-one support provided by WE:ARE team members, and via partnerships with various local agencies, depending on individual needs. Information available at weareuk.org

physical safety had been obtained, women said they could begin moving towards *'emotional safety'*, or *'psychological safety'*, developed via the acquisition of knowledge of abuser tactics and behaviour and an understanding of the impact of abuse on an individual. Recovery via the development of internal resources and assertiveness skills was also highlighted [13].

When women self-refer to WE:ARE, they may be just out of an abusive relationship, or long-term separated. They commonly arrive feeling anxious and confused, experiencing feelings of self-doubt ('Was it abuse?' 'Am I the problem?'), imposter syndrome ('What I've experienced can't be as bad as what others have experienced'), guilt or self-blame. The journey to emotional safety therefore begins with women being supported to 'name' and acknowledge the abuse that took place so that the individual can process what has happened to them.

The first programme in the WE:ARE pathway is Pat Craven's Freedom Programme [18]. Sessions explore abusive tactics, controlling behaviours and belief systems of the 'dominator' [21] (see Fig. 13.2). Women begin to recognise similarities between session content and their own experiences. They become able to name abusive tactics and the psychology of abuse, which helps dissipate the confusion they had previously experienced and leads to a recognition that they are not to blame for what has happened. They begin to realise that what they believed to be true— that they are stupid, worthless, useless, ugly—because that is what they had constantly been told, is not, and they can work towards building confidence and self-worth. Additionally, women have reported that new knowledge of abuser tactics leads to an ability to recognise 'red flags' early on in future potential partners. Once completed or when women feel ready, they are invited to move on to the 'You and

THE DOMINATOR IS HIS NAME
CONTROLLING WOMEN IS HIS GAME

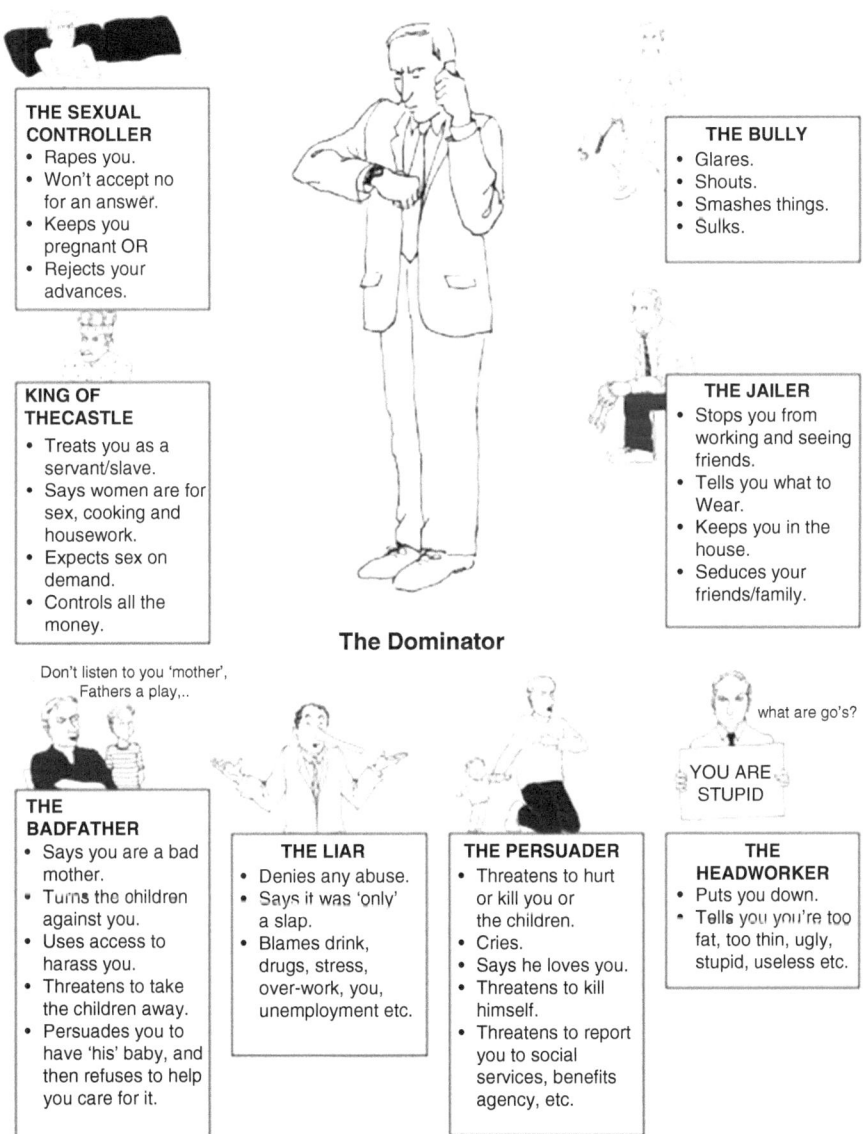

THE SEXUAL CONTROLLER
- Rapes you.
- Won't accept no for an answer.
- Keeps you pregnant OR
- Rejects your advances.

THE BULLY
- Glares.
- Shouts.
- Smashes things.
- Sulks.

KING OF THE CASTLE
- Treats you as a servant/slave.
- Says women are for sex, cooking and housework.
- Expects sex on demand.
- Controls all the money.

THE JAILER
- Stops you from working and seeing friends.
- Tells you what to Wear.
- Keeps you in the house.
- Seduces your friends/family.

The Dominator

Don't listen to you 'mother', Fathers a play,...

what are go's?

YOU ARE STUPID

THE BADFATHER
- Says you are a bad mother.
- Turns the children against you.
- Uses access to harass you.
- Threatens to take the children away.
- Persuades you to have 'his' baby, and then refuses to help you care for it.

THE LIAR
- Denies any abuse.
- Says it was 'only' a slap.
- Blames drink, drugs, stress, over-work, you, unemployment etc.

THE PERSUADER
- Threatens to hurt or kill you or the children.
- Cries.
- Says he loves you.
- Threatens to kill himself.
- Threatens to report you to social services, benefits agency, etc.

THE HEADWORKER
- Puts you down.
- Tells you you're too fat, too thin, ugly, stupid, useless etc.

Fig. 13.2 The Dominator. (With permission from: Craven, P, 'Living With The Dominator' Freedom Publishing, 2008)

Me, Mum' Programme (if they have children) and/or the 'Own My Life' Programme. Both build on women's new foundation of knowledge, by exploring how the abuse may have impacted them and how they can support themselves moving forward.

'You and Me, Mum' [19] empowers and supports mothers in addressing the needs of their children after DVA. Sessions involve developing an understanding of the impact of domestic abuse on the mother–child relationship and developing strategies to promote healing, understanding the child's needs, roles and behaviours and exploring key Protective Behaviour messages to keep both mother and child safe from further harm [19]. Women report significantly improved *'emotional attachment'* (P25) with their children, and a deeper understanding of how they can heal together.

'Own My Life' incorporates a more holistic view of abuse and recovery; using a feminist approach, it educates women about the impact of abuse on an individual, within the context of patriarchal power structures and dominance of women in society [20]. Sessions build women's trauma-literacy, enabling them to understand ways they have responded to abuse (i.e. coping or survival strategies such as placation, or self-blame), how to recognise triggers, and developing positive coping mechanisms to replace previous survival tactics which no longer serve them. Issues are explored within the context of male entitlement and controlling behaviour, socio-political education around what drives abuser behaviour, and identifying misogyny and patriarchy in media, history and across society [20].

Interestingly, women reported that unpicking abuse in this way and being able to put their experiences into words 'equips and empowers' them to represent themselves in high-pressure situations with those they labelled *'professionals'* (P33, P11) (e.g. social workers, judges, police); women could confidently articulate their experiences and the complex dynamics of abusive relationships and its impact on them and their children, in (e.g.) family court or meetings with social workers. Representing themselves when needed contributed to new assertiveness skills, self-confidence and a feeling of control over their lives [13].

WE:ARE is a trauma-informed service; programme content and delivery methods emphasise the physical, psychological and emotional safety of those attending sessions. Upon initial arrival, some women struggle to sit in a room of people they do not know, in an unfamiliar space. They might be thinking 'is he looking thought the window', 'will he walk in', 'does someone here know me' and 'do I have to open up': all very real and rational fears. Attending for the first time can be potentially traumatic, so it is vital to create a welcoming environment promoting a sense of safety; recognise signs of trauma in women who attend and any staff or volunteers; understand the coping mechanisms adopted in response to past traumas and ensure that women have a choice about attending and how long they want to stay.

Women are invited to attend an initial WE:ARE session with no obligation to stay and no intrusive questions asked. The Freedom Programme is run continuously so that women can join or leave at any point and are consistently welcomed back until they are ready to participate fully. Thus, individuals control the process and are empowered to manage their own safety, as they develop a familiarity with the setting. They become able to stay in the room for longer periods, as they manage their own physiology, and can take in information, eventually managing to fully interact with session content. Additionally, sessions are interactive and innovative with facilitators using a range of tools and props to articulate complicated concepts in easy-to-understand ways. Movement, games and creative activities help release stress and provide fun and laughter once stolen from women's lives and now reclaimed. Each programme session has a therapeutic activity afterwards (yoga, Zumba or art), providing an opportunity for reflection, decompression and socialising. The WE:ARE evaluation highlighted the importance of an informal and friendly approach, contrasting it to other 'professionals', whom, women felt, often spoke *at* them.

One final consideration relating to the first element of the Thrivership Model is that of physical safety. Many women are forced to flee to escape abuse, despite a preference to stay in their homes. Unfortunately, refuge spaces available in England and Wales still fall short (by 1684) of the Council of Europe's minimum recommendation, and most declined referrals to refuges in 2019 (64.1%) were due to lack of capacity [22]. Furthermore, abuser isolation tactics often lead to a loss of social network, meaning women may not have friends or family to stay with, leaving them vulnerable to further abuse, or homelessness. To support women towards physical safety, WE:ARE host weekly drop-in sessions at their base where women can access agencies such as Cranstoun, who provide one-to-one advisory services, developing individualised safety and housing plans—Women's Aid have developed The Survivor's Handbook [23] providing focused guidance in this area—and undertaking risk and need assessments using the Domestic Abuse, Stalking and Honour-Based Violence (DASH) model [24].

Reflective Exercise 1

For each of the 'dominator' personas in Fig. 13.2, consider and make a note of:

- Four more tactics each might use.
- Two beliefs that might exist behind each persona.
- Two belief reinforcements (e.g. If police do not arrest following reporting; influence of the media).
- Two beliefs that the women being abused might begin to share.
- How these tactics and behaviours might impact on the person being abused (e.g. her behaviour, health, her beliefs, emotions and relationships with others).

13.4 Sharing the Story

'...by talking about it you realise that actually you are believed, and actually that is a big deal...'—P18

Overwhelmingly, participants in the Thrivership Study reported that discussing their experiences with someone was a significant part of their thrivership journey. 'Sharing the story' in this way was commonly mentioned within the context of a

Fig. 13.3 Dear Friend Letter

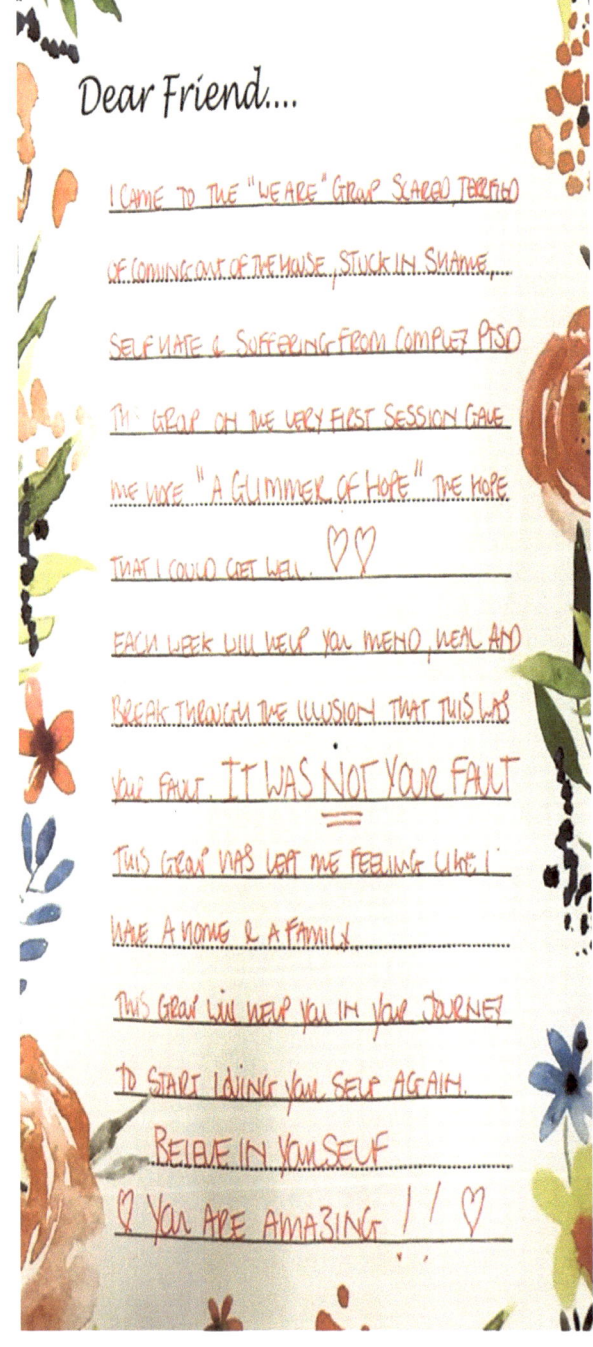

Dear Friend....

I CAME TO THE "WE ARE" GROUP SCARED, TERRIFIED OF COMING OUT OF THE HOUSE, STUCK IN SHAME, SELF HATE & SUFFERING FROM COMPLEX PTSD THIS GROUP ON THE VERY FIRST SESSION GAVE ME MORE "A GLIMMER OF HOPE" THE HOPE THAT I COULD GET WELL. ♡♡

EACH WEEK WILL HELP YOU MEND, HEAL AND BREAK THROUGH THE ILLUSION THAT THIS WAS YOUR FAULT. IT WAS NOT YOUR FAULT

THIS GROUP HAS LEFT ME FEELING LIKE I HAVE A HOME & A FAMILY

THIS GROUP WILL HELP YOU IN YOUR JOURNEY TO START LOVING YOUR SELF AGAIN.

BELIEVE IN YOURSELF

♡ YOU ARE AMAZING ! / ♡

'peer group' of other women who had also experienced DVA, which provided a new, positive social network and contributed to a feeling of mutuality. Sharing with others gave them ownership over the past and a chance to heal. Crucial to this component is the availability of services (e.g. support groups, counsellors) and a culture within which women feel they can share their story free from judgement [13].

Psychological trauma commonly leaves those affected feeling disempowered and disconnected from others; the recovery process, therefore, should be based upon empowerment of the survivor and restoration of positive relationships [25]. Abusers often use isolation as a key tactic, separating their partners from friends and family to maintain control, and the resulting loneliness can harm a person's health and well-being, their confidence and their ability to trust others. Even once an individual has left the abuser, this isolation can continue due to habit, depression, shame or as a coping mechanism. WE:ARE attendees reported that the group setting of programme delivery made them recognise that they were not alone in their experiences, as they may have thought previously. Receiving group support alongside other survivors led to women feeling 'believed' and having their experiences validated as others understood and could empathise. Furthermore, being part of a group of women with shared experiences provides a source of friendship, belonging and support, bringing an end to isolation. After-programme activities and larger social events such as twice-yearly celebration days, all encourage further socialising outside of programme sessions, increasing the new sense of community as new social networks are formed, which continue long term. Once women have completed WE:ARE programmes, they are invited to write a 'Dear Friend' letter (see Fig. 13.3). Letters provide an opportunity for the writer to anonymously share their story of recovery, giving hope and encouragement to those thinking of coming along for the first time. Letters are on display at the project base, on social media and on WE:ARE's YouTube channel.

WE:ARE utilise a Protective Behaviours 'one-step removed' approach to explore sensitive topics to avoid triggers and re-traumatisation of individuals involved in group sessions; utilising the fictional character 'Anne' (instead of 'I' or 'me', cf. Exercise 2), alongside fictitious scenarios and case studies, during group sessions, allows participants to take part in discussions without directly talking about their own situation. Personal information is principally kept for workbooks or worksheets, providing a private tool for women to relate sessions back to their own experiences.

Group settings are incredibly effective, but triggers or emotional contagion remain a risk, even when using a Protective Behaviours approach. Sessions must be managed closely by trained and empathetic practitioners, with additional support provided if needed. Group sessions may not be for everyone, and some individuals may be better supported on a one-to-one basis; women who need in-depth, focused support at WE:ARE are referred to a partner agency domestic abuse key worker who provides individualised sessions for up to 6 months.

13.5   A Social Response

'My next-door neighbour was a GP…and the judge quoted him saying 'if you don't know to look for domestic violence you won't see it'. And I actually thought that was a really good point…'—P20

In the Thrivership Study, women reported mixed experiences with 'professionals' (e.g. police officers, social workers and health workers) during their recovery, though negative interactions were common, and hindered individuals' recovery often leaving them feeling further victimised. These interactions included misdiagnosis with (e.g.) Borderline Personality Disorder, rather than symptoms being recognised as reactions to trauma—a common misconception [26]; police dismissing concerns or reports by victims; and social workers criticising mother's parenting skills and blaming them for the impact of the abuse on children. Women said a 'social response' to DVA is needed, with a predominant focus on education of 'professionals' [13].

Negative interactions like those highlighted indicate a lack of awareness and understanding of abuse and its impact on individuals affected. Thus, providing those who may encounter survivors through their work with the appropriate knowledge and information around the complex dynamics of domestic abuse, how to recognise abuse, and the pathway of support available to survivors, can minimise the likelihood of negative interactions and improve support. For example, social workers must recognise that victims have their resources and 'space for action' limited [27] by the central tactics of coercive control [28]; leaving an abusive relationship is therefore not straightforward, nor is it necessarily the safest option, as leaving is the most dangerous point in an abusive relationship. Additionally, women who have experienced DVA are at a threefold risk increase of developing depression, anxiety or schizophrenia, than women who have not [29]; may be dependent on nicotine, alcohol or drugs [30] or may exhibit physical signs like bruises or broken bones. Thus, primary healthcare professionals are well-placed to identify cases and be a valuable resource for victims [31]. Schemes such as IRIS (Identification & Referral to Improve Safety) have been shown to be successful [32] in providing general practices with comprehensive training on DVA assessment, interventions and responding to concern [33].

WE:ARE deliver educational workshops for sector workers providing attendees with improved knowledge of how support programmes contribute to a woman's healing, and the dynamics of abuse and its impact. Often using the fictional character of 'Anne' in interactive activities, attendees are encouraged to develop an understanding of how perpetrator's actions impact Anne's health, well-being and behaviour, by considering: 'what does it look like, feel like, sound like, to be Anne?', 'What are her self-blaming thoughts, do they match what you are thinking about her?, 'How might she be feeling?', 'What survival strategies might she use to cope with the abuse?', 'Think about your own coping strategies when under intense stress', 'Imagine being blamed for doing the best you can at that time—how would that feel?', 'Name Anne's many strengths'.

WE:ARE advocate that lived-experience individuals are the experts on their own lives, and by learning from them we can better provide for survivors. Indeed, NICE guidance recommends sector consultation with survivors and encourages local strategic partnerships with involvement of front-line practitioners and service users [34]. In 2020, WE:ARE launched the 'Collaborative Communicators' project which provides training for former programme attendees who are thriving, to develop public speaking, assertiveness and communication skills, so that they can then go on to deliver educational workshops for front-line workers. Furthermore, women can train to co-facilitate Own My Life programme sessions for future groups, using their new skills and knowledge to help other survivors. By training lived-experience individuals to become advocates in this way, sector workers can learn from the ultimate experts whilst the individual is empowered by her new experiences.

Alongside learning from organisations like WE:ARE, key agency workers who work with survivors can participate in their local Multi-Agency Risk Assessment Conference (MARAC); a victim-focused information sharing and risk management meeting attended where high-risk cases are discussed [35]. Additionally, organisations such as SafeLives and Women's Aid offer focused training around abuse for police forces, MARACs, front-line workers, IDVAs (Independent Domestic Violence Advisor) and facilitators, and in 2019 the University of Sheffield launched their 'Supporting Victims of Domestic Violence' online course for health and social care workers.

Finally, we would like to highlight that thrivership is a personal, fragile process that does not happen overnight. Women participating in the Thrivership Study spoke of a common expectation from family, friends and wider society that they should recover almost immediately after leaving an abusive partner. This is an unrealistic expectation; it takes time to heal from the damage caused by abuse. Recovery is a 'fluid' (P21), long term and non-linear journey, with a vulnerability to triggers that can cause fluctuation between individuals identifying as a 'victim', 'survivor' and 'thriver' [13], and individuals should not feel pressured to recover by a certain point. They require ongoing, flexible support. WE:ARE run the Freedom Programme on a continuous basis and deliver sessions for all three programmes on consecutive days, meaning women can progress to the next programme immediately. Furthermore, women can return to the organisation to re-take programmes (or if they simply need someone to talk to) for as long as is needed for them to feel that they are thriving. Moreover, WE:ARE provide a free of charge crèche on-site, and free course workbooks, to improve accessibility to programs for under-resourced individuals. Similar additional considerations could be providing transport funds for attendees and delivering evening or online programmes for those working during the day.

13.6   Conclusion

This chapter has provided insight into how women who have experienced DVA can be empowered to thrive long term. Using the work of WE:ARE as a 'best practice' example, we have indicated how the core elements of the Thrivership Model (Fig. 13.1) can be implemented in practice by DVA services, and how those who work in Health and Social Care may learn from it. To this end, there have been several key messages throughout the chapter. The first relates to the provision of safety, as the first step towards thrivership; in order to be empowered towards emotional safety, survivors need access to knowledge and tools about abuse and its impact, so that they can make sense of their experiences and move forward. We have provided examples of programs that are effective in this area, and how they can be used in conjunction with one another, and within the context of trauma-informed care, to achieve this.

Secondly, we have explored how empowerment can result from survivors having the opportunity to 'share the story' of abuse, and how this can be done safely and successfully within a group setting using a Protective Behaviours approach. Access to a group of other survivors provides an end to isolation, and bonding via mutuality of shared experiences, so that women no longer feel alone. Lastly, we have looked at how education of others—particularly those who are likely to encounter survivors or victims—can contribute to a social response to abuse, leading to better informed care and support. Even better is when thrivers are empowered to provide this education themselves; learning from thrivers in this way offers access to their knowledge pool and facilitates the empathy needed from professionals who work with them and wider society. We encourage readers to use the references to immerse themselves further in what is an important public health issue that affects people at all levels of society, worldwide.

References

1. Bradbury-Jones C, Appleton JV, Clark M, Paavilaine EA. A profile of gender-based violence research in Europe: findings from a focused mapping review and synthesis. Trauma Violence Abuse. 2017;4:470–83. https://doi.org/10.1177/1524838017719234.
2. World Health Organization. Understanding and addressing violence against women. 2012. https://apps.who.int/iris/bitstream/handle/10665/77433/WHO_RHR_12.35_eng.pdf?sequence=1. Accessed 4 Jul 2019.

3. World Health Organization. Violence against women. 2017. https://www.who.int/news-room/fact-sheets/detail/violence-against-women. Accessed 3 Jan 2018.
4. Crown Prosecution Service. Domestic abuse. 2017. https://www.cps.gov.uk/domestic-abuse. Accessed 25 Apr 2019.
5. Women's Aid. What is domestic abuse? 2019. https://www.womensaid.org.uk/information-support/what-is-domestic-abuse/. Accessed 23 Apr 2020.
6. Office for National Statistics. Domestic abuse victim characteristics, England and Wales: year ending March 2019. 2019. https://www.ons.gov.uk/peoplepopulationandcommunity/crimean-djustice/articles/domesticabusevictimcharacteristicsenglandandwales/yearendingmarch2019. Accessed 23 Apr 2020.
7. Singh Chandan J, Thomas T, Bradbury-Jones C, Taylor J, Bandyopadhyay S, Nirantharakumar K. Risk of cardiometabolic disease and all-cause mortality in female survivors of domestic abuse. J Am Heart Assoc. 2020. https://doi.org/10.1161/JAHA.119.014580.
8. García-Moreno C, Zimmerman C, Morris-Gehring A, Heise L, Amin A, Abrahams N, Montoya O, Bhate-Deosthali P, Kilonzo N, Watts C. Addressing violence against women: a call to action. Lancet. 2015;385(9978):1685–95. https://doi.org/10.1016/S0140-6736(14)61830-4.
9. García-Moreno C, Jansen HAFM, Ellsberg M, Heise L, Watts CH. Prevalence of intimate partner violence: findings from the WHO multi-country study on women's health and domestic violence. Lancet. 2006;368:1260–9. https://doi.org/10.1016/S0140-6736(06)69523-8.
10. Campbell JC. Health consequences of intimate partner violence. Lancet. 2002;359(9314):1331–6. https://doi.org/10.1016/S0140-6736(02)08336-8.
11. Oliver R, Alexander B, Roe S, Wlasny M. Home Office. The economic and social costs of domestic abuse. 2019. https://assets.publishing.service.gov.uk/government/uploads/system/uploads/attachment_data/file/772180/horr107.pdf. Accessed 23 Apr 2020.
12. Lakshmi P. The economic costs of violence against women: remarks by UN assistant secretary-general and deputy executive director of UN women, at the high-level discussion on the "economic cost of violence against women". September 21, 2016. https://www.unwomen.org/en/news/stories/2016/9/speech-by-lakshmi-puri-on-economic-costs-of-violence-against-women.
13. Heywood I, Sammut D, Bradbury-Jones C. A qualitative exploration of 'thrivership' among women who have experienced domestic violence and abuse: development of a new model. BMC Womens Health. 2019. https://doi.org/10.1186/s12905-019-0789-z.
14. Merritt-Gray M, Wuest J. Counteracting abuse and breaking free: the process of leaving revealed through women's voices. Health Care Women Int. 1995;16(5):399–412. https://doi.org/10.1080/07399339509516194.
15. Allen K, Wozniak D. The language of healing: women's voices in healing and recovering from domestic violence. Soc Work Ment Health. 2010;9(1):37–55. https://doi.org/10.1080/15332985.2010.494540.
16. Concise Oxford English Dictionary. Thrive. Oxford: Oxford University Press; 2011.
17. Poorman P. Perceptions of thriving by women who have experienced abuse or status-related oppression. Psychol Women Q. 2002;26(1):51–62. https://doi.org/10.1111/1471-6402.00043.
18. The Freedom Programme. What is the Freedom Programme? 2018. https://www.freedompro-gramme.co.uk/. Accessed 23 Apr 2020.
19. Women's Aid. You and me, mum: facilitation programme. 2019. https://www.womensaid.org.uk/what-we-do/training/facilitator-training/mum-facilitation-programme/. Accessed 17 Apr 2020.
20. Own My Life Course. Why? Core values. 2018. https://www.ownmylifecourse.org/why. Accessed 23 Apr 2020.
21. Craven P. Living with the dominator: Freedom Publishing; 2008.
22. Women's Aid. The domestic abuse report 2020: the annual audit. Bristol: Women's Aid; 2020.
23. Women's Aid. The survivor's handbook. 2009. https://www.womensaid.org.uk/the-survivors-handbook/print-and-audio-versions/. Accessed 16 Apr 2020.
24. DASH Risk Model. What is the aim of the DASH Risk Identification and Assessment Model? 2009. https://www.dashriskchecklist.co.uk/dash/. Accessed 26 Apr 2020.
25. Herman JL. Trauma and recovery; the aftermath of violence—from domestic abuse to political terror. New York: Basic Books; 1997.

26. Mind. Post-traumatic stress disorder (PTSD). https://www.mind.org.uk/information-sup-port/types-of-mental-health-problems/post-traumatic-stress-disorder-ptsd/complex-ptsd/. Accessed 23 Apr 2020.
27. Kelly L, Sharp N, Klein R. Finding the costs of freedom: how women and children rebuild their lives after domestic violence. Solace Women's Aid; 2003.
28. Stark E. Domestic violence report. Coercive control: the entrapment of women in personal life. Oxford: Oxford University Press; 2009.
29. Chandan J, Thomas T, Bradbury-Jones C, Russell R, Bandyopadhyay S, Nirantharakumar K, Taylor J. Female survivors of intimate partner violence and risk of depression, anxiety and serious mental illness. Br J Psychiatry. 2019:1–6. https://doi.org/10.1192/bjp.2019.124.
30. Long J, Harper K, Harvey H. The Femicide Census: 2017 findings. 2020. https://1q7dqy2unor827bqjls0c4rn-wpengine.netdna-ssl.com/wp-content/uploads/2018/12/Femicide-Census-of-2017.pdf. Accessed 23 Apr 2020.
31. Evans MA, Feder GS. Help-seeking amongst women survivors of domestic violence: a qualitative study of pathways towards formal and informal support. Health Expect. 2015;19(1):62–73. https://doi.org/10.1111/hex.12330.
32. Bradbury-Jones C, Clark M, Taylor J. Abused women's experiences of a primary care identification and referral intervention: a case study analysis. J Adv Nurs. 2016;73(12):3189–99. https://doi.org/10.1111/jan.13250.
33. IRISi. How the IRIS programme can support your practice and patients. https://irisi.org/iris/how-can-iris-help/. Accessed 17 Apr 2020.
34. NICE. Domestic violence and abuse: multi-agency working. 2014. https://www.nice.org.uk/guidance/ph50/chapter/1-Recommendations. Accessed 23 Apr 2020.
35. Safe Lives. For MARACs. https://safelives.org.uk/training/maracs. Accessed 17 Apr 2020.

Laura L. Jones and Juliet Albert

14.1 Introduction

In this chapter, we will mainly draw on UK-based examples of female genital mutilation (FGM) research and practice as this is where we are based and so are most familiar. We anticipate that the knowledge and principles of good practice gained from engaging with the information below will be transferable to a range of different settings. Providing a safe space where those affected by FGM can be heard is key, whatever your role and wherever you are based. It is however important to recognise that there can be local, national and international variation in FGM legislation, policy and guidelines and so you will need to familiarise yourself with these in the place where you are working.

14.2 What Terminology Should You Use When Discussing FGM?

The practice of FGM is known by a range of different terms including female circumcision, female genital cutting and female genital excision [1]. The terms 'cut', 'closed' and, to some extent increasingly, FGM are used by diaspora communities living in the UK; however, they may not always be understood as women and girls may use other traditional terms specific to their community such as Sunna, Tahoor and Khitan [2]. The National FGM Centre has published a list of traditional terms which is helpful when working with affected communities [3].

L. L. Jones (✉)
University of Birmingham, Birmingham, UK
e-mail: L.L.Jones@bham.ac.uk

J. Albert
Imperial College Healthcare NHS Trust, London, UK
e-mail: juliet.albert@nhs.net

© Springer Nature Switzerland AG 2021   217
C. Bradbury-Jones, L. Isham (eds.), *Understanding Gender-Based Violence*,
https://doi.org/10.1007/978-3-030-65006-3_14

The World Health Organisation (WHO) uses the term FGM (as will we herein) to make it clear that the practice is a serious violation of human rights, differentiating it from male circumcision, and emphasising the harmfulness of the act [4]. The term female genital cutting is advocated by some affected communities and agencies working with these communities as they may perceive that the term 'mutilation' is stigmatising and can impact efforts to support eradication of the practice. The WHO strongly advocates that the term female circumcision not be used as it implies that male and female circumcision are comparable, which is not the case, creating confusion and potentially undermining understanding of the significant consequences of FGM for women and girls [4].

The key when discussing FGM with affected women and communities is to try to avoid using judgmental and value-laden language. It is often helpful to ask what term they would prefer to use and ensure that you both understand what that term means.

Reflection 1: Thinking About Terminology

- What term(s) have you heard FGM referred to as before, if any?
- What term(s) might you use in your own practice going forward? Might this change depending on who you are talking to?
- Why is it important to think carefully about the term(s) that you use?

14.3   What Is FGM?

Female genital mutilation involves the partial or total removal of, or injury to, the external female genitalia for non-medical reasons [5]. A joint statement from WHO/UNICEF/UNFPA published in 1997 categorised FGM into four main types (types 1–4; Fig. 14.1) [6]. A further seven subtypes (types 1a, b; 2a–c; 3a, b) were subsequently identified to capture more closely the potential for significant variation in practice [6, 7]. It is important to recognise that there are limitations to the typology of FGM. However,

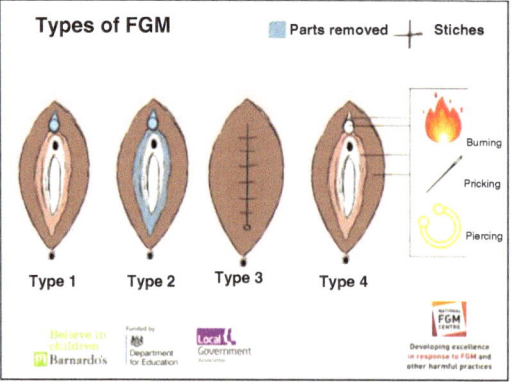

Type 1 (Clitoridectomy): Partial or total removal of the clitoral hood and/or clitoral glans.

Type 2 (Excision): Partial or total removal of the clitoral glans and inner labia and/or outer labia

Type 3 (Infibulation): Usually includes partial or total removal of the clitoral glans and inner labia and/or outer labia, with inner and/or outer labia sewn/fused together leaving a small hole.

Type 4 (Other harmful procedures): Any other injury to the genitalia including piercing, scraping, burning, stretching or pricking.

Fig. 14.1 Classification of the different types of female genital mutilation (adapted and used with permission from the National FGM Centre [9, 10])

evidence would suggest that, in general, the amount of genital tissue removed increases from type 1 to type 3, with type 3 (also known as infibulation) the most extensive [8].

14.3.1 What Is Deinfibulation?

Women and girls with type 3 FGM (infibulation) may require surgery, known as deinfibulation (or opening surgery), to divide the scar tissue covering the vaginal opening [5]. In England, the NHS publishes a list of National FGM Specialist Clinics with information about each clinic and how they can be contacted—many of these offer deinfibulation [11]. The WHO has suggested that deinfibulation improves health and well-being [12] and recommends it to prevent and/or treat obstetric complications [4]. However, the evidence to support these statements is relatively limited and of low quality highlighting the need for further research in this area.

There is no agreement as to when it is best for a survivor to be deinfibulated [12–14], although a large UK qualitative study [15] is currently ongoing to address this issue. The Royal College of Obstetricians and Gynaecologists (RCOG) guidelines suggest that deinfibulation can take place at a number of different time points in a woman's life: prior to pregnancy (preferably before first sexual intercourse), during the antenatal period, in the first stage of labour and at the point of delivery [16]. The WHO FGM clinical handbook states that women and girls with type 3 should be counselled, as early as possible, around deinfibulation including before and/or during pregnancy to support informed decision-making about whether and when to have the procedure [4].

14.3.2 What Is Reinfibulation?

Reinfibulation is the practice of re-stitching the external genitalia of women with type 3 FGM following childbirth or gynaecological procedures [17, 18]. It is difficult to accurately estimate the number of women who are re-infibulated as girls, and women may experience several cycles of infibulation and re-infibulation (typically during or following childbirth) [17]. In 2010, Serour suggested that 50–80% of women and girls living with type 3 may undergo reinfibulation [17]. Reinfibulation is reportedly practiced predominantly to enhance male sexual pleasure [19] and is a further violation of the girl's or woman's human rights [4].

Refection 2: What Is FGM?

- Could you give a definition of FGM if asked?
- How would you describe the four different types?
- Which type is the most extensive?
- When do you think the best time is for deinfibulation? Is there one?
- Would your explanation of what FGM is change depending on who you were talking to?

14.4   How Big Is the Problem of FGM Globally?

Female genital mutilation is an increasing global concern as a result of international migration and mobility [20]. It has been practiced for millennia [21] and is most closely associated with 31 predominantly African countries [22]. In 2020, UNICEF reported that it may be performed in as many as 50 countries including in Eastern Europe, Latin America, South-Eastern Asia and the Middle East and amongst diaspora communities in Western Europe, North America and Australia [22]. The National FGM Centre has developed an interactive map providing information such as FGM prevalence rates, terminology and legislation for different countries across the world—this is a helpful resource when discussing FGM with diverse patient/client populations [23]. Whilst it is difficult to know the exact number of women and girls who have undergone FGM due to a lack of robust representative data, it is estimated that at least 200 million live with the consequences of FGM globally [20, 22]. This equates to roughly 5% of the total global female population (~3.86 billion) [24]. It is anticipated that this number will rise significantly over the next 15 years as the world population grows and more girls undergo the procedure [20].

Female genital mutilation is a form of violence against women and girls and is a violation of their human rights [25]. The practice now forms part of the United Nations 2015 Sustainable Development Goals (SDG) [26]. Sustainable Development Goal 5 aims to achieve gender equality and empower all women and girls [26]. One of the targets associated with Goal 5 (SDG 5.3) is to eradicate FGM by 2030 [26]. UNICEF recently highlighted that FGM is becoming slightly less common in some countries where it was historically universal (for example in Djibouti, Egypt, Ethiopia and Sudan); however, in other countries little has changed over the last 30 years (for example in Somalia, Guinea and Gambia) [22]. To meet the SDG of eradicating FGM by 2030, it is estimated that even in the countries where the prevalence is reducing, progress would need to be at least 10 times greater than it is currently [22].

14.4.1 How Big Is the Problem of FGM Nationally and Locally?

As highlighted earlier, it can be very challenging to accurately estimate the prevalence of women and girls who have undergone FGM living in a particular country—this is also true for UK FGM diaspora [27, 28]. Using 2011 census data, MacFarlane and Dorkenoo estimated that at least 137,000 women and girls were living with the consequences of FGM in England and Wales at that point in time [29]. Between 2008 and 2011, it was estimated that survivors of FGM accounted for 1.5% of all women giving birth in England and Wales [29]. Van Baelen et al. also used 2011 Census data to estimate European prevalence of foreign-born women and girls over the age of 10 years with FGM reporting that 178,781 were living in the UK [30]. Irrespective of the exact numbers, the research of MacFarlane and Dorkenoo suggested that FGM was present in all local authorities in England and Wales [29] and so it is likely that FGM is an issue that all health and social care professionals may come across at some point.

Since 2015, NHS Digital has collected detailed data about FGM within the patient population through the Female Genital Mutilation Enhanced Dataset (FGMED) from English NHS acute trusts, mental health trusts and GP practices [31]. These data are reportedly used to better inform FGM prevalence estimates at a population level and support service planning and provision in England [32]. Between 2015 and 2019, the FGMED identified 20,470 previously unrecorded cases of FGM and 40,030 health care attendances relating to, or involving notification of, FGM in England [27]. It is important to interpret these data with caution as suggested by NHS Digital and others such as Karlsen et al. who concluded that they are deeply problematic [28]. For example, since inception only 62% of NHS Trusts and 2% of general practices have submitted data to the FGMED [27].

Other sources of FGM-related data include the Department for Education annual Children in Need (CIN) statistics which report where FGM has been identified at the end of an assessment in each English local authority area [33]. In 2018/2019, FGM was identified in 0.2% (approximately 1000 cases) of assessments [34]. As part of the Family Court statistics, the Ministry of Justice publishes the number of FGM Protection Orders (FGMPO) (see "What are FGM Protection Orders and how can they help" section for further information) issued in England and Wales each quarter [35]. Between July 2015 when FGMPOs were introduced and December 2019, 547 orders have been granted [36]. From April 2019, police forces in England and Wales are mandated to record honour-based abuse crimes, including FGM [37].

Reflection 3: How Big Is the Problem of FGM?

- How many women and girls are thought to have been cut around the world?
- Why do you think that it is difficult to collect reliable data on FGM?
- Where can you access information about the prevalence of FGM by country?
- What data are collected around FGM and where might you find them in the sector where you work (for example health, social, education, police)?
- How likely is it that you will meet women and girls affected by FGM as part of your everyday practice?

14.5   What Are the Immediate, Short-Term and Long-Term Consequences of FGM?

There are no health benefits of FGM, and all women and girls who have experienced FGM are likely to report some physical and psychological complications [4]. Women and girls with more extensive FGM appear to experience more severe complications [8, 38]. A large number of FGM-related health consequences have been identified that can be immediate, short term and/or long term [4]. Figure 14.2 provides an overview of some of these consequences.

Immediate	Shorter term	Longer term
• Severe pain and injury to genital tissues • Haemorrhage and haemorrhagic shock • Acute urinary retention • Urinary, vaginal, uterine infections • Septicaemia • Trauma to adjacent tissues • Transmission of blood borne viruses (Hepatitis B, HIV) • Death • Fracture of bones (from being held down during the practice)	• Delayed wound healing • Scarring/keloid formation • Pelvic infection • Epidermoid cysts/abscesses • Neuroma	• Reproductive tract infections • Haematocolpos-impaired flow of menstrual blood • Dysmenorrhoea-painful menstruation • Dysuria-painful and difficult urination • Dyspareunia-difficult or painful sexual intercourse • Morbidity and mortality during pregnancy and childbirth • Pelvic inflammatory disease/infertility • Psycho-sexual and-social trauma • Mental health issues • Increased risk of HIV transmission • Death

Fig. 14.2 Summary of the key immediate, short- and long-term impacts of female genital mutilation (collated and adapted from [4, 8, 10, 38–40, 42, 44, 47, 48])

The impacts of FGM reach far wider than just physical health, and whilst challenging to categorise, in general, include psychological, psychosexual, social and economic consequences [8, 39–48]. Female genital mutilation is associated with adverse mental health outcomes [38]. For example, compared to women without FGM those with FGM are at an increased risk of developing psychological disorders such as post-traumatic stress disorder, anxiety and low self-esteem [47, 48]. Impaired sexual function is commonly reported amongst women with FGM, including increased pain during intercourse, reduced ability to become physiologically stimulated, lower desire and sexual satisfaction when compared to uncut women [47, 48].

The economic impacts of FGM can be significant at individual, societal and governmental levels [49]. The physical consequences of FGM such as pain and infection can reduce girls' school attendance, performance and employment opportunities [50]. Survivors are more likely to enter into a child (<18 years of age) or early marriage [51]. Girls typically bear children shortly after their early marriage and have high overall fertility rates further limiting their education and longer term prospects [52]. In 2020, the WHO, using a novel FGM Cost Calculator [53], estimated that the annual financial cost of healthcare for FGM survivors was 1.4 billion US dollars globally [54]. It is predicted that by 2050, these costs could increase by up to 50% if the practice of FGM is not abandoned [54]. In 2016, the annual cost of NHS care for FGM survivors in the UK was estimated at £100 million [23], this is similarly likely to increase going forward as a result of growing migration of FGM diaspora to the UK.

It is important to consider that not just women experience the consequences of the FGM, men also report issues including psychological dissatisfaction and sexual frustration, with some articulating that they perceive themselves to also be victims of the practice [55–57].

14.6   Who Performs FGM and How Is It Done?

Female genital mutilation is usually performed by designated 'traditional cutters' who are almost exclusively older women within the community [18]. However, the UNFPA has reported that FGM may also be carried out by other female relatives, traditional birth attendants, traditional health practitioners, herbalists or even male barbers [18]. Cutters may use a range of different instruments to perform FGM (e.g. razor blades, scissors, and sharpened rocks, shards of glass), often in unhygienic conditions and without pain relief [18]. Girls who experience type 3 FGM may have their legs bound for a period of time (7–14 days) after the procedure to facilitate scar formation [18].

There is also evidence that FGM (and reinfibulation) is being performed in clinical settings, at home or elsewhere by doctors, midwives, nurses and/or other trained healthcare professionals [4, 18]. This is known as 'medicalised' FGM and is often carried out using surgical tools, antiseptics and anaesthetics with the incorrect perception that this will mitigate complications and reduce harm [4, 58, 59]. Drawing on population-level survey data from 26 countries, 21% of women aged 15–49 years (~16 million) reported being cut by a healthcare provider [58, 60]. The vast majority (93%) of women who report being cut by a healthcare provider live in Egypt, Sudan and Nigeria [58, 60]. In 2010, a joint interagency global strategy was published to stop healthcare providers from performing FGM [59]. Despite the increasing global criticism, legal regulation and overarching consensus to end FGM, rates of medicalised FGM appear to be increasing [58–60].

14.7   Is FGM Associated with Other Forms of VAWG?

Female genital mutilation is a violation of the human rights of women and girls [25]. The practice is deeply entrenched in gender inequalities and discrimination [5, 18] and as highlighted previously is a form of violence against women and girls (VAWG) [61]. Unlike some other forms of VAWG, females are not only subjected to FGM but they are typically the ones who subject other women and girls to the violence and may help to ensure the continuation of the practice [61]. For some women and girls, FGM may constitute a singular instance of violence against them. For others, however, it might be associated with other forms of honour-based violence and domestic abuse [62]. One example of this is where women (and potentially girls) are subjected to both FGM and forced marriage [63].

14.8 Why Is FGM Practiced?

A large number of reasons or justifications for why FGM is practiced have been identified and these can vary between affected communities and cultures [4, 5]. The UNFPA [18] and the WHO [4] provide comprehensive summaries of the reasons why FGM is practiced including: psychosexual, sociological, cultural, hygiene and aesthetics, religious and socio-economic factors. It is important to know that FGM is a socio-cultural practice and is not supported or required by religious groups or scripture [4, 5, 18]. Figure 14.3 provides an overview of the main reasons identified for why FGM is practiced.

Reflection 5: Who, How and Why Is FGM Practiced?

- Who performs FGM in most cases?
- Can you explain what medicalised FGM is?
- Can you identify five reasons why FGM is practiced?
- Is FGM associated with other forms of violence against women and girls?

Sociological and cultural reasons

- Historical and cultural tradition
- Respect for elders in the community
- Social convention
- Acceptance and status in the community
- Bound in strong societal pressures to conform
- Community identity
- Gender inequalities-issues of male coercion and control
- Myths (e.g. an uncut clitoris will grow into a penis, FGM enhances fertility and promotes child survival)
- Rite of passage from childhood to womanhood

Psychosexual reasons

- Control a woman's sexuality
- Preservation of virginity prior to marriage
- Ensure fidelity after marriage
- Increase male sexual pleasure
- Protects a girl's and her family's honour

Socioeconomic factors

- Prerequisite for marriage and right to inherit
- Income generation for traditional cutters

Hygiene, aesthetic and femininity reasons

- Cut genitals perceived as clean and beautiful
- Spiritual purity
- More hygienic
- Clitoris seen as masculine and so removal increases perceived femininity

Marriageability

- Preparation and eligibility for marriage
- Men only marry cut women

Religious reasons

- Religious obligation

Fig. 14.3 Summary of the key reasons why female genital mutilation is practised (collated and adapted from [4, 18])

14.9 What Is the Legal Context Around FGM, Specifically in the UK?

This section covers the FGM legislative context that shapes professional practice. Female genital mutilation is illegal in at least 59 countries including the UK [18]. The countries of the UK (England, Scotland, Wales and Northern Ireland) have different legislation around FGM. We will try to point these differences out but there is a need to be familiar and keep up to date with the laws and local policies/guidelines in the country within which you are working. Female genital mutilation has been illegal in the UK since 1985 as a result of the Prohibition of Female Circumcision Act 1985 [64]. Figure 14.4 provides an overview of the key information and offences associated with the different FGM Acts but more detailed

Prohibition of Female Circumcision Act 1985	Female Genital Mutilation Act 2003 and Prohibition of Female Genital Mutilation (Scotland) Act 2005	Serious Crime Act 2015 and Female Genital Mutilation (Protection and Guidance) (Scotland) Act 2020
Act UK wide	Combination of Acts UK wide	Combination of Acts UK wide
It was an offence for any person to: Excise, infibulate or otherwise mutilate the whole or any part of the labia majora or labia minora or clitoris of another person; or, Aid, abet, counsel or procure the performance by another person of any of those acts on that other person's own body. **A person guilty of this offence was liable to:** On conviction on indictment, to a fine or to imprisonment for a term not exceeding five years or to both.	**Offence of FGM*:** A person is guilty of an offence if he excises, infibulates or otherwise mutilates the whole or any part of a girl's labia majora, labia minora or clitoris. **Offence of assisting a girl to mutilate her own genitalia:** A person is guilty of an offence if he aids, abets, counsels or procures a girl to excise, infibulate or otherwise mutilate the whole or any part of her own labia majora, labia minora or clitoris. **Offence of assisting a non-UK person to mutilate overseas a girl's genitalia:** A person is guilty of an offence if he aids, abets, counsels or procures a person who is not a UK national or UK resident to do a relevant act of FGM outside the UK. **Offence of failing to protect girl from risk of genital mutilation:** If a genital mutilation offence is committed against a girl under the age of 16, each person who is responsible for the girl at the relevant time is guilty of an offence.	**The 2003 and 2005 FGM Acts now includes:** An offence of failing to protect a girl from the risk of FGM. Extra-territorial jurisdiction over offences of FGM committed abroad by UK nationals and those habitually, as well as, permanently resident in the UK. Lifelong anonymity for victims of FGM. FGM Protection Orders which can be used to protect and safeguard victims and potential victims of FGM.

Fig. 14.4 Summary overview of the key information and offences associated with the different female genital mutilation acts in the UK (collated and adapted from [64–70]). *By definition this includes reinfibulation of a girl or woman following the birth of a baby

information should be reviewed regularly and as a starting point can be accessed via the following references [64–70].

14.9.1 What Is the Offence of 'Failing to Protect a Girl from FGM'?

As part of the Serious Crime Act 2015, a new offence was introduced focussing on the responsibility that parents have to protect their daughter(s) from FGM and the associated criminal liability should they fail to take adequate preventive action [71]. The rationale for the introduction of this offence was that if it is established that a girl has been subjected to FGM, then her parents have failed to protect her from the violence [71]. Christou and Fowles have written an excellent in-depth article on failing to protect girls from FGM that explores the issues from a legal perspective [71].

14.9.2 What Are FGM Protection Orders and How Can They Help?

Female genital mutilation protection orders are a civil order that can be made to protect a girl or woman who is at risk of FGM or who has been subjected to the practice [65]. An FGMPO may include, for example, ordering the surrender of passports to prevent a girl from being taken abroad where she may be at risk of FGM [65, 72]. Confidential applications can be made to the court by the individual at risk/ has had FGM, a local authority or another person with permission from the court such as a family member or teacher [65, 72]. More information about applying for FGMPOs, conditions of the orders and breaches can be found here [65, 72, 73].

14.9.3 What Does FGM Mandatory Reporting Duty Involve and Who Does It Apply To?

In England and Wales, all regulated health and social care professionals and teachers are mandated by law to report 'known' cases of FGM in girls under 18 years of age, identified as part of their work, to the police [62, 65]. 'Known' cases are those where a girl herself discloses that she has undergone FGM or where a professional observes evidence on a girl's genitals that she may have been cut [65]. This legal duty has been in place since October 2015 [62]. Mandatory reporting is a personal duty which means that the professional who identifies the FGM or receives the disclosure must make the report—it cannot be transferred [62]. The Department of Health and NHS England have created an excellent resource pack to support regulated professionals with FGM mandatory reporting duty [74], including a decision-making infographic that can be followed if you are worried about a girl in relation to FGM [75]. If you are concerned that a girl or woman is at imminent risk or has very recently been subjected to FGM, you should contact the police immediately via 999.

Whilst the duty only applies to regulated professionals, those who are not regulated should follow appropriate safeguarding action [76, 77] in relation to suspected cases of FGM in girls [62]. Mandatory reporting does not apply in the following circumstances: (a) an adult woman over the age of 18 years discloses that she has had FGM, (b) a parent or guardian discloses that his/her child has had FGM, (c) a professional thinks a girl might have had FGM but she has not disclosed and they have not seen any signs/symptoms and (d) a professional is aware that a case has already been reported by a regulated professional in their organisation. In these situations, local safeguarding action needs to be followed.

14.9.4 What Does FGM Mandatory Recording Involve?

In addition to the FGM mandatory reporting duty, there are two further requirements for NHS organisations and professionals in relation to recording and sharing FGM risks and information in England [78]. These include the FGMED (see earlier section on "How Big Is the Problem of FGM Nationally and Locally?") [32] and the FGM information sharing system (FGM-IS) [79]. The FGM-IS is a digital system that allows NHS professionals to share information where there is a history of FGM in the family of a girl under the age of 18 years [78, 79]. This system facilitates early intervention and ongoing safeguarding of girls who might be at risk of FGM [78, 79].

Reflection 6: FGM Legal Context in the UK?

- Could you briefly outline the law in England and Wales to a colleague?
- What is mandatory reporting and who does it apply to?
- Could you explain what a 'known' case means in relation to FGM mandatory reporting?
- What is mandatory recording?

14.10 Why Is It Important That We Use a Multi-Faceted and Multi-Agency Approach to Safeguarding Around FGM?

To effectively address the complexities around FGM, legislation is needed in combination with, for example (a) education and training of professionals, (b) improved service provisions, (c) commitment from the government and (d) engagement with and empowerment of diaspora communities [80, 81]. Due to the nature of their (potentially) regular interactions with affected girls and women, professionals such as those working in health, social care and education may be well placed to provide education, support and services around FGM [80, 81].

Safeguarding and supporting women and girls affected by FGM can be challenging for a number of reasons. Firstly, it can be difficult to identify girls that are at risk of FGM, as well as those that have undergone FGM. Secondly, there is no one homogenous FGM-affected community as such, rather there are diverse number of peoples from different parts of the world all with their own cultural and social norms and traditions. Thirdly, FGM is often perceived as a 'taboo' subject that is surrounded by shame, stigma and secrecy [82].

In 2016, the Departments for Education and Health and Social Care in collaboration with the Home Office issued 'Multi-agency Statutory Guidance of Female Genital Mutilation' for those working in England and Wales [65]. The multi-agency guidance has three key functions to provide: (a) information on FGM, (b) strategic guidance on FGM and (c) advice and support to front-line professionals [65]. This is further supported by specific guidance on FGM risk and safeguarding for healthcare professionals which includes an excellent FGM safeguarding risk assessment framework [83]. For social care professionals, the National FGM Centre has created a good practice guide and assessment tool to support social workers to assess risk, gather further information and actions to consider [84]. It is important to know that these different pieces of guidance should be considered in line with local policies on safeguarding children and vulnerable adults, for example [76, 77].

14.11 What Are the Key Factors to Consider When Assessing if a Girl or Woman Is at Risk of or Has Recently Undergone FGM?

The vast majority (~80%) of women over the age of 18 who are affected by FGM are identified when they access maternity services [32]. It can be more difficult to identify girls under the age of 18 and non-pregnant women, although they might present throughout the NHS or in social care. In some cases, women and girls may directly disclose that they have undergone FGM to a professional. In rare cases, they might be identified by chance, such as by a nurse if a woman presented for a cervical smear test or by a paediatrician if a child required catheterisation.

It is important to consider a wide range of factors when assessing whether a girl or woman is at risk of FGM including whether she has a family history of FGM and if she is from an FGM affected community [65]. Figure 14.5 provides a summary of potential risk factors of which to be aware. In addition to knowing about potential risk of harm, professionals need to also consider the signs that a girl or woman might have recently undergone FGM [65]. Figure 14.6 provides a summary of potential indicators to be aware of. It is likely that a number of these factors and/or indicators, in combination, will alert a professional to consider if FGM is an issue.

14.11.1 How Can You Ask About FGM Appropriately?

Female genital mutilation can be hard to talk about even as an experienced professional. It can take time to build confidence and skills in how to raise the issue of FGM sensitively and without judgement. NHS Choices have made a video resource

Factors to consider when assessing whether a girl or woman may be at risk of FGM

- Girl's mother has undergone FGM
- Girl has other family members (e.g. older siblings and/or cousins) that have undergone FGM
- Girl's father comes from a FGM affected community
- Family indicate strong influence of elders and/or elders are involved in raising girls
- Woman/family believe FGM is important to their cultural and/or religious identity
- Persons responsible for the girl (e.g. parents) lack knowledge and awareness of the harms of FGM or the UK law
- Girl discloses that she is to have a procedure or attend an event to 'become a woman'
- Girl discusses plans to take a long holiday to a FGM affected country
- Persons responsible for the girl (e.g. parents) disclose that they or a relative are planning to take the girl out of the UK for an extended period

- Parents or family members express concern that the girl might be at risk of FGM
- Parents or family are not engaging with professionals (e.g. health, education, social care)
- Parents or family are known to professionals (e.g. social workers) in relation to other safeguarding concerns
- Girl requests help from a professional (e.g. a teacher) or adult as she is worried that she may be subjected to FGM
- Girl talks about FGM in conversation with other (the context of the discussions is important to consider)
- Girl from affected community is withdrawn from PSHE education and/or from lessons covering FGM
- Girl is unexpectedly absent from school
- Girl has attended a clinic for travel related vaccinations and/or anti-malarial prescription

Fig. 14.5 Factors to consider when assessing whether a girl or woman may be at risk of FGM (adapted from [65])

Indicators that a girl or woman may have recently undergone FGM

- Girl/woman asks for help
- Girl/woman tells a professional that they have undergone FGM
- Mother/family member discloses that a girl has undergone FGM
- Girl/family is already known to professionals (e.g. social workers) in relation to other safeguarding concerns
- Girl/woman has difficulty walking, sitting or standing or looks uncomfortable
- Girl/women finds it hard to sit still for long periods of time when this was not a problem previously
- Girl/woman spends longer that normal using the toilet due to difficulties urinating
- Girl/woman has frequent urinary, menstrual or stomach issues

- Girl spends long periods of time away from the classroom during the day with bladder and/or menstrual difficulties
- Girl avoids physical exercise or is excused from physical education lessons without a medical letter
- Prolonged or repeated absences from school, college or work
- Increased emotional and psychological needs (e.g. withdrawal or depression) or significant changes in behaviour
- Girl/woman reluctant to undergo medical examinations
- Girl/woman asks for help but is not explicit about the reason
- Girl/woman talks about pain or discomfort between her legs

Fig. 14.6 Indicators that a woman or girl may have recently undergone FGM (adapted from [65])

[85] where survivors talk about their personal experiences of FGM which might be a helpful starting point. The setting (e.g. clinic, home, school) within which the issue of FGM has become apparent and who (e.g. a child vs. an adult) is involved in the conversation are important contextual considerations for the professional [65]. A failure to discuss FGM appropriately may lead to loss of trust in the relationship, distress to the individual(s) and ultimately may result in a girl or woman undergoing FGM when it could potentially have been prevented. Figure 14.7 provides a

Ensuring sensitivity and appropriateness of the conversation

- Your primary concern is the care of the girl/woman affected by FGM
- Treat her as an individual
- Respect her dignity
- Be open and honest–tell her what is happening and why
- Act with integrity
- If needed, use an accredited and trained female interpreter
- Do not allow family members or members of the community known to the girl/woman to act as an interpreters
- Allow enough time for the conversation

Building rapport during the conversation

- Do not be afraid to ask about FGM
- Try to use culturally sensitive language
- Be aware of the different terms that are used for FGM
- Allow the girl/woman to speak
- Only ask one question at a time
- Leave time between questions
- Don't interrupt her story
- Be encouraging
- Seek her permission to discuss very sensitive topics (e.g. how, when, where she was cut)
- Have access to resources and information about services to support the conversation

At the start of the conversation

- Try to start the conversation sensitively
- Be aware of your own views on FGM
- Try not to be judgmental
- Try to be aware of the context within which the girl/woman is presenting to you
- Remember that not all girls/women know that they have undergone FGM, especially if it took place when they were young
- Try not to make assumptions based on her ethnicity, religion and/or country of origin

Example conversations starters

- *"I notice that you come from a country where some girls/women may have been cut. How do you feel about this?"*
- *"You have mentioned cutting and the traditions in your community. Is there anything else you want to tell me about this?"*
- *"How does your partner/husband feel about girls/women being cut?"*
- *"How does your family feel about girls/women being cut?"*
- *"In your community, at what age are females usually cut?"*
- *"I can see in your notes that you have been cut. Would you like to talk about this?"*

Fig. 14.7 Summary of the standards and advice in the multi-agency statutory guidance to support professionals to engage in sensitive and appropriate conversations around FGM (adapted from [65])

summary of the standards and advice in the multi-agency statutory guidance [65] to support professionals to engage in sensitive and appropriate conversations, supplemented by our own experiences of interacting with women and girls affected by FGM. Examples of other questions that you can ask as part of a structured risk assessment can be found in the FGM Safeguarding Risk Assessment Guidance for healthcare professionals [83] and in the FGM Good Practice Guidance and Assessment Tool for Social Workers [84].

14.12 What Do You Need to Know About Safeguarding, Referrals and Information Sharing Around FGM?

Professionals have reported confusion, following the introduction of mandatory data recording and reporting around when referrals need to be made to other services such as Children's Social Services [83]. There are four groups to think about when safeguarding around FGM: (a) children and vulnerable adults who have undergone FGM, (b) children and vulnerable adults who are at risk of FGM, (c) women who are not pregnant and do not have daughters and (d) women who are pregnant and/or have daughters. Figure 14.8 provides a summary of the guidance produced by the Department of Health about what to do for each of these groups [83]. The FGM Risk and Safeguarding guidance also includes a useful list of the information sharing processes and responsibilities of different professional groups [83].

Children (and vulnerable adults) who are thought to have undergone FGM

- HISTORIC CASE-If a girl (< 18 years) discloses to a regulated professional that she has *had* FGM, or if the professional observes that she has *had* FGM but this is an HISTORIC case they should make a referral to children's social care. This will be discussed at a Multi-Agency Safeguarding Hub. Police may need to become involved to confirm the circumstances when FGM was carried out; to ensure no other siblings/children are at risk of FGM; and a specialist paediatrician may be required to confirm FGM has taken place. If other children are considered at risk see section below. In England and Wales ONLY: if a girl (< 18 years) discloses to a regulated professional that she has had FGM, or if the professional observes that she has had FGM, they are mandated to report to the police via 101.
- RECENTLY CUT-If a girl (<18 years)is identified as having recently been cut (i.e. bleeding from the genital area) this is child abuse and a crime and the Police would need to be contacted via 999 and the child taken to Accident and Emergency. The on call consultant paediatrician; local safeguarding leads and children's services will be involved as part of a multi-agency response.
- If a vulnerable adult is identified or suspected as having had FGM, professional needs to follow existing safeguarding procedures for vulnerable adults
- If an adult discloses that a girl has *had* FGM – this is a report of child abuse and a crime. Follow local safeguarding processes (which usually means a referral to Social Services). This may require a report to the police for further investigation.
- Always consider the wider family context of girls who might have had FGM.

Children (and vulnerable adults) who are thought to be at risk of FGM

- URGENT-If a child (or vulnerable adult) is *suspected* of being at serious or imminent risk of FGM then an urgent referral should be made to Children's Services and the Police should be contacted immediately via 999 - as there is a risk that the child or other children may be taken out of the country and Border Force may need to be involved.
- NON-URGENT -If a child (or vulnerable adult) is considered to be at risk of FGM but that risk is NO I thought to be serious or imminent then local safeguarding procedures (e.g. a discussion with the local safeguarding lead and sharing of information between agencies) should be followed to facilitate potential intervention.

Adult women who are not pregnant and/or do not have daughters

- *No requirement* for automatic referral of adult women with FGM to Adult Social Services or the Police
- Need to remember that it might be the first time the adult woman has talked about FGM
- Assess each case individually and consider referral to support services such as NHS FGM Clinic or FGM community groups
- Respect the wishes of the adult woman but inform her of her right to make a police criminal report against her perpetrators
- Explore with the adult woman about risk of FGM for other females e.g. cousins, younger sisters etc.

Fig. 14.8 Summary guidance on safeguarding, referral and information sharing around FGM (adapted from [83])

Women who are pregnant and/or adult women who have daughters

- All pregnant women should be asked if they have FGM at booking. If they disclose FGM they should attend a safeguarding appointment for an FGM risk assessment. This discussion should include the woman's extended family, including woman's partner and partner's extended family.
- If low risk of carrying out FGM on a female infant, share information with GP and health visitor
- If high risk a social care referral must be made and a multi-agency strategy meeting to decide upon a plan to safeguard any female infant and other female children in the household. (May require an FGM Protection Order or child to be taken into care).
- Whenever a woman with FGM gives birth to a female infant or if the female infant's father is from an FGM practising community-this information must be shared with relevant healthcare professionals such as GP and health visitor (and if in England complete FGM-IS).
- If an adult woman discloses that her daughter(s) <18 years has(ve) *already undergone* FGM a social care referral must be made. This will establish where and when FGM took place and whether other female children in the family, such as younger siblings or the female children of siblings are at risk (see HISTORIC CASE in section above).
- If an adult woman discloses that her adult daughter(s) (> 18 years) has(ve) *already undergone* FGM you may not need to make a social care referral. You need to establish where and when FGM took place and whether other female children in the family or the female children of siblings are at risk.
- Always explore with the adult woman about risk of FGM for other daughters, cousins and wider family context, in particular male partners and their extended family must also be considered
- Depending on the outcome of the discussion, information should be recorded and shared with multi-agency partners as necessary

Fig. 14.8 (continued)

Department of Health FGM Risk Assessment Checklist

Have you:

- Discussed FGM with the girl/women and their family
- Completed an FGM risk assessment template
- Recorded your actions and the outcome of the assessment on the patient's healthcare record
- Followed your local safeguarding process and made a referral to children's social care, if appropriate
- Reported a known case of FGM to a child under 18 to the police under the FGM mandatory reporting duty, if appropriate
- Shared relevant information with other health professionals including the GP, health visitor, school nurse, your local safeguarding lead
- Provided a copy of the patient leaflet 'More information about FGM' (available for free in 11 languages)

Fig. 14.9 Department of Health FGM Risk Assessment Checklist (adapted from [86])

The Department of Health guidance also provides information and templates for practitioners on how to make an initial assessment of risk for women (including those who are pregnant/have recently given birth) and children who come from FGM-affected communities (see Annex 1 in [83]). Figure 14.9 highlights the Department of Health's FGM Risk Assessment Checklist [86] which can be used as a quick reference guide to ensure that you have followed each of the safeguarding steps as a health professional. If you are unsure about what you need to do with regard to FGM, you can contact the NSPCC helpline on 0800 0283550 or via email on fgmhelp@nspcc.org.uk for advice.

14.13   Applying Your Learning to a Real-Life Case Study

Having read the chapter to this point, Fig. 14.10 provides you with a real-life example of safeguarding a pregnant FGM survivor. What would you have done as the midwife in this situation?

Key Concepts

This list provides a summary of the key concepts and anticipated outcomes having read the chapter.

- FGM involves the partial or total removal of, or injury to, the external female genitalia for non-medical reasons.
- FGM is a form of violence against women and girls and is a violation of their human rights.
- FGM is an increasingly global concern thought to be practiced in more than 50 countries.
- Globally, at least 200 million women and girls are living with the consequences.
- There are no health benefits of FGM, and all women and girls who have experienced FGM are likely to report some health problems including physical and psychological complications.
- FGM is usually performed by traditional cutters but rates of medicalised cutting are increasing.
- FGM is performed for a range of different reasons including cultural, religious and psychosexual.
- FGM is illegal in at least 59 countries, including the UK.
- Regulated health and social care professionals and teachers in England and Wales are mandated by law to report 'known' cases of FGM to the police.
- Safeguarding around FGM can be challenging and requires a multi-faceted and multi-agency approach.
- The key for front-line professionals is that they are able to assess if FGM might occur and if FGM has occurred.
- A range of guidance is available, including risk assessment tools, to support front-line professionals to recognise and respond appropriately to FGM.
- Together, professionals can make a difference to the lives of girls and women affected by FGM.

Case study scenario

A woman who is 30 weeks pregnant (SM) disclosed to the FGM team (specialist midwife, health advocate and counsellor) during her FGM clinic appointment that she was being pressurised by her mother to return home to her country of origin with her new born baby girl. Upon her return, her daughter would be cut.

SM was born in Ethiopia. She suffered FGM age five years old. She has two children, both male, and is pregnant with her third child, a girl. She is currently separated from her husband and he has a new partner who is also pregnant. SM has previously suffered from severe postnatal depression. SM was deinfibulated during the birth of her first child but was found to have been reinfibulated at the time of birth of her second child. SM disclosed that this was carried out whilst on holiday in Ethiopia and that her mother had suggested that she needed to be closed again because "the hole was too big". SM has problems with urinary incontinence and pain during sexual intercourse.

SM has previously had a designated social worker because of issues around domestic violence and poor mental health but her case is currently closed.

If you were the midwife in this situation, what would you have done?

Case study answer

The FGM midwife convened an emergency strategy meeting so that a discussion could be undertaken involving SM's social worker, maternity safeguarding lead, FGM specialist midwife and FGM health advocate. The FGM midwife recommended the local authority take out an FGM Protection Order. There was discussion around whether the new-born baby girl would be under imminent risk of FGM which the team agreed was the case. The Department of Health safeguarding guidance was used to help assess the level of the risk to the unborn baby girl.

The multi-agency professionals accessed the 28 Too Many resources on the age when girls are usually cut in Ethiopia and the world prevalence map from the National FGM Centre. The midwife needed to balance the risk of potential harms to the baby with her concerns about losing trust with SM. SM was involved in the subsequent conversations as transparency is very important as long as this did not put the baby at further risk.

In addition, SM is vulnerable and there were concerns regarding her mental health and ability to cope with three children as a single parent. She has already agreed to reinfibulation previously and informed professionals that her mother is very dominating. She says that she is keen to go and stay with her mother as soon as the baby is born. Her partner is not a protective factor as he is with a new partner who is also pregnant. SM was cut at five years of age but FGM can take place at any age in Ethiopia. Although FGM is illegal in Ethiopia, the law is not enforced and the practice continues.

An FGM risk assessment was carried out by the social worker. The local authority decided to take out an FGM Protection Order. The protection order was granted and the judge agreed to retain the baby's passport with Children's Social Care until she is 18 years of age. Relevant data were recorded and information shared as appropriate.

Fig. 14.10 Real-life case study of safeguarding around FGM

References

1. 28TooMany. Terminology and FGM. https://www.28toomany.org/thematic/terminology-and-fgm/. Accessed 7 May 2020.
2. NHS. Female genital mutilation (FGM). 2019. https://www.nhs.uk/conditions/female-genital-mutilation-fgm/. Accessed 7 May 2020.
3. National FGM Centre. Traditional terms for female genital mutilation. http://nationalfgm-centre.org.uk/wp-content/uploads/2017/12/FGM-Terminology-for-Website.pdf. Accessed 7 May 2020.
4. World Health Organization. Care of women and girls living with female genital mutilation: a clinical handbook, Geneva. 2018. https://www.who.int/reproductivehealth/publications/health-care-girls-women-living-with-FGM/en/.
5. World Health Organization. Female genital mutilation 2016. http://www.who.int/mediacentre/factsheets/fs241/en/. Accessed 21 Dec 2016.

6. World Health Organization. Female genital mutilation: a Joint WHO/UNICEF/UNFPA Statement. World Health Organization, Geneva. 1997. http://apps.who.int/iris/bitstream/10665/41903/1/9241561866.pdf. Accessed 20 April 2017.
7. World Health Organization. Sexual and reproductive health: classification of female genital mutilation. 2007. http://www.who.int/reproductivehealth/topics/fgm/overview/en/. Accessed 19 April 2017.
8. Banks E, Meirik O, Farley T, Akande O, Bathija H, Ali M. Female genital mutilation and obstetric outcome: WHO collaborative prospective study in six African countries. Lancet. 2006;367(9525):1835–41. https://doi.org/10.1016/S0140-6736(06)68805-3.
9. National FGM Centre. Female genital mutilation. 2020. http://nationalfgmcentre.org.uk/fgm/. Accessed 11 May 2020.
10. National FGM Centre. Potential health consequences of female genital mutilation. 2020. http://nationalfgmcentre.org.uk/wp-content/uploads/2019/02/FGM-and-Health-Consequences-Infographic-1.pdf. Accessed 11 May 2020.
11. NHS. National FGM Support Clinics—Female genital mutilation (FGM). 2019. https://www.nhs.uk/conditions/female-genital-mutilation-fgm/national-fgm-support-clinics/. Accessed 24 May 2020.
12. World Health Organization. Guidelines on the management of health complications from female genital mutilation. 2016. https://www.ncbi.nlm.nih.gov/books/NBK368491/.
13. Abdulcadir J, Rodriguez MI, Say L. Research gaps in the care of women with female genital mutilation: an analysis. BJOG. 2015;122(3):294–303. https://doi.org/10.1111/1471-0528.13217.
14. Esu E, Okoye I, Arikpo I, Ejemot-Nwadiaro R, Meremikwu MM. Providing information to improve body image and care-seeking behavior of women and girls living with female genital mutilation: a systematic review and meta-analysis. Int J Gynaecol Obstet. 2017;136(Suppl 1):72–8. https://doi.org/10.1002/ijgo.12058.
15. Jones L, Danks E, Clarke J, Alidu L, Costello B, Jolly K, et al. Exploring the views of female genital mutilation survivors, their male partners and healthcare professionals on the timing of deinfibulation surgery and NHS FGM care provision (the FGM sister study): protocol for a qualitative study. BMJ Open. 2019;9(10):e034140. https://doi.org/10.1136/bmjopen-2019-034140.
16. Royal College of Obstetricians & Gynaecologists. Female Genital Mutilation and its Management: Green-top Guideline No. 53. 2015. https://www.rcog.org.uk/globalassets/documents/guidelines/gtg-53-fgm.pdf. Accessed 21 Dec 2016.
17. Serour GI. The issue of reinfibulation. Int J Gynaecol Obstet. 2010;109(2):93–6. https://doi.org/10.1016/j.ijgo.2010.01.001.
18. United Nations Population Fund (UNPF). Female genital mutilation (FGM) frequently asked questions. 2015. http://www.unfpa.org/resources/female-genital-mutilation-fgm-frequently-asked-questions. Accessed 21 December 2016.
19. Berggren V, Abdel Salam G, Bergstrom S, Johansson E, Edberg AK. An explorative study of Sudanese midwives' motives, perceptions and experiences of re-infibulation after birth. Midwifery. 2004;20(4):299–311. https://doi.org/10.1016/j.midw.2004.05.001.
20. United Nations Children's Fund (UNICEF). Female genital mutilation/cutting: a global concern. 2016. https://www.unicef.org/media/files/FGMC_2016_brochure_final_UNICEF_SPREAD.pdf. Accessed 21 Dec 2016.
21. 28 Too Many. What are the origins and reasons for FGM? 2013. https://www.28toomany.org/blog/what-are-the-origins-and-reasons-for-fgm-blog-by-28-too-manys-research-coordinator/#:~:text=Some%20researchers%20have%20traced%20theBritish%20Museum%20dated%20163%20BC. Accessed 8 Oct 2020.
22. United Nations Children's Fund. Female genital mutilation: a new generation calls for ending an old practice. New York: UNICEF; 2020.
23. National FGM Centre. World FGM Map: Interactive Map. 2020. http://nationalfgmcentre.org.uk/world-fgm-prevalence-map/. Accessed 5 Jun 2020.
24. Worldometer. Worldometer—real time world statistics. https://www.worldometers.info/. Accessed 24 May 2020.

25. World Health Organization. Eliminating Female genital mutilation: An interagency statement (OHCHR, UNAIDS, UNDP, UNECA, UNESCO, UNFPA, UNHCR, UNICEF, UNIFEM, WHO). 2008. http://apps.who.int/iris/bitstream/10665/43839/1/9789241596442_eng.pdf. Accessed 19 Apr 2017.
26. United Nations. Transforming our world: the 2030 agenda for sustainable development A/RES/70/1. 2015. https://sustainabledevelopment.un.org/content/documents/21252030%20Agenda%20for%20Sustainable%20Development%20web.pdf. Accessed 11 May 2020.
27. Karlsen S, Howard J, Carever N, Mogilnicka M, Pantazis C. Establishing FGC/M prevalence in the UK. [Report]. In press. 2019.
28. Karlsen S, Mogilnicka M, Carver N, Pantazis C. Female genital mutilation: empirical evidence supports concerns about statistics and safeguarding. BMJ. 2019;364:l915. https://doi.org/10.1136/bmj.l915.
29. Macfarlane AJ, Dorkenoo E. Estimating the numbers of women and girls with female genital mutilation in England and wales. J Epidemiol Commun Health. 2015;69(A61).
30. Van Baelen L, Ortensi L, Leye E. Estimates of first-generation women and girls with female genital mutilation in the European Union, Norway and Switzerland. Eur J Contracept Reprod Health Care. 2016;21(6):474–82.
31. NHS Digital. SCCI2026: Female Genital Mutilation Enhanced Dataset. 2018. https://digital.nhs.uk/data-and-information/information-standards/information-standards-and-data-collections-including-extractions/publications-and-notifications/standards-and-collections/scci2026-female-genital-mutilation-enhanced-dataset#current-release. Accessed 18 May 2020.
32. NHS Digital. Female Genital Mutilation Datasets. 2020. https://digital.nhs.uk/data-and-information/clinical-audits-and-registries/female-genital-mutilation-datasets. Accessed 18 May 2020.
33. Department for Education. Statistics: children in need and child protection. 2019. https://www.gov.uk/government/collections/statistics-children-in-need. Accessed 24 May 2020.
34. Department for Education. Characteristics of children in need: 2018 to 2019. 2020. https://www.gov.uk/government/statistics/characteristics-of-children-in-need-2018-to-2019. Accessed 24 May 2020.
35. Ministry of Justice. Family court statistics quarterly: a collection giving National Statistics on activity in the family courts of England and Wales. 2019. https://www.gov.uk/government/collections/family-court-statistics-quarterly. Accessed 24 May 2020.
36. Ministry of Justice. Family Court Statistics Quarterly, England and Wales, October to December 2019 including 2019 annual trends. 2020. https://assets.publishing.service.gov.uk/government/uploads/system/uploads/attachment_data/file/874822/FCSQ_October_to_December_final.pdf. Accessed 24 May 2020.
37. Home Office. Annual data requirement from police forces in England and Wales. 2019. https://www.gov.uk/government/publications/annual-data-requirement-from-police-forces-in-england-and-wales. Accessed 24 May 2020.
38. Abdalla SM, Galea S. Is female genital mutilation/cutting associated with adverse mental health consequences? A systematic review of the evidence. BMJ Glob Health. 2019;4(4):e001553. https://doi.org/10.1136/bmjgh-2019-001553.
39. Berg RC, Underland V. The obstetric consequences of female genital mutilation/cutting: a systematic review and meta-analysis. Obstet Gynecol Int. 2013;2013:496564. https://doi.org/10.1155/2013/496564.
40. Berg RC, Underland V, Odgaard-Jensen J, Fretheim A, Vist GE. Effects of female genital cutting on physical health outcomes: a systematic review and meta-analysis. BMJ Open. 2014;4(11):e006316. https://doi.org/10.1136/bmjopen-2014-006316.
41. Bishai D, Bonnenfant YT, Darwish M, Adam T, Bathija H, Johansen E, et al. Estimating the obstetric costs of female genital mutilation in six African countries. Bull World Health Organ. 2010;88(4):281–8. https://doi.org/10.2471/BLT.09.064808.
42. Iavazzo C, Sardi TA, Gkegkes ID. Female genital mutilation and infections: a systematic review of the clinical evidence. Arch Gynecol Obstet. 2013;287(6):1137–49. https://doi.org/10.1007/s00404-012-2708-5.

43. Knipscheer J, Vloeberghs E, van der Kwaak A, van den Muijsenbergh M. Mental health problems associated with female genital mutilation. BJPsych Bull. 2015;39(6):273–7. https://doi.org/10.1192/pb.bp.114.047944.
44. Mpinga EK, Macias A, Hasselgard-Rowe J, Kandala NB, Felicien TK, Verloo H, et al. Female genital mutilation: a systematic review of research on its economic and social impacts across four decades. Glob Health Action. 2016;9:31489. https://doi.org/10.3402/gha.v9.31489.
45. Obermeyer CM. The consequences of female circumcision for health and sexuality: an update on the evidence. Cult Health Sex. 2005;7(5):443–61. https://doi.org/10.1080/14789940500181495.
46. Stein K, Hindin MJ, Chou D, Say L. Prioritizing and synthesizing evidence to improve the health care of girls and women living with female genital mutilation: an overview of the process. Int J Gynaecol Obstet. 2017;136(Suppl 1):3–12. https://doi.org/10.1002/ijgo.12050.
47. Berg RC, Denison E, Fretheim A. Psychological, social and sexual consequences of female genital mutilation/cutting (FGM/C): a systematic review of quantitative studies. Oslo, Norway: NIPH Systematic Reviews; 2010.
48. Buggio L, Facchin F, Chiappa L, Barbara G, Brambilla M, Vercellini P. Psychosexual consequences of female genital mutilation and the impact of reconstructive surgery: a narrative review. Health Equity. 2019;3(1):36–46. https://doi.org/10.1089/heq.2018.0036.
49. Refaei M, Aghababaei S, Pourreza A, Masoumi SZ. Socioeconomic and reproductive health outcomes of female genital mutilation. Arch Iran Med. 2016;19(11):805–11.
50. World Economic Forum. What is the economic cost of FGM? 2020. https://www.weforum.org/agenda/2020/02/female-genital-mutilation-economics-world-health-organization/. Accessed 4 Jun 2020.
51. Population Council. Exploring the association between female genital mutilation/cutting and early/child marriage. 2018. https://www.popcouncil.org/uploads/pdfs/2018RH_FGMC-ChildMarriage.pdf. Accessed 24 May 2020.
52. Nour NM. Health consequences of child marriage in Africa. Emerg Infect Dis. 2006;12(11):1644–9. https://doi.org/10.3201/eid1211.060510.
53. World Health Organization. Female genital mutilation cost calculator. 2020. https://srhr.org/fgmcost/. Accessed 18 May 2020.
54. World Health Organization. The economic cost of female genital mutilation. 2020. https://www.who.int/news-room/detail/06-02-2020-economic-cost-of-female-genital-mutilation. Accessed 18 May 2020.
55. Varol N, Turkmani S, Black K, Hall J, Dawson A. The role of men in abandonment of female genital mutilation: a systematic review. BMC Public Health. 2015;15:1034. https://doi.org/10.1186/s12889-015-2373-2.
56. Berggren V, Musa Ahmed S, Hernlund Y, Johansson E, Habbani B, Edberg A. Being victims or beneficiaries? Perspectives on female genital cutting and reinfibulation in Sudan. Afr J Reprod Health. 2006;10(2):24–36.
57. Fahmy A, El-Mouelhy MT, Ragab AR. Female genital mutilation/cutting and issues of sexuality in Egypt. Reprod Health Matters. 2010;18(36):181–90. https://doi.org/10.1016/S0968-8080(10)36535-9.
58. Kimani S, Shell-Duncan B. Medicalized female genital mutilation/cutting: contentious practices and persistent debates. Curr Sex Health Rep. 2018;10(1):25–34. https://doi.org/10.1007/s11930-018-0140-y.
59. World Health Organization. Global strategy to stop health-care providers from performing female genital mutilation. 2010. https://www.who.int/reproductivehealth/publications/fgm/rhr_10_9/en/. Accessed 24 May 2020.
60. Shell-Duncan B, Njue C, Moore Z. Trends in medicalisation of female genital mutilation/cutting: what do the data reveal? October 2018 (Update). In: Evidence to end FGM/C Research to help women thrive. Population Council, New York 2018. https://www.popcouncil.org/uploads/pdfs/2018RH_MedicalizationFGMC_update.pdf. Accessed 24 May 2020.
61. United Nations Women. Policy note. Female genital mutilation/cutting and violence against women and girls: strengthening the policy linkages between different forms of violence. In: Ending violence against women section. New York. 2017. https://www.unwomen.org/-/media/

headquarters/attachments/sections/library/publications/2017/policy-note-female-genital-mutilation-cutting-and-violence-against-women-and-girls-en.pdf?la=en&vs=905. Accessed 27 May 2020.

62. Department for Education and Home Office. Mandatory reporting of female genital mutilation—procedural information. 2016. https://assets.publishing.service.gov.uk/government/uploads/system/uploads/attachment_data/file/573782/FGM_Mandatory_Reporting_-_procedural_information_nov16_FINAL.pdf. Accessed 2 Jun 2020.

63. Foreign and Commonwealth Office, and Home Office. Guidance: forced marriage. 2020. https://www.gov.uk/guidance/forced-marriage#guidance-for-professionals. Accessed 4 Jun 2020.

64. The National Archives (legislation.gov.uk). Prohibition of Female Circumcision Act 1985. 1985. http://www.legislation.gov.uk/ukpga/1985/38/section/1?view=extent. Accessed 1 Jun 2020.

65. Department for Education, Department of Health and Social Care, and Home Office. Multi-agency statutory guidance on female genital mutilation. 2016. https://assets.publishing.service.gov.uk/government/uploads/system/uploads/attachment_data/file/800306/6-1914-HO-Multi_Agency_Statutory_Guidance.pdf. Accessed 1 Jun 2020.

66. The National Archives (legislation.gov.uk). Female Genital Mutilation Act 2003. 2003. http://www.legislation.gov.uk/ukpga/2003/31/contents. Accessed 1 Jun 2020.

67. The National Archives (legislation.gov.uk). Prohibition of Female Genital Mutilation (Scotland) Act 2005. 2005. http://www.legislation.gov.uk/asp/2005/8/contents. Accessed 1 Jun 2020.

68. The National Archives (legislation.gov.uk). Serious Crime Act 2015. 2015. http://www.legislation.gov.uk/ukpga/2015/9/pdfs/ukpga_20150009_en.pdf. Accessed 1 Jun 2020.

69. The National Archives (legislation.gov.uk). Female Genital Mutilation (Protection and Guidance) (Scotland) Act 2020. 2020. http://www.legislation.gov.uk/asp/2020/9/contents/enacted. Accessed 1 Jun 2020.

70. Ministry of Justice/Home Office. Serious Crime Act 2015 Factsheet—female genital mutilation. 2015. https://assets.publishing.service.gov.uk/government/uploads/system/uploads/attachment_data/file/416323/Fact_sheet_-_FGM_-_Act.pdf. Accessed 1 Jun 2020.

71. Christou TA, Fowles S. Failure to protect girls from female genital mutilation. J Criminal Law. 2015;79(5):344–57. https://doi.org/10.1177/0022018315603593.

72. HM Government. Female Genital Mutilation (FGM) Protection Orders. 2016. https://assets.publishing.service.gov.uk/government/uploads/system/uploads/attachment_data/file/573786/FGMPO_-_Fact_Sheet_-__1-12-2016_FINAL.pdf. Accessed 1 Jun 2020.

73. HM Government. Get a female genital mutilation protection order. https://www.gov.uk/female-genital-mutilation-protection-order. Accessed 1 Jun 2020.

74. Department of Health and Social Care. FGM: mandatory reporting in healthcare. 2017. https://www.gov.uk/government/publications/fgm-mandatory-reporting-in-healthcare. Accessed 1 Jun 2020.

75. Department of Health and Social Care. Female Genital Mutilation (FGM) Mandatory reporting duty. 2017. https://assets.publishing.service.gov.uk/government/uploads/system/uploads/attachment_data/file/525405/FGM_mandatory_reporting_map_A.pdf. Accessed 1 Jun 2020.

76. Department for Education. Statutory guidance: working together to safeguard children. 2019. https://www.gov.uk/government/publications/working-together-to-safeguard-children%2D%2D2. Accessed 2 Jun 2020.

77. Social Care Wales. Statutory guidance: working together to safeguard people. 2017. https://socialcare.wales/hub/statutory-guidance. Accessed 2 Jun 2020.

78. Home Office. Female genital mutilation: resource pack. 2020. https://www.gov.uk/government/publications/female-genital-mutilation-resource-pack/female-genital-mutilation-resource-pack. Accessed 2 Jun 2020.

79. NHS Digital. Female genital mutilation—information sharing. 2020. https://digital.nhs.uk/services/female-genital-mutilation-information-sharing. Accessed 2 Jun 2020.

80. Hussain S, Rymer J. Tackling female genital mutilation in the UK. Obstetr Gynaecol. 2017;19:273–8. https://doi.org/10.1111/tog.12394.
81. Mohammad S. Legislative action to eradicate FGM in the UK. In: Momoh C, editor. Female genital mutilation. Oxford: Radcliffe; 2005.
82. Elneil S. Female sexual dysfunction in female genital mutilation. Trop Doct. 2016;46(1):2–11. https://doi.org/10.1177/0049475515621644.
83. Department of Health. Female genital mutilation risk and safeguarding: guidance for professionals 2016. https://assets.publishing.service.gov.uk/government/uploads/system/uploads/attachment_data/file/525390/FGM_safeguarding_report_A.pdf. Accessed 4 Jun 2020.
84. National FGM Centre. FGM Good Practice Guidance and Assessment Tool for Social Workers. 2016. http://nationalfgmcentre.org.uk/wp content/uploads/2018/03/FGM-Best-Practice-Guidance-for-Social-Workers-1.pdf. Accessed 4 Jun 2020.
85. NHS Choices. Women talking about their personal experiences of female genital mutilation (FGM). 2015. https://www.youtube.com/watch?v=531RXHalKuI. Accessed 5 Jun 2020.
86. Department of Health. FGM Safeguarding and Risk Assessment: Quick guide for health professionals. 2017. https://assets.publishing.service.gov.uk/government/uploads/system/uploads/attachment_data/file/585083/FGM_safeguarding_and_risk_assessment.pdf. Accessed 15 Jul 2020.

Ruth Tweedale

*"No woman had a voice in the design of the legal institutions
that rule the social order under which women, as well as
men, live."*

Catharine A. McKinnon [1].

15.1 Introduction

As part of the radical feminist legal analysis, this chapter will consider whether 'the law is male' [2–5] specifically with respect to the Family Justice System of England and Wales (FJS). The FJS is the legal system for arbitrating on family law issues (see Box 15.1). The focus will be on child arrangement proceedings (private family law proceedings) where the mother has been abused by the father of the child(ren) subject to the litigation. The aforementioned court cases involve disputes between parents concerning 'contact' and 'residence', formerly known as 'access' and 'custody' [6]. This chapter evaluates to what extent the FJS provides justice for women victims of domestic violence and their children and offers an analysis of the often-hidden forces that lead to the imposition of unsafe contact orders in the FJS.

Social workers and health professionals play a key role in supporting women victims of domestic violence and their children. Health professionals can be first responders to victims of domestic violence as often they are the only people that the victims can see without the perpetrator present and therefore have an important role in recording evidence. Where domestic violence is raised as an issue in private children proceedings, a social worker is usually appointed and their report into the child's best interests is considered of great weight in family court proceedings. This

R. Tweedale (✉)
University of Greenwich, London, UK

© Springer Nature Switzerland AG 2021
C. Bradbury-Jones, L. Isham (eds.), *Understanding Gender-Based Violence*,
https://doi.org/10.1007/978-3-030-65006-3_15

type of social worker is called a CAFCASS (Child and Family Court Advisory Support Service) officer, see [7]. Research indicates that social workers' focus is all too often towards the promotion of 'post separation family relationships' at the expense of children's welfare in child arrangement cases with domestic violence (see [8, 9]). It is hoped this chapter will provide a critical basis and offer an insight into child contact proceedings and this in turn will support you, as a health or social work professional, in your career and ensure you are better equipped to centre children and women victims of domestic violence in your practice.

15.2   What Is the Problem?

It is argued that both historically and currently, the law not only favours men, but it actively disadvantages women [3, 5]. Until somewhat recently, domestic violence was not just considered a private matter between 'man and wife', but deemed beyond the remit of the law. Furthermore, it was considered a man's right to chastise his wife. Up until the 1990s, it was not a criminal offence for a man to rape his wife. This resulted from the origin of the law on rape failing to conceptualise rape as a violation of women's rights. Rather, it was conceptualised as a property crime: a crime against a husband for the interference with his chattel: wife (*R v R [1991] 4 All ER 481*) [10].

Over the last 20 years, feminist research and activism have led to increased awareness of domestic violence as a human rights issue as well as a child welfare concern [11, 12]. With this, England and Wales have seen the development of a purposeful legal and policy framework for tackling child arrangement cases where the father has been abusive to the mother. Despite the known risks to the safety of women and children, it is still extremely rare for a family court to deny violent fathers unsupervised visiting contact with their child. Of applications made by non-resident parents, the vast majority being fathers for child contact, less than 1% are refused despite issues of harm having been identified in over half the cases [13, 14].

Box 15.1 The Family Justice System
The FJS is the body of law and policy administered by the family court. The cases before the court are adjudicated by judges and magistrates. Decisions are made on issues such as divorce, finances on divorce, child contact, domestic violence injunctions and care proceedings.
(a) Private proceedings issues tend to be disputes between parents when they cannot agree on issues concerning the ubbringing of their child: mainly child contact—formerly known as access, child residence - formerly known as 'custody'; frequency of parental contact, conditions of supervision (direct or indirect) or establishing an order for no contact (very rare.) Social workers are often involved in private law proceedings in their role as CAFCASS officers.
(b) Public law proceedings cases involve child protection social service departments' intervention to remove children from their parents' care (make a care or interim care order) due to the potential risk of 'serious harm'.

Question

Is it a father's right to have contact with his child/children?

15.3   What Is the Radical Feminist Legal Perspective?

'When one gets to know women close up and without men present, it is remarkable the
extent to which their so-called biology, not to mention their socialization, has failed'.
Catharine A. MacKinnon [15]

A 'radical feminist' lens is being used here to critique the law. It is used as the academic genre in which I have always considered feminism, which is a critique of the law in terms of how it affects different women 'as women' [5]. This is described by MacKinnon as 'Feminism Unmodified' [15]. A wide range of feminisms exist such as 'liberal feminism' or 'socialist feminism'. It is contended that these categories of feminism serve to divide and conquer and must be considered within the overall power dynamic of oppression of women in a patriarchal society. Furthermore, it is believed that the labelling serves the ideological purpose of opening up a space to attack feminism from within [16].

Although the words sex and gender are often used interchangeably, it is fundamental to understand that sex and gender are not the same thing. Sex is the biological group into which we are born: male or female (and a small minority of people who are intersex); gender is the set of rules, characteristics, norms, 'choices' and behaviours into which we are socialised. Gender traits are usually attributed to femininity and masculinity which are socially constructed, hierarchised and enforced. Millett describes gender differences to be 'essentially cultural, rather than biological bases' [17]. The radical feminist perspective is that gender reinforces women's subordination so that women are socialised into subordinate roles. Women learn to be 'caring', passive, quiet, emotional support for men, nurturers of children and in today's society: stupid, vain and looks obsessed [17]. This oppressive gender system operates to subordinate women not only through social customs but also through politics and law [18].

Radical feminist or 'structural feminist' theory argues that society is organised to ensure that male power and dominance exists over women [19]. That society is patriarchal is therefore an inevitable consequence of its design. From early civilisation, the patriarchal structure relied on the oppression of women to maintain order. This continues today with gender constructs playing a seminal role in this oppression. As explained by Dworkin, the definition of patriarchy is 'instructive', as 'pater' means owner, possessor or master [20]. The prime social unit of patriarchy is the family. Interestingly, the word family comes from the Oscan[1] *famel*, which means servant, slave or possession [21]. Therefore, the FJS, a mechanism of state power, is a pressure point for analysing to what extent the law interacts to enforce patriarchal oppression within the family.

---

[1] Oscan is a sister language to Latin https://www.britannica.com/topic/Oscan-language

Feminist legal theorists such as Bartlett argues that the law plays a crucial role in the construction and enforcement of gender norms [5]. It can never be overstated that women had no say in: the design of the system of government, the basis of constitutional democracy, the foundations of the law and the justice structures within which society operates [1]. The laws and customs which form the foundation of our legal and democratic system were put in place before women had a vote or were able to sit in parliament. It is therefore no coincidence that the law may not serve women on an equal footing with men. The law is inherently male; therefore, an invisible bias exists towards men [5]. Where the law obviously discriminates, this can be challenged. The late Ruth Bader Ginsburg was very successful in challenging such explicit gender bias in the US Supreme Court [3].

The effect of a patriarchal society is that every aspect of a woman's life is impacted by patriarchal requirements. This furthers the idea that a woman's body is public—consider the treatment of mothers of newborn babies: they are deemed 'exhibitionists' if they breastfeed in public; they are labeled as failures and unnatural if unable to breastfeed; they are categorised as selfish or a 'bad' mother if they choose not to breastfeed. But women's abuse by men is private and not something to discuss or make a fuss about. Radical feminists do not consider all women as weak and all men as powerful. Rather, the patriarchal system protects, supports and bolsters men as a class of people whilst oppressing and suppressing women as a class of people [18].

'Gender' or sex-based violence is central for patriarchy to maintain control. Domestic violence is part of the continuum of male violence against women. It operates as an oppressive force to serve the patriarchy. Domestic violence is both a cause and consequence of women's inequality. Male violence against women is often misunderstood as 'individually motivated, with few social consequences, though with trauma caused to a few women', when gender-based violence has all the trappings of an oppressive social structure [22]. Hence, it should not be considered and isolated outside of the patriarchal structure [22]. Radical feminist legal scholars argue that 'domestic violence' is an assertion of male power [23]. It appears that this is prevalent in the FJS—as a body of the State—and serves not only to minimise women's fears for their safety but also to legitimise abusers, for instance, ordering contact with violent fathers provides state sanctioned validation of men's past and continued abuse of women and children.

Bartlett, Smart and McKinnon propose that it is a fair assumption that the law is 'male' and not gender-neutral [1, 5, 24]. Therefore, repeated issues in the FJS need to be considered in this light with added consideration as to whether the FJS fundamentally does not serve 'women' [5]. Scholars such as Smart use the term 'malevolence' of the patriarchal system, which makes it resistant to women's concerns, as a result of women's inequality [24]. Therefore, this evaluation of the FJS is from the standpoint that women (as a class of people in society) are subordinated and oppressed by men (as a class of people in society) through inter alia patriarchal violence: i.e. domestic violence: and patriarchal structures, i.e. the FJS [1].

Questions

1. Can the radical feminist lens be applied to health and social work?
2. What legal reforms would you propose to alleviate sex discrimination in health and social work practice?

15.4 Historical Context and Birth of Women's Rights to Their Children

It is vital to trace the history and development of women's rights in the family, when asking 'the woman question' in order to establish how far women's equality has come [19].

Feminism has wide historical connotations. The foundations of today's liberal democratic legal system and the basis of the rule of law were developed from Roman and Christian patriarchal traditions. In Roman times, a husband was legally vested as 'the law enforcer within the family' to this end, he had the right to sentence a woman to death with no repercussions [25]. The roots of domestic violence in Western society can be founded in this right of men to 'physically and socially dominate women' [25].

Historically, the law on children and disputes between parents unequivocally favoured men [3]. Up until the late twentieth century, domestic violence between married couples was considered a private matter and beyond the realms of the law and the 'public sphere'. Throughout the nineteenth century, domestic violence or 'wife beating' was prevalent and there was widespread belief amongst men and women that it was a man's right to discipline his wife. Before 1858, women could not apply for or get a divorce from her husband. Up until this point, when women married, due to the doctrine of coverture, her 'legal personhood' disappeared. In explaining the law in Victorian England, the eminent legal scholar Sir William Blackstone stated: *'In the eyes of the law a husband and wife are one, and that one is the husband'* [26].

Coverture determined that spouses could not bring legal proceedings against one another as they were considered one legal entity; thus, women could not divorce [27]. Furthermore, women had no legal rights to their children [26]. Until the late 1800s, married women's rights to their own children were worse than non-existent.[2] Only fathers had rights and ownership of their children. This was surmised by the Attorney General Lord Lyndhurst (1824–26) who stated that the court would not interfere with 'the sacred right of the father over his children' [27].

In 1839, a law named the 'Custody of Infants Act' (the 1839 Act) was passed further to feminist activism. This was led by Caroline Norton who was a victim of domestic violence [28]. This act was hailed as the birth of the modern FJS and an important milestone in women's rights. The 1839 Act legislated, for the first time, that mothers could make a court application for custody of her child. If a woman made a successful application, she was granted rights to nurture her child and retain

---

[2]For example when a father died the surviving mother was not the automatic legal guardian of children. Under 1646 Abolition of Tenures Act, fathers had sole power to designate a testamentary guardian and could entirely exclude the mother from seeing her children and this prevailed until the

custody. However, once the child reached the age of seven, all the mother's rights would cease and the child could be taken from her and returned to the father (or to a relative of the father) [29]. The Victorian era is renowned for espousing the virtues of women's roles in the home as mothers. The 'patriarchal vision of the good pious wife and mother' [27] was deemed to be flattering to women—a kind of 'romantic paternalism'. Yet in reality, it did not put women on a 'pedestal but in a cage' [3].

Despite the 1839 Act, it remained incredibly difficult for women to win custody of her children. This was due to the wide discretion of the courts in decision-making and the entrenched entitlement of men to ownership of his children. Wright's review of the case law of this time indicates that the courts, when accessing a mother in a custody case, would focus on the performance of her marital duties and, effectively, her obedience to gender stereotypes [27]. Bartlett describes this as 'the appropriateness of the role of women assumed by the law' [5]. Judicial concerns about the breakdown of family patriarchy, the absolute rights of men over women and children and the enforcement of appropriate role of women ensured that the 1839 Act became nothing more than a slight expansion of common law rules.

The court's wide discretion did not, however, vest them with the power to deprive fathers of ownership of his children unless he had forfeited his rights through endangerment of 'life and limb'. Described as the forfeiture test, it only succeeded where the father had raped a child or was homosexual [27]. The case law from this era shows that no mother won on the merits of her own case for custody of her child, but rather on the demerits of her husband's case [27]. Effectively, at this time, father's rights were paramount; whereas today, S1.1 of the Children Act 1989 prioritises the child's rights [30].

Wright describes the 1839 Act as 'terribly important not for what it did accomplish but for what it did not accomplish' [27]. In a patriarchal society, there is the potential for feminist activism to succeed but the patriarchal forces can use it to work in a counterproductive manner, by repackaging or reforming the black letter law (that is, well-established legal rules that are no longer subject to reasonable dispute in a common law system) into a more palatable and contemporarily acceptable version of the same thing. Seigal describes this as 'preservation through transformation' [31].

Discussion Questions

- What is the historical context of health and social work?
- How has practice developed to recognise domestic violence as an issue of harm for children?
- Have there been any examples of 'preservation by transformation'?

15.5 Development of Law and Policy Framework for Tackling Child Contact and Domestic Violence

'The legal impediments associated with being a woman, early on, were so blatant' (Bartlett, 1990) [5].

Reflecting on the desperate state of women's rights in the family during the Victorian era, it may be surprising and certainly disappointing that it is only within the last 20 years that domestic violence has been recognised in law as a child welfare issue in private law children proceedings. The previous two decades have, however, seen many advances in law and policy governing child arrangement disputes between parents where domestic violence is an issue.

As a starting point for social work and healthcare students, it is vital to dispel some myths on 'custody battles'. The first is the false perception that parents are highly litigious when it comes to disputes over their children. The vast majority of parents reach agreement on arrangements between themselves for **residence**: where their child or children will live and for **child contact:** how often the child will see the non-resident parent—usually the father. Ministry of Justice data shows that only 10% of parents who separate become involved in child contact proceedings [32]. This is not widely known. The importance of this is that the cases that appear before the family court are the 'tough cases'.

The vast majority of applications for child arrangement orders are made by fathers seeking a child arrangement order for contact in relation to children who are living with the mothers [9, 33, 34]. This does not mean that the mother has stopped the father seeing his child. Usually the father is seeking to change the current arrangements. It is also important to identify that most women who have experienced domestic violence want their child to have contact with their father, but they want it to be safe [35].

In over half of all child arrangement cases in the family court, there are allegations of harm. The majority of these involve domestic violence perpetrated by the father onto the mother [33]. It is commonly misconstrued that the courts favour mothers; the reality is that in less than 1% [13, 14] of applications by non-resident parents, the vast majority of which are fathers for child contact, over half the cases, which involve issues of harm, are refused [14].

If a child arrangement order is made by the court for a violent father to have contact with his child, the mother is the subject of the order and is required to make the child available for contact. Research indicates that in relatively few cases do mothers refuse to allow fathers contact [36].

15.6   The Modern Family Justice System

The key piece of legislation governing disputes between parents regarding children is the Children Act, 1989 (CA, 1989). When the legislation was first introduced, at its core was the 'paramountcy principal'. This means that the child's best interests must be paramount in any decisions the court makes about the upbringing of a child, for example when making child arrangement orders for contact or residence. From its introduction, the CA (1989) distanced itself from the concept of parental rights to children. The language changed to 'parental responsibility' for children. At its core is the 'welfare principal' which placed the child's welfare (physical and emotional) as the overriding factor for the court; this would supersede the notions of parent: maternal or paternal rights. The Children Act is viewed as a model piece of legislation, promoting the requirement that all rights would emanate from the child and going further than the UN Convention on the Rights of the Child 1989 in its child centred focus.

Question

How can social workers and health professionals best understand what is in the child's best interest?

The Court of Appeal decision *Re L; Re V; Re M; Re H 2000 2 FLR 334 (Re LVMH)* established for the first time that domestic violence was an issue which courts needed to consider when making decisions about child arrangements. Prior to this, although it was often considered by judges, there was no guidance on this. Additionally, there was no recourse for mothers if a court refused to take account of women and children's emotional and physical well-being if they had experienced domestic violence. Domestic violence was routinely separated from father's parenting abilities. Re L is hailed as a landmark decision. For the first time, judges were provided with guidance on dealing with women's allegations of domestic violence in child arrangement disputes. The guidance, for example required the court to adjudicate on the domestic violence in an adversarial court hearing called a 'finding of fact' to establish if the violence alleged had occurred.

More progress for women and children victims of domestic violence came with the amendment to Section 1. (3) of the Children Act (1989) and the Adoption and Children Act (2002) to include in the definition of 'harm': seeing or hearing harm to another. This was in recognition and as guidance to judges that the definition of harm specifically caused by seeing or hearing domestic violence perpetrated by their father onto their mother [37].

Question

What are the detrimental short- and long-term consequences for children being exposed to violence perpetrated by their father onto their mother?

Practitioner Point to Note

Enforcement of child arrangement orders: If a child arrangement order is made by the court for a violent father to have contact with his child, the mother is the subject of the order and is required to make the child available for contact. If she does not obey the order, she can face sanctions and women have been committed to prison for not complying with contact or had children removed from their care and placed with the father. In the case of *A (see A Child)* **[2007] EWCA Civ 899,** the court ordered a transfer of residency because of the mother's repeated failure to comply with the contact order and a diagnosis that she had bipolar disorder. The eight-year-old boy was moved 300 miles away to live with his father, despite the child's strong desire to stay living with his mother. The order was only reversed by the courts when the boy became suicidal at the prospect of living with his father and an emergency hearing allowed him to reside at his mother's. The court has the option of less punitive sanctions, such as unpaid work and compensation for financial loss. In the context of domestic violence, this means women can be required to bring their child to stay with an abusive father even if she has serious concerns for her child's welfare. Research indicates that relatively few contact orders are breached and that the focus for actors in the FJS should be to prioritise finding sustainable, child-centred solutions for enforcement and to avail appropriate safeguarding and use of perpetrator intervention programmes (see [38]).

In 2006, Women's Aid issued a report into the killing of 29 children by their own fathers, where he was a known perpetrator, and the homicides occurred during court sanctioned contact visits [39]. The findings of this report prompted a review of judicial practice and in 2008, guidance. As a consequence of the report and feminist campaigning, more progress ensued with Re LVHM being extended and formalised. It was added to the Family Procedure Rules for the Family Courts, as Practice Direction 12J—Child Arrangements and Contact Order: Domestic Violence and Harm. PD12J dictates—the legal process to be followed in contact proceedings where domestic violence is an issue.

An independent Family Justice Review [40] took place in 2012 to examine issues of children and the law. Pressure was mounted by 'father's rights' groups to amend the CA (1989) to include a presumption of 'shared parenting' [37]. The CA (1989) was amended with the insertion of S1.2 (A), a legal presumption that unless the contrary is shown it is to be assumed that the child's best interests will be furthered by the involvement of both parents in the child's life. This amendment highlights the reality that the perceived progress for women leads to misogynistic backlash. This is based on the idea that equality has been achieved; therefore, any legislation that specifically protects women (or is seen in some way to favour women) is deemed discriminatory against men [41–43]. In the UK, the increased legal protections for domestic violence in the family courts correlates with a rise in 'father's rights' activism [42]. This led to the significant change in the Children Act (1989). Walby argues that backlash such as this does not merely signify an attempt to hinder feminist progress, but it is also an attempt to 'reaffirm patriarchal domination of women' [44].

Box 15.2 Children Act 1989 S1.2 (A)

A court, in the circumstances mentioned in subsection (4)(a) or (7), is as respects each parent within subsection (6)(a) to presume, unless the contrary is shown, that involvement of that parent in the life of the child concerned will further the child's welfare.

(2B)In subsection (2A) "involvement" means involvement of some kind, either direct or indirect, but not any particular division of a child's time.

Point to note for practitioners

There is a misconception that the presumption in S1.2 (A) means that a violent father should have visiting contact. This is not the case, the presumption will apply to the vast majority of eligible applications, because in all but the most serious cases there will be some form of involvement that does not have to be face to face visiting contact with the non-resident parent which could be without risk. For example, if visitng contact with a father is deemed a risk to child and/or mother, an order for indirect contact could be made for example to send their child a birthday and Christmas card to the solicitors firm of the mother to be passed on (so as to protect the confidentiality to ensure the mother and child's whereabouts are not disclosed to the perpetrator).

Box 15.3

Practitioner point to note: there are 'overriding' legal principles to be applied by the court in decision-making on contact that social workers and health professionals should be mindful of:

1. The court has very wide powers in any application made under the Children Act 1989 (CA 1989). It can make orders for which neither party has applied and impose their own solution.

2. The delay principle (Section 1(2) CA 1989) also specifies that any delay in determining questions relating to a child's upbringing is 'likely to prejudice the welfare of the child'. This requires courts to consider making interim orders prior to reaching a final decision, or emergency orders during the proceedings.

3. The 'no order' principle (Section 1 (5) CA 1989) sets out that the court should only make an order in respect of a child where it is necessary, the purpose being not to impose unnecessary formal arrangements regarding children where there are no significant disputes. For example, if the non-resident parent is not disputing residence, the court will not make a child arrangement order for residence.

15.7 How Successful Have Legal Advances Been in Reversing Centuries of Men's Complete Ownership of Women and Children?

Hard fought advances have been made in the design of law and policy in order to protect women and children from male violence. These advances have been designed to help the process of implementing safe contact arrangements. The Family Justice

Systen (FJS) applies the Children Act 1989 (CA 89), which provides courts with a wide discretion in decision-making on child arrangements. However, despite the known risks of domestic violence to women and children, the FJS seems to be immune to women's valid safety concerns (for themselves and their children) [45]. The consequences have been fatal with 48 child homicides over a 20-year period during court sanctioned child contact. Additionally, with women being systematically killed by their male partners/ex-partners at a rate of two women per week [46], evidence shows that around 30% of domestic homicides involve child contact disputes (Metropolitan Police Service 2004).

Research reiterates repeated failures in the FJS response to women and children's experiences of domestic violence over the last 20 years [46, 47, 48]. These include:

- Judicial minimisation of women's experiences of domestic violence [49] with judges equating domestic violence only with physical 'incidents' of violence [50] whilst women's actual experiences of domestic violence were reflective of a well-documented pattern of coercive control [51].
- Contact is emphasised as 'the desired outcome' whatever the circumstances. This is underpinned by an assumption that men's violence towards the mother can be separated from their parenting ability [35].
- Unsupervised contact being ordered to violent fathers in almost all cases.
- Perpetrators' use of the child contact process to continue to abuse their victim and assert power and control [52, 53].
- Patchy judicial compliance with rules on dealing with child contact and domestic violence (as set out in Practice Direction 12J) [45, 54].

The FJS applies the law as set out in the Children Act (1989). This provides judges with wide discretion in decision-making. Despite the known risks of domestic violence to women and children, there are clear patterns in case outcomes that indicate a 'contact at all costs' approach. In 2016, Women's Aid published the report 19 Child Homicides. Although aforementioned legal advancements were designed to avoid the approval of unsafe contact arrangements, an additional 19 children were killed during court sanctioned contact arrangements by fathers known to be violent and dangerous. In response to this, the President of the family court, Mr. Justice Cobb, reissued Practice Direction 12J in December 2017 [55]. Apparently strengthening the Practice Direction, for example that the court must be satisfied that any contact order does not expose 'the other parent' and/or the child to risk of harm, rather than considering the risk to just the child.' Justice Cobb issued a statement to family law judges that: the presumption contained in section 1 (2 (A) (see Box 15.2) of the CA 1989 does not operate to require 'contact at all costs' in all cases. The Women's Aid report highlighted that the adherence to the PD12J was at best patchy and that the introduction of S1.2 (A) may have led to judges awarding contact routinely without considering fully the impact of domestic violence and their requirements to follow PD 12J [56].

Bartlett, Smart and McKinnon propose that patterns such as these disproportionately impact women negatively, because the law is 'male' and not gender-neutral [15, 24, 57]. It is argued that modern laws such as the Children Act (1989) allow women access to all the rights previously restricted for men, the right to make applications to court with respect to her child. A 'man' is, however, the default standard to which all things are measured. Scholars such as MacKinnon argue that 'gender-neutrality' is actually holding women to the male standard; therefore, it strives to achieve equality for women on the basis that the current legislation is at worst futile, and moreover, it is likely to be counterproductive in achieving equality of outcomes for women [15].

To reflect back on the 1839 Act, which did little to progress women's rights, it is compelling to consider whether the advancements in law and policy are simply 'preservation through transformation'. As Wooley describes, 'changing legislation on the books' can be very different to 'law in action'. While the outcomes for women and her children remain largely unchanged, the law is repackaged in a way that seems to offer protection [25]. Crucially, it is important to note that gender norms continue to prevail in today's FJS, as with the Victorian era. Violent fathers are not generally required to prove their parenting skills. It is for mothers to prove that a father's violence has happened and that it is relevant to the court's decision on child contact. Conversely, mothers parenting abilities are routinely called into question, for example in regard to her ability to protect the child from an abusive partner, or her parenting skills in terms of her mental health as a result of abuse perpetrated by the father [58].

Learning Points for Social Workers and Health Professionals

Women in child contact proceedings are legitimately terrified

It is important that professionals are aware that women in child contact proceedings where domestic violence is an issue are often not calm, and moreover, are all too often are still experiencing abuse. They are often terrified of being in the same room as the perpetrator but, the overwhelming fear, is for their children. Women can often come across as 'hysterical' simply because the most important things in the world to them is at risk.

There is no stereotypical perpetrator

Perpetrators are often seasoned and experienced manipulators. It is commonly misconstrued that domestic violence is a loss of control and a fit of anger, or that it is caused by alcohol or drugs-it is not, it is decisive and contrived behaviour designed to assert power and dominance over the victim. Often perpetrators present extremely well to the court and to professionals. They are very often charming, successful and articulate. Perpetrators also ascend class and race. In my experience, the most serious perpetrators do not lose their temper in front of professionals.

Children must be listened to both when they want to see their father and when they do not

Research indicates that children are routinely listened to when they express a desire to see their father. However, professionals, particularly CAFCASS and family social workers, must listen when children say they do not want to see their father [8].

The FJS as explained is a system set up by men for men

Women victims of domestic violence are all too often not 'good witnesses'. Domestic violence is not a series of incidents for women but is an all-encompassing nightmare. The FJS when considering allegations of domestic violence considers this as a series of incidents. But the lived experience is an ordeal. Women experience high levels of trauma and mental health consequences as a result of domestic violence, and this makes it difficult to remember what happened when giving evidence at court or when being interviewed by CAFCASS.

Women are telling the truth and perpetrators are lying

From my experience as Senior Legal Officer at Rights of Women working with victims of abuse on a daily basis, one thing was starkly clear, women do not lie about domestic violence (every rule has exception). Women want their child to have a relationship with their father but they want it to be safe. This is because women overwhelmingly want what is best for their child and we are consistently told that children are damaged by not having their father in their life. I have found very little evidence to support this assertion.

Professionals (particularly social workers) hold a lot of power in the FJS

I hope from this chapter you have an understanding of the radical feminist critique and that you can apply this to your practice to ensure that you support the best outcomes for women and children. That you can be part of the solution to ensuring that violent men's abuse of the mother of their child is **not** validated by provision of a contact order that ignores the health and safety concerns that the mother has for her child and for herself and moreover, that women and children are heard and their experiences validated and accounted for in judicial decision-making. The role of a CAFCASS officer in child arrangement proceedings is a very powerful one.

15.8   Conclusion

'Women are not passive victims of oppressive structures. They have struggled to change both their immediate circumstances and the wider social structures.' Sylvia Walby [22]

It may seem like a bleak outlook, but it is only in understanding the flaws in the patriarchal system and unearthing the deep-seated problems that we can begin to bring about change. The FJS is quite clearly not protecting women and children from domestic violence. Moreover, it is rubberstamping male violence by disregarding or minimising it when making decisions on child arrangements. Perhaps it is time to overhaul the man-made adversarial court system and to hold the FJS to account. But, fundamentally as women we need to support each other, believe each other, respect each other and protect each other within this system that is operating against us. And as men, you must support women, believe women, respect women and protect women.

References

1. MacKinnon CA. Reflections on sex equality under Law. Yale Law J. 1991 Mar;100(5):1281.
2. MacKinnon CA. Women's lives, men's laws. Cambridge, MA: Belknap Press of Harvard University Press; 2005.
3. Law SA, Hennessey P. Is the law male: the case of family Law, 69 chi. vol. 345, L. Rev. 1993.
4. Levit N, Verchick RRM. Feminist legal theory: a primer. New York: New York University Press; 2006. 235 p.
5. Bartlett K. Feminist legal methods. Harv Law Rev. 1989;103:829.
6. Herring J. Family law. London: Pearson Education; 2019. 933 p.
7. Home—Cafcass—Children and Family Court Advisory and Support Service [Internet]. [cited 10 Oct 2020]. https://www.cafcass.gov.uk/.
8. Macdonald GS. Hearing children's voices? Including children's perspectives on their experiences of domestic violence in welfare reports prepared for the English courts in private family law proceedings. Child Abuse Negl. 2017;65(September 2013):1–13.
9. Humphreys C, Harrison C. Focusing on safety-domestic violence and the role of child contact centres. Child Fam Law Q. 2003;1.
10. Herring J. Criminal law: text, cases, and materials. 888 p.
11. Sturge C. LAW-BRISTOL- DG-F, 2000 undefined. Contact and domestic violence—The Experts' Report. Jordan Publ Ltd.
12. Macdonald GS. Domestic violence and private family court proceedings: promoting child welfare or promoting contact? Violence Against Women. 2016;22(7):832–52.
13. Statistics J. Annual report 2003. Family matters. Table 2003;5.
14. Ministry of Justice. Swift and sure justice: the Government's plans for reform of the criminal justice system. London: The Stationery Office; 2012.
15. MacKinnon C. Feminism unmodified: discourses on life and law. Cambridge, MA: Harvard University Press; 1987.
16. Thompson D. Radical Feminism today. Sydney: Sage; 2001.
17. Millet K. Sexual politics. New York: Ballantine; 1978.
18. Jensen R. The end of patriarchy: radical feminism for men. North Melbourne: Spinifex Press; 2017.
19. Mackinnon CA. Feminism, Marxism, method, and the state: toward feminist jurisprudence, vol. 8. Source: Signs; 1983.
20. Dworkin A. Our blood. London: The Women's Press; 1974.
21. Harper D. Online Etymology Dictionary [Internet]. [cited 23 Jul 2019]. https://www.etymonline.com/search?q=family.
22. Walby S. Theorizing patriarchy. Oxford: Blackwell; 1990.
23. MacKinnon CA. Chapter 8: the Liberal state. In: Toward a Feminist Thoery of the State. Cambridge, MA: Harvard University Press; 1989.
24. Smart. Feminism and the Power of Law. 2001.
25. Woolley ML. Marital Rape: a unique blend of domestic violence and non-marital rape issues. Hast Women. 2007:269.
26. Sir William Blackstone. Commentaries on the Laws of England in Four Books, vol. 1. London; 1753.
27. Wright DC. The crisis of child custody: a history of the birth of family law in England. Columbia J Gend Law. 2002;11(2):175.
28. Wroath J, Edwards A. Until they are seven: the origins of women's legal rights. Hook: Waterside Press; 2008. 160 p.
29. John W. Until they are seven: the origins of women's legal rights. Winchester: Waterside Press; 1998.
30. Children Act 1989.
31. Siegel R. The rule of love: wife beating as prerogative and privacy (1995–1996). Yale Law J. 2010;105(8):2117–207.

32. Blackwell and Dawe. Non-resident Parent Contact. 2003.
33. Hunt J, Macleod A. Outcomes of applications to court for contact orders after parental separation or divorce briefing note. Fam Law. 2008;(September).
34. Ministry of Justice. Judicial and Court Statistics 2010. London: MOJ, Table 2.4 Ministry of Justice, (2011) data released further to a FOI request by Rights of Women, 2011.
35. Coy MPKSETR. Picking up the pieces: domestic violence and child contact. London; 2012.
36. Trinder L, Hunt J, Macleod A, Pearce J, Woodward H. Problem-solving or punishment? Enforcing contact orders. 2013.
37. Women's Aid. Domestic abuse, child contact and the family courts. Bristol; 2016.
38. Trinder L, Hunt J, Macleod A, Pearce J, Woodward H. Enforcing contact orders: problem solving or punishment? Exeter Law School Commissioned: Nuffield Foundation; 2013. https://www.Enforcement20report20final20Dec202013.pdf (https://www.kinstacdn.com).
39. Saunders H. Twenty-nine child homicides: lessons still to be learnt on domestic violence and child protection contents. Bristol; 2006.
40. Norgrove D. Family justice review: final report—GOV.UK. 2012.
41. Dragiewicz M. Patriarchy reasserted: fathers' rights and anti-VAWA activism. Fem Criminol. 2008;3(2):121–44.
42. Jordan A. Conceptualizing backlash: (UK) men's rights groups, anti-feminism, and post feminism. Can J Women Law. 2016;28(1):18–44.
43. Chambers C. Masculine domination, radical feminism and change. Fem Theory. 2005;6(3):325–46.
44. Walby S. "Backlash" In historical context—research portal. Lancaster University, Taylor Fr; 1993.
45. Barnett AE. Contact at all costs? Domestic violence, child contact and the practices of the family courts and professionals. 2014;(March).
46. Long J, Harper K, Harvey H, Smith KI. The Femicide census: profiles of women killed by men. 2017.
47. Radford ML, Radford GP. Power, knowledge, and fear: Feminism, Foucault, and the stereotype of the female librarian. Libr Q. 2009;67(3):250–66.
48. Holt S. Domestic violence and the paradox of post-separation mothering.
49. Naughton CM, O'Donnell AT, Greenwood RM, Muldoon OT. 'Ordinary decent domestic violence': a discursive analysis of family law judges' interviews. Discourse Soc. 2015;26(3):349–65.
50. Carline A, Easteal P. Shades of grey—domestic and sexual violence against women: Law reform and society. London: Taylor and Francis; 2014. p. 1–271.
51. Stark E. Insults, injury, and injustice. Violence Against Women. 2004;10(11):1302–30.
52. Thiara RK, Gill AK. Domestic violence, child contact and post-separation violence: issues for south Asian and African-Caribbean women and children. The Learning Exchange; 2012.
53. Thiara RK. Domestic violence, child contact, post-separation violence: experiences of South Asian and African-Caribbean women and children.
54. Douglas H, Walsh T. Mothers, domestic violence, and child protection. Violence Against Women. 2010;16(5):489–508.
55. The Honourable Mr. Justice Cobb, 'Review of Practice Direction 12J FPR 2010 Child Arrangement and Contact Orders: Domestic Violence and Harm: Report To The President Of The Family Division.' 2017.
56. Birchall J, Choudhry S. What about my right not to be abused? Domestic abuse, human rights and the family courts. Bristol: Women's Aid; 2018. p. 1–60.
57. Bartlett KT. Tradition, change, and the idea of progress in feminist legal thought. Wis L Rev. 1995;1995.
58. Hester M. The three planet model: towards an understanding of contradictions in approaches to women and Children's safety in contexts of domestic violence. Br J Soc Work. 2011;41:837–53.

Engaging in Gender-Based Violence Research: Adopting a Feminist and Participatory Perspective

16

Sanne Weber and Siân Thomas

Researching gender-based violence (GBV) is a complex task, presenting practical, ethical and emotional challenges for all those involved in the research process. This chapter explores how feminist and participatory approaches can help researchers to overcome these challenges. Researchers do not usually choose to study GBV for purely academic reasons—'the point is to end it' [1, p. 183]. Healthcare and social work professionals bring significant practice skills and knowledge to the research process, but may also face additional obstacles when building a research relationship with service users. This chapter will help you think through such obstacles, based on the basic assumptions and ethical principles underlying feminist and participatory research methods. The chapter also highlights the potential for creative research methods to enable participants to share their experiences in a more meaningful way. While the principles discussed are relevant to researching GBV in general, the chapter includes specific reference to cross-cultural research and examples of projects conducted in China, Guatemala and South Africa.

16.1 Researching GBV in Healthcare and Social Work

Research in the fields of healthcare and social work spans a disciplinary range across medical and social sciences and draws on diverse methodological approaches, both quantitative and qualitative. As a practitioner, you may become involved in research in different ways and at different points in your career. Research activities might include dissertations as part of academic programmes, institutional or service-orientated research, policy evaluation and projects undertaken as an independent or academic researcher. The existing research into best practice in GBV research

S. Weber (✉) · S. Thomas
University of Birmingham, Birmingham, UK
e-mail: S.Weber@bham.ac.uk; S.N.Thomas@bham.ac.uk

© Springer Nature Switzerland AG 2021
C. Bradbury-Jones, L. Isham (eds.), *Understanding Gender-Based Violence*,
https://doi.org/10.1007/978-3-030-65006-3_16

highlights a number of common themes, including the importance of protecting confidentiality, ensuring support is in place for participants, building relationships of trust and ensuring participant safety [2]. All forms of GBV research require an understanding of the potential risk to participants and researchers [3]. Survivors of GBV 'can be doubly disempowered in the research process, first as research subjects and second as part of a stigmatised and marginalised community' [4, p. 443]. The risk of repercussions and stigmatisation from perpetrators or the wider community if survivors are known to have disclosed their experiences must be recognised and managed within the research process. However, it is also important to involve survivors in this assessment and acknowledge their autonomy and ability to make their own decisions [5]. Even when you are using secondary data which has previously been collected for another purpose, it is important to ensure confidentiality and well-being. For example, police records or data from other agencies could contain identifying details which could put survivors at risk if made public.

The use of quantitative data is increasingly valued as a way of establishing the prevalence of GBV and evaluating the effectiveness of prevention and support interventions [6]. Quantitative methods are often associated with a positivist research philosophy (see Box 16.1) and an aspiration to objectivity. However, the lack of consistent definitions of GBV, non-response bias for survey data and barriers to disclosure mean that it is difficult to build a picture of how prevalent GBV really is, particularly when researchers intend to compare across different contexts [7]. Furthermore, the perception that numbers are objective masks the assumptions and interpretations that have gone into the research process, for example decisions about which acts are included within the definition of GBV [8]. Making these

---

Box 16.1 Thinking About Research Philosophies and Epistemologies
Research philosophies or epistemologies

The term *epistemology* refers to the theory or philosophy of knowledge: i.e. what can we know about reality?

It is different from the related term *ontology*, which refers to the philosophy of reality: i.e. what is reality?

There are different epistemologies, including:

Positivism refers to the traditional way of viewing knowledge. It assumes that there is a reality 'out there' that can be uncovered. The researcher can study this reality without influencing it or being influenced by it, by testing a hypothesis which ultimately leads to objective knowledge.

Constructivism assumes that reality is socially constructed, and therefore differs by community or social context. The researcher is part of the creation and uncovering of this reality, which he or she interprets.

Critical theory, including feminist theory, believes that reality is shaped by social and political forces which have come to be seen as natural. The researcher's role is to expose these structures, including gendered norms and inequality, in order to transform them.

interpretations explicit can give additional insights into the experiences that under-lie the numerical data [9]. In the case of GBV research using secondary sources, two key considerations are how violence is defined and which sources are used to gather information. For example, using secondary data such as police or health records will only give information on how many people have reported a crime to the police or sought medical treatment. Such reporting would not include forms of violence that were not recognised as a crime or acts that did not result in physical injury; nor would it account for the well-established levels of underreporting of GBV [10]. Moreover, quantitative research is less able to give detailed insight into the diversity of survivors' experiences or the contexts in which the violence has occurred. Rather than dismiss quantitative data, however, we need to think instead about how it can be better collected and used, in combination with other data, to build a more holistic picture of survivors' experiences [11].

Qualitative approaches can provide some solutions to the gaps in quantitative data, but present their own challenges. Interviews and focus groups can provide opportunities for survivors to share their stories in their own words and provide a richer insight into the impact of their experiences. While focus groups can be useful for gaining insights into normative expectations around GBV within the group, more personal and sensitive questions are often better suited to individual inter-views [12]. However, it is important to bear in mind that the definition of a sensitive topic will vary between participants and should be understood relationally, based on what feels safe to discuss in the space of the interview [13]. In order for participants to make an informed decision about what they want to share, ethical practice requires us to be clear with participants about how they will benefit from the study and also about potential risks, such as the limits of confidentiality, the potential for them to be identifiable from their data, the potential negative impacts of taking part in the research and how their data will be managed [14].

Physical and emotional safety are key requirements for participants to take part in GBV research. Disclosing traumatic experiences, which may still be ongoing, can potentially be both painful and cathartic [15]. It is important that survivors feel in control of how they share their story and what details they choose to include. For the researcher, this means thinking carefully about how much information is

---

Box 16.2 Thinking About Terminology
'Victims' or 'survivors'?

We have used the term 'survivors' to talk about people who have experi-enced GBV, but there is ongoing debate about the best term to use, and indi-vidual survivors may also have differing views. The term 'victim' is often used in relation to the criminal justice system, or by those who want to empha-sise the impact of violence, while 'survivor' tends to be used by those who wish instead to emphasise the resilience and agency of those who have expe-rienced GBV. The term 'victim-survivors' is also used by some to emphasise this duality of experience.

actually needed in order to avoid re-traumatisation [16]. For example, if a study is focusing on the impact of rape, it is likely to be sufficient to talk about the impact on day-to-day life without needing to ask for detailed disclosures about the assault. Balancing the risks and benefits of the research ethically between the researcher and participants is also important [12].

In addition to the emotional impact on survivors, researchers can also face the risk of emotional distress or secondary traumatisation from exposure to repeated accounts of traumatic experiences, whether this is through interviewing survivors directly or from reading or transcribing their testimony [17, 18]. Given the prevalence of GBV, it is also likely that many researchers will themselves have experienced some form of violence, which can exacerbate the emotional impact of hearing survivors' stories [17]. It is important that researchers have access to training and ongoing support to work through these emotional responses [19].

Initial contact with research participants is often made through gatekeepers, individuals or support organisations with whom survivors have already built up a trusting relationship [20]. This also provides reassurance to the survivor that it is safe to participate and to the researcher that there is support in place if a participant finds the emotional impact of the research difficult to manage. However, there can also be disadvantages, in particular with gatekeepers preselecting a particular group of participants to take part rather than enabling each service user to decide for themselves [20]. Where gatekeepers are community leaders, who may be men and potentially perpetrators themselves, it may be necessary to provide only general information about the study in advance, without mentioning the focus on GBV, and only share fuller details with individual participants in a confidential setting where they can make an informed choice about participation [21].

Many healthcare and social work researchers fulfil a 'dual role' as both practitioners and researchers, whether this is with their own clients or with others who are accessing similar services. Regulated practitioners will need to keep their professional code of ethics and safeguarding processes in mind alongside their consideration of research ethics. This dual role can bring benefits, particularly in terms of accessing participants and having knowledge of the presenting issues, relevant skills to manage risk and disclosure and an awareness of appropriate support services for onward referrals where needed [22, p. 15]. However, it can also be challenging to negotiate the boundary between the two roles and to ensure that expectations are managed and participants can make informed decisions about consent [23]. Practitioners who are working with participants from outside their institution can feel powerless when focusing solely on the research role and being unable to intervene in a professional capacity. If you are working with other practitioners as your participants, there may be a need to report practice concerns that you encounter during your research which could make participants reluctant to share their challenges or concerns about practitioners. Many of these concerns about ethics, safety and well-being of those involved in GBV research can be addressed through feminist and participatory research approaches.

16.2   Feminist Research: Principles and Benefits

There are many different strands of feminist research, which share certain key interests. In the first place, feminist research is interested in uncovering knowledge that is often taken for granted. 'Traditional', positivist research (see Box 16.1) has long taken the male worldview as its standard, assuming that reality and knowledge about it are the same for everyone [24]. Women's experiences, or even 'their very existence', are often insufficiently recognised in positivist research [25, p. 15]. Feminist research instead aims to produce knowledge that promotes the transformation of different forms of oppression that women and other oppressed groups experience. The production of knowledge is therefore a political process and practice [24, 26, 27].

Feminist research aims to uncover gendered and other forms of inequality through analysing and questioning the oppression inherent in everyday experiences. Therefore, the personal is political [26, 28]. Emotions are treated with suspicion or even discredited in positivist research, since emotions risk distorting 'true knowledge'. This shows the gendered ways in which research itself is constructed. In Western culture, men are conventionally associated with reason and women with emotions. Men are therefore seen as dispassionate, objective and value-free investigators, whereas knowledge claims of women—and people of colour—have historically often been discredited [29]. Nevertheless, emotions can be a site for the construction of knowledge, especially when studying a topic like violence, since people *feel* violated, abandoned, angry or hurt. Moreover, people experience and interpret violence in different ways. Feminist research considers these different and multiple truths and aims to disrupt essentialising categories and binaries that fail to do justice to the complexity of human experiences [30]. This also means being attentive to silence; survivors can be silenced by others, or refuse to speak to protect themselves or others [30].

Feminist research questions the assumption of a single objective truth about the social world, which is embedded in social structures in which researchers and their research are located. The term 'situated knowledges' is often used to indicate that knowledge is always partial, subjective, relational and multiple [24, 31]. Instead of assuming that the researcher is neutral and independent from the objects researched and therefore able to produce value-free research, feminist research explicitly recognises the role of the researcher within the research process. Since researchers are always situated in social, historic and economic structures, feminist researchers scrutinise how their own background and identity, as well as their emotions, biases and values affect the research, and vice versa. This reflexivity enables the production of more transparent and accountable knowledge [24, 27]. For practitioners, the reflexivity required within the research process fits well with the skills of critical reflection developed through qualifying programmes and applied in direct practice.

Another issue of concern to feminist research is power, in relation to the power inequalities between men and women and other oppressed groups in society, and also within the research process. In contrast to positivist research, which has often been critiqued for objectifying and exploiting its research participants for a higher scientific goal, feminist research is concerned with diminishing the power imbalance between researcher and participants which results from differences in ethnic, economic, class and educational backgrounds [24, 26, 27]. These power imbalances are of particular concern in cross-cultural GBV research.

Reflective Exercise

Using your own experience: Think about your own training and experience as a practitioner. What skills have you developed that will be useful to you as a researcher? What areas do you need to learn more about?

Reflecting on positionality: Think about your identity. How might that influence your choice of research topic and your understanding of the information you collect?

Understanding power relations: Consider what the challenges might be of conducting research in a cross-cultural context. What kind of power inequalities might you encounter (think about gender, race, socioeconomic groups, professional status etc.)? What could you do to redress these power imbalances?

16.3   Researching Gender-Based Violence Across Cultures

There are additional challenges involved in conducting GBV research across cultures, whether this is working with cultural difference within a country or carrying out a research project internationally. In fact, black and postcolonial feminists have been crucial in pointing out how feminism itself has long ignored 'other' female voices, and how white feminists have often taken on neocolonial roles in 'speaking for' marginalised or 'Third World' participants [32–34]. To prevent such inequalities, researchers require a critical consciousness about their own privilege, which can be based on their ethnic or geographical origin [33, 35]. This is particularly vital where a researcher from a dominant or more privileged group is researching the experiences of people within a more marginalised or disadvantaged community [36]. Researchers must seek to actively challenge inequality within the research process and 'not unintentionally replicate oppressive dynamics and patterns of power and control' that survivors have experienced from perpetrators [37, p. 508]. In addition, it is important to avoid 'exoticising' forms of violence that are located in non-Western cultures while failing to recognise that all GBV takes place within a particular cultural context [38, p. 102].

Box 16.3 Some Reflections on Theory

Postcolonial studies examine the impacts and ongoing legacies of colonialism on previously colonised societies. They critique ongoing Western influence and cultural imposition in different fields (including academia), arguing for more diverse forms of knowledge instead.

Postcolonial feminists have exposed inequalities and Euro-centrism within feminism, calling for more diversity and against oppression within feminism.

Box 16.4 Example of Feminist Participatory and Creative Research in a Cross-Cultural Context

Western researchers Brinton Lykes and Allison Crosby have worked with indigenous survivors of conflict-era sexual violence in **Guatemala**, using a variety of methods, including drama, creative storytelling and drawings, combined with indigenous practices such as rituals and ceremonies. The research helped to understand participants' understandings of and needs for reparation for the crimes they suffered, resulting in a demand for integral reparations presented to the Inter-American Commission on Human Rights [43].

The involvement of interpreters in the research process brings an additional layer of complexity. On the one hand, there is potential for interpreters to act as cultural as well as linguistic mediators, and for the shared language barrier to help redress power imbalances between researcher and participant [39]. On the other, bringing another person into the research process can impact the dynamics of the relationship, particularly if the participant does not want to share their experiences in front of someone from a similar community [40]. In addition to cultural factors, researchers need to keep in mind the impact and intersections of other identity characteristics on survivors' experiences of violence and ability to engage safely with the research process [41, 42]. Many definitions and interventions focused on GBV assume a female victim and male perpetrator within a heterosexual relationship, rather than recognising the myriad forms which violence can take. Experiences of violence will also be mediated through intersecting characteristics such as class, race, sexuality, (dis)ability, educational levels, family status and religion, in addition to gender [8, 42]. It is important for researchers to recognise this diversity of experience through all stages of the research process in order to promote inclusivity and meaningful representation. Giving participants more control over the research process, through participatory research approaches, can be a way of responding to this challenge.

16.4   Participatory Research: Principles and Benefits

Like feminist research, participatory research approaches have a strong focus on the potential of research as a political tool for social change. Rather than a set of particular methods, it refers to a way of doing research as a collaborative process [44]. It is based on a bottom-up approach, making participants' priorities and perspectives central to the research, to produce knowledge as the result of a collaboration between researcher and participants [45]. It aims to democratise research processes and diminish power inequalities between researchers and participants. By using specific methods, it promotes co-constructive knowledge production processes with the ultimate goal of social action (Table 16.1) [44].

Table 16.1 The differences between participatory and non-participatory research

	Non-participatory	Participatory
Aims	Focus on understanding a situation and finding or testing solutions	Focus on understanding a situation from the perspective of those most affected and finding or testing solutions based on their interests
Process	Research methods are chosen by researchers	Research process aims to bring about change
Ownership	Researchers set research agenda; participants are research subjects	Research agenda is set in partnership between researchers and participants
Beneficiaries	Researchers are main beneficiaries of the research process	Participants and wider communities are main beneficiaries

Participatory research is of a political nature, both in terms of its process and outcome. The participatory research process intends to raise consciousness and increase participants' critical awareness of their situation and of the problems and inequality they face [46, 47]. It enables research participants to produce and maintain ownership over their own knowledge, using it as an instrument to produce change [46]. This is based on the assumption that knowledge is socially constructed and embedded. Not limited to academic knowledge, it also includes experiential knowledge of non-academics. The legitimisation of popular knowledge disrupts the traditional, positivist process of knowledge production which is controlled by 'experts', often white and male, who generate 'expert knowledge' about participants that they themselves have no control over [48]. Like feminist research, participatory research thus aims to emancipate marginalised groups, helping them to transform their lives.

Participatory research methods have long been used by geographers and development researchers and practitioners. They include mapping exercises, the drawing of timelines, problem trees and other tools to identify and collectively analyse the specific problems at stake [45]. Another strand of participatory research involves creative research methods. An often-used method is Photovoice, which allows participants to document their reality through photographs, to then collectively construct a narrative about their problems and the steps needed to overcome these [49]. Other visual methods include film, drawing or collage making. Mapping can also be used as a creative method. Body mapping, for example, enables participants to artistically represent their physical and mental health [43]. Corporal forms of expression such as dramatization, or verbal techniques such as storytelling, poetry, narrative writing or oral histories are other examples of creative methods [43]. The creative product which results from the research process, for example a film, play, exhibition or book, can help the participants to show their situation and needs to policymakers [49]. These products offer more diverse forms of presenting knowledge and experiences than traditional written academic texts [28, 34].

Box 16.5 Example of the Diverse Outputs of a Feminist Participatory and Creative Research Project
The MoVE project in **South Africa** has deployed various participatory creative and arts-based methods to enable migrant sex workers to represent their own experiences. Drawings, photovoice, zines (small self-published works), narrative writing, poetry, body mapping and posters have been used to enable sex workers to speak for themselves and disrupt harmful and negative stereotypes about them [28].

Reflexive Exercise

Exercise:

- What do you think the risks could be of researching the situation of migrant sex workers using traditional, non-participatory methods?
- Do you think the use of participatory and creative methods will lead to different research results? Do you think the research will have a different impact, and if so, how and why?
- Do you think there can be risks or challenges from using participatory and creative methods in this research?

16.5 Feminist Participatory Research Practice to Research Gender-Based Violence

As described, feminist and participatory research approaches have a shared goal of transforming inequality and oppression. Yet there are more reasons that make feminist approaches to participatory research particularly appropriate for researching GBV. First of all, the involvement of survivors as co-researchers is ethically important. Without including those whose lives are being debated in national and international academic and policy debates, knowledge will always be incomplete or superficial [28]. Furthermore, participatory strategies can have important individual and collective impacts on research participants. GBV survivors are often portrayed as vulnerable and fragile. Participatory and creative methods can help change such negative stereotypes by allowing participants to give their own account of their situation. The recognition and validation of their experiences, through their own self-representation rather than being spoken for or about, can give an important impulse to participants' well-being [28]. The collective knowledge production process contributes to developing skills and building solidarity among the participants, helping them to take action to actively change their situation, which is an important element of the social justice goals of feminist and participatory research [43].

It is also important to recognise that survivors of GBV can experience research fatigue. They may have been interviewed many times, asked indecent or intrusive

Box 16.6 Example of the Potential for Impact of Feminist Participatory and Creative Research
Caroline Wang developed the Photovoice method, initially working with a women's reproductive health programme in **China**. Photography was used to identify the reproductive health needs of community women and their everyday lives. The photographs taken formed the basis for discussions and participatory data analysis in groups, eventually helping the participants to frame and participate in policy discussions [49].

questions and seen few direct, tangible results from their participation [50]. Feminist research is mindful of these risks by centring the research participants and diminishing power relations. Participatory creative methods give participants the tools to express their own experiences, rather than relying on pre-established questionnaires, thus helping to avoid stirring up painful memories which can be re-traumatising [51]. Feminist participatory and creative research can help to make research a positive experience for participants by enabling them to engage in creative practices that are enjoyable and enable them to work together in a group towards a shared goal [28, 43, 51].

16.6 Concluding Remarks

This chapter has described the benefits of combining a feminist and participatory approach when researching GBV. These methods enable research to be more beneficial for participants by giving them more power over the research process, avoiding risks of re-traumatisation and developing tools for social justice. Creative methods can reinforce these benefits, making research an enjoyable experience for participants and exploring more diverse ways of expressing and representing sensitive, complex and diverse experiences, which are often hard to express in written texts. Participatory and creative methods can draw on practitioner-researchers' existing values of engagement and reflexivity to break down power inequalities and place survivors' voices and experiences at the centre of the research process.

In spite of these benefits, there are some things to consider when exploring these methods. They tend to be more time and resource-consuming than more traditional methods and require careful planning. It is also important to realise that not all research participants are interested in longer term and more intensive research participation [44, 45]. When using visual methods, it is important to be mindful of the risk of co-creating images which hyper-visualise or objectify women as victims of violence and reduce them to this role, rather than showing their agency [43]. Finally, in spite of the explicit intention to reduce power inequalities between researcher and participants, it is often hard to eliminate these inequalities completely [28, 43]. Therefore, critically analysing your own positionality and influence on the research is crucial to guarantee that the research process is carried out effectively *with* rather than *on* survivors of GBV, enabling it to contribute to the transformation of their reality.

References

1. True J. The political economy of violence against women. Oxford: Oxford University Press; 2012.
2. Thomas SN, Weber S, Bradbury-Jones C. Using participatory and creative methods to research gender-based violence in the global south and with indigenous communities: findings from a scoping review. Trauma Violence Abuse. 2020.
3. Taylor J, Bradbury-Jones C. Sensitive issues in healthcare research: the protection paradox. J Res Nurs. 2011;16(4):303–6.
4. Malpass A, Sales K, Feder G. Reducing symbolic violence in the research encounter: collaborating with a survivor of domestic abuse in a qualitative study in UK primary care. Sociol Health Illn. 2016;38(3):442–58.
5. Ponic P, Jategaonkar N. Balancing safety and action: ethical protocols for photovoice research with women who have experienced violence. Arts Health. 2012;4(3):189–202.
6. Adams V. Metrics: what counts in global health. Durham, NC: Duke University Press; 2016.
7. Ellsberg M, Heise L, Pena R, Agurto S, Winkvist A. Researching domestic violence against women: methodological and ethical considerations. Stud Fam Plann. 2001;32(1):1–16.
8. Merry SE. The seductions of quantification: measuring human rights, gender violence, and sex trafficking. Chicago: University of Chicago Press; 2016.
9. Ryan L, Golden A. "Tick the box please": a reflexive approach to doing quantitative social research. Sociology. 2006;40(6):1191–200.
10. Alhabib S, Nur U, Jones R. Domestic violence against women: systematic review of prevalence studies. J Fam Violence. 2009;25(4):369–82.
11. Hughes C, Cohen RL. Feminists really do count: the complexity of feminist methodologies. Soc Res Method. 2010;13(3):189–96.
12. Ellsberg M, Heise L. Researching violence against women: a practical guide for researchers and activists. Washington, DC: World Health Organisation/PATH; 2005.
13. Hyden M. Narrating sensitive topics. In: Andrews M, Squire C, Tamboukou M, editors. Doing narrative research. London: Sage; 2008. p. 121–36.
14. Westmarland N, Bows H. Researching gender, violence and abuse: theory, methods, action. Abingdon: Routledge; 2019.
15. Sikweyiya Y, Jewkes R. Perceptions and experiences of research participants on gender-based violence community based survey: implications for ethical guidelines. PLoS One. 2012;7(4):e35495.
16. Hossain M, McAlpine A. Gender-based violence research methodologies in humanitarian settings: an evidence review and recommendations. Cardiff: Elrha; 2017.
17. McGarry J, Ali P. Researching domestic violence and abuse in healthcare settings: challenges and issues. J Res Nurs. 2016;21(5–6):465–76.
18. World Health Organization (WHO). Ethical and safety recommendations for intervention research on violence against women. In: Building on lessons from the WHO publication 'Putting women first: Ethical and safety recommendations for research on domestic violence against women'. Geneva: WHO; 2016.
19. Ellsberg M, Potts A. Ethical considerations for research and evaluation on ending violence against women and girls: guidance paper prepared by the global Women's institute (GWI) for the Department of Foreign Affairs and Trade. Canberra: DFAT; 2018.
20. Van der Heijden I, Harries J, Abrahams N. Ethical considerations for disability-inclusive gender-based violence research: reflections from a south African qualitative case study. Glob Public Health. 2019;14(5):737–49.

21. Jewkes R, Wagman J. Generating needed evidence while protecting women research partici-pants in a study of domestic violence in South Africa: a fine balance. In: Lavery JV, Wahl ER, Grady C, Emanuel EJ, editors. Ethical issues in international biomedical research: a case book. Oxford: Oxford University Press; 2007. p. 350–5.

22. Skinner T, Hester M, Malos E. Methodology, feminism and gender violence. In: Skinner T, Hester M, Malos E, editors. Researching gender violence: feminist methodology in action. Cullompton: Willan; 2005. p. 1–22.

23. Judkins-Cohn TM, Kielwasser-Withrow K, Owen M, Ward J. Ethical principles of informed consent: exploring nurses' dual role of care provider and researcher. J Contin Educ Nurs. 2014;45(1):35–42.

24. Letherby G. Feminist research in theory and practice. Buckingham: Open University Press; 2003.

25. Roberts H. Women and their doctors: power and powerlessness in the research process. In: Roberts H, editor. Doing feminist research. London: Routledge & Kegan Paul; 1993. p. 7–29.

26. Stanley L, Wise S. Breaking out again: feminist ontology and epistemology. 2nd ed. London: Routledge; 1993.

27. Nagy Hesse-Biber S. Feminist research: exploring, interrogating, and transforming the inter-connections of epistemology, methodology and method. In: Nagy Hesse-Biber S, editor. The handbook of feminist research. 2nd ed. Los Angeles: Sage; 2012. p. 2–26.

28. Oliveira E. The personal is political: a feminist reflection on a journey into participatory arts-based research with sex worker migrants in South Africa. Gender Dev. 2019;27(3):523–40.

29. Jaggar AM. Love and knowledge: emotion in feminist epistemology. Inquiry. 1989;32(2):151–76.

30. Krystalli R. Narrating violence: feminist dilemmas and approaches. In: Shepherd LJ, editor. Handbook on gender and violence. Cheltenham: Edward Elgar; 2019. p. 173–88.

31. Haraway DJ. Situated knowledges: the science question in feminism and the privilege of par-tial perspective. Fem Stud. 1988;14(3):575–99.

32. hooks, b. Yearning: race, gender, and cultural politics. Boston: South End Press; 1990.

33. Lorde A. The Master's tools will never dismantle the Master's house. In: Sister outsider: essays and speeches. Berkeley: Crossing Press; 2007. p. 110–4.

34. Tuhiwai Smith L. Decolonizing methodologies. 2nd ed. London: Zed Books; 2012.

35. Ahmed S. A phenomenology of whiteness. Fem Theory. 2007;8(2):149–68.

36. Mannell J, Guta A. The ethics of researching intimate partner violence in global health: a case study from global health research. Glob Public Health. 2018;13(8):1035–49.

37. Nnawulezi N, Lippy C, Serrata J, Rodriguez R. Doing equitable work in inequitable condi-tions: an introduction to a special issue on transformative research methods in gender-based violence. J Fam Violence. 2018;33:507–13.

38. Narayan U. Dislocating cultures: identities, traditions, and third world feminism. Abingdon: Routledge; 1997.

39. Palmary I. "In your experience": research as gendered cultural translation. Gend Place Cult. 2011;18(1):99–113.

40. Vara R, Patel N. Working with interpreters in qualitative psychological research: methodologi-cal and ethical issues. Qual Res Psychol. 2011;9(1):75–87.

41. Crenshaw K. Mapping the margins: intersectionality, identity politics, and violence against women of color. Stanford Law Rev. 1991;43(6):1241–99.

42. Connell R. Gender, health and theory: conceptualising the issue, in local and world perspec-tive. Soc Sci Med. 2012;74:1675–83.

43. Lykes MB, Scheib H. The artistry of emancipatory practice: photovoice, creative techniques, and feminist anti-racist participatory action research. In: Bradbury H, editor. The SAGE hand-book of action research. 3rd ed. London: Sage; 2017. p. 130–41.

44. Cornwall A, Jewkes R. What is participatory research? Soc Sci Med. 1995;41(12):1667–76.

45. Kesby M, Kindon S, Pain R. "Participatory" approaches and diagramming techniques. In: Flowerdew R, Martin D, editors. Methods in human geography. A guide for students doing a research project. 2nd ed. Harlow: Pearson Education; 2005. p. 144–66.

46. Fals-Borda O. The application of participatory action-research in Latin America. Int Sociol. 1987;2(4):329–47.
47. Freire P. Pedagogy of the oppressed. 2nd ed. London: Penguin Books; 1996.
48. Gaventa J, Cornwall A. Power and knowledge. In: Reason P, Bradbury H, editors. The SAGE handbook of action research: participative inquiry and practice. 2nd ed. London: Sage; 2008. p. 172–89.
49. Wang C, Burris MA. Photovoice: concept, methodology, and use for participatory needs assessment. Health Educ Behav. 1997;24(3):369–87.
50. Clark T. "We're over-researched here!": exploring accounts of research fatigue within qualitative research engagements. Sociology. 2008;42(5):953–70.
51. Weber S. Participatory visual research with displaced persons: "listening" to post-conflict experiences through the visual. J Refug Stud. 2019;32(3):417–35.

Louise Isham and Caroline Bradbury-Jones

This edited book brings together the voices and insights of survivors, practitioners, educators and researchers working to prevent and minimise the harms of gender-based violence. As editors, our intention was to develop a collection that could be used by readers seeking to learn more about specific topics. We also wanted to highlight the critical and practical value of recognising the gendered dimensions of violence and abuse given the limited focus this perspective receives in contemporary education and training for health and social work professionals. In this collection, the authors address issues relating to gendered dimensions of some forms of violence, such as intimate partner violence (IPV), sexual violence in intimate and community settings, stalking and harassment and female genital mutilation (FGM). Other chapters explore the interconnections between gendered harms and inequalities, for example across the refugee experience, the manifestation of trauma over the life course and the different ways that we engage with boys and girls who display harmful sexual behaviour. Throughout the chapters, authors share their experiecnes and insights from working in different contexts: for example within emergency settings, the courts and the class or training room. Our hope is that readers will find chapters that speak to their current work and interests and also find it valuable to learn about issues in less familiar (but often related) fields.

Throughout the chapters, the authors elicit questions and considerations that are of particular relevance to health and social work practitioners. We asked contributors to think about what messages they wanted to share with this audience and reflect on the strengths and challenges of these professions when responding to gendered violence. They rose to this task, by reflecting on the findings of research

L. Isham (✉)
Institute of Applied Health Research, University of Birmingham, Birmingham, UK
e-mail: l.j.isham@bham.ac.uk

C. Bradbury-Jones
Institute of Clinical Sciences, College of Medical and Dental Sciences, University of Birmingham, Birmingham, UK
e-mail: c.bradbury-jones@bham.ac.uk

© Springer Nature Switzerland AG 2021
C. Bradbury-Jones, L. Isham (eds.), *Understanding Gender-Based Violence*,
https://doi.org/10.1007/978-3-030-65006-3_17

carried out with and for survivors, showcasing areas of innovation in the field of gender-based violence and by raising awareness of 'hidden' or neglected issues. The chapters' breadth and depth speak to the knowledge and expertise of the contributors, as well as the growing scope and vitality of work being carried out to prevent and minimise the harms of gendered violence. It also speaks to the different ways that practitioners, working across disciplines and in different organisational contexts, can play a critical role in supporting those affected by gendered violence. Some of the principal themes that run through the book are captured in the following short discussion.

17.1 Amplifying the Knowledge, Experience and Voice of Victim-Survivors

A theme that runs throughout this collection is the need to place victim-survivors at the heart of responses to addressing gendered inequalities and violence. This call is rooted in an acknowledgement that the accounts of victim-survivors have too often not been heard, believed and given the credibility and respect they deserve. These silences and acts of misrecognition have been shaped by the normalisation and permissibility of violence against people who are considered to have less value and worth than others and who are often women and children. Laura Jones and Juliet Albert's chapter unpacks, for example how these intersecting factors can normalise the practice of FGM in some communities, obscuring recognition of the physical and psychological trauma it can cause to victim-survivors. Sarah Rockowitz et al.'s chapter on sexual violence in Kenya similarly illustrates the myriad historical, social and cultural factors that have contributed to impunity for those who commit sexual crimes. As many of the contributors highlight, judgements about value and worth are rooted in cultural practices and social precedents; they are also upheld and reinforced by systems of law, economics, education and healthcare that seek to maintain power and privilege based on gendered, race, class and embodied lines.

The complexity of this ecosystem may seem daunting and perhaps frustrating for those seeking to affect change. However, by amplifying the voices and leadership of victim-survivors, the contributors demonstrate that new ways of knowing and responding to violence and abuse can develop. This is particularly critical when supporting victim-survivors whose needs are rendered structurally and symbolically invisible by their physical and social environment. Claire Sullivan and colleagues powerfully explain how, for example, the contemporary refugee experience can create and sustain violence beyond conflict and transit spaces. Similarly, Simon Sawyer's chapter on emergency responses underlines that there is a role for health and social work practitioners to play in situations of crisis and emergency that may not be initially framed as situations of gendered violence. What these chapters emphasise is the value, however challenging and complex the circumstances, to work with and for victim-survivors. Other chapters help readers to see how this work could be carried out. Isobel Heywood and Jacky Mulveen's chapter, for example showcases the work of a grassroots survivor-led organisation and how creative and participatory approaches can support recovery. Kathryn Hodges and Lyndsey Harris' chapter also underlines the importance of adopting a survivor-led approach for women who experience multiple forms of disadvantage. Their 'complex care model' highlights how, by understanding the things that have happened to women, on their own terms, practitioners can work alongside them as they make decisions and potentially seek help and support. These chapters illustrate that working in a survivor-focused way can be transformative and highly effective. It can also be challenging when professionals lack training, skills and organisational support.

17.2 Thinking, Responding and Educating Differently

Although adopting a gendered perspective is increasingly recognised as a useful, even necessary, way of understanding some forms of violence and abuse, this is by no means a universal view and has certainly not been the case historically. There remain important gaps in our knowledge about some of the impacts of gender-based violence and the needs and experiences of survivors when seeking help, as detailed in Kathleen Baird's chapter on the impact of IPV in pregnancy. Training and education can play a critical role in shaping practitioners' understanding and building their skills. Elizabeth McLinden and colleagues set out how gender-based violence has risen on many educators' agenda; however, they also identify that whilst good pockets of practice and training exist, there needs to be greater emphasis on upskilling and supporting non-specialist professionals throughout their careers. This is particularly important given the emotional impact of supporting victim-survivors and the emotional sensitivity and investment that is required of practitioners to do this work well. It is thus an important time for health and social work organisations to consider how they can create and sustain cultures where professionals can meaningfully identify and respond to victim-survivors, including those in their own workforce, in the long term.

One of the strengths of this collection is its plurality of voices from different disciplines and from contributors working across practice, research and advocacy fields. With this variation comes different ways of thinking about and responding to gendered inequalities and violence. This invites the reader to consider their own understandings as well as the relative strengths and limitations of different perspectives. For example, Ben Donagh's chapter, exploring the experiences of children affected by domestic violence, considers different theories and concepts that could be used to explain, assess and inform work with the family. The chapter also highlights the contribution of experiential knowledge and practice reflection. In addition, Stuart Allardyce and colleagues' chapter powerfully illustrates how adopting a gender-sensitive approach generates new insights that can inform and improve work with children affected by harmful sexual behaviour. Aided by some of the reflective exercises in the collection, readers are invited to draw links between theory, practice and research and to consider their personal views and experiences of gender. The different answers these questions evoke also help to explain why such stark differences of opinion remain about the relative value of adopting a 'gendered lens'.

17.3 The Contribution of Feminist Thought, Activism and Practice

That gender-based violence has gained currency across such a range of professions and disciplines over the last 10–20 years speaks to its transition from a marginal to a mainstream issue. Without wishing to any way over-state the degree of 'progress' made or the extent of suffering caused by gender based vioelcne across the globe, it is possible to recognise that some legislative changes, policy reforms and shifting public attitudes have played a role in raising awareness of and improving responses to GBV. As Finn Mackay succinctly argues in the opening chapter, this shift in awareness is also in large part a testament to feminist advocacy, campaigning and scholarship. As she also notes, this legacy is unfortunately not consistently acknowledged or understood and misconceptions about feminism persist and evolve.

The contribution of feminism to challenging cultural norms, lobbying for legal and policy reform, and leading innovation is hard to overstate and important to recognise [2, 3]. Feminist-informed practice also offers a critical and values-based approach that health and social work professionals may find helpful in their work with and for victim-survivors. Echoing some of the themes in Isobel Heywood and Jacky Mulveen's chapter on feminist empowerment work, Sanne Weber and Siân Thomas demonstrate how feminist approaches to gender-based violence research can facilitate creative, partnership working that attends to the potential power asymmetries of knowledge production. This in turn creates spaces for different forms of knowledge that benefit victim-survivors and are sensitive to the colonial and patriarchal legacies of academia. Ruth Tweedale's chapter on domestic violence law in England and Wales similarly highlights some of the tensions and contradictions of supporting women and children affected by abuse within an inherently patriarchal legal system. These chapters offer readers ways of re-imagining institutional and social spaces and increasing our sensitivity to the subtle and systemic expressions of gender inequality.

We are not advocating that all practitioners need to adopt a feminist approach when supporting those affecting by gendered violence. Indeed, this may feel difficult or even disingenuous for practitioners who work within social or health systems that, at a structural level, do not protect and promote gender equality and/or who have a troubled history supporting victim-survivors of violence and abuse. However, it is important to recognise the intellectual, political and creative contribution of feminist thought and activism to the way we understand, talk about and respond to gendered violence.

17.4 Building Alliances, Sharing Knowledge and Working in Partnership

A fourth theme of this book is the need to prioritise the building of alliances and partnerships. The contributors powerfully illustrate that the complex nature of gender-based violence means attempts to address it need to be similarly multi-faceted. The need to work across professional and disciplinary boundaries, in a determinedly survivor-focused way, is clearly illustrated in Mickey Sperlich et al.'s chapter. The authors explore how adopting a trauma-informed approach can support survivors recover and thrive at different stages of their life course. Anna Nikupeteri and Merja Laitinen's chapter on post-separation stalking similarly demonstrates the importance of strategic and effective partnerships between health, social work and criminal justice professionals. Their work also highlights the harms that can be done to survivors when systems and services do not work together. However, it is important to take as a starting point that organisations and practitioners with specialist knowledge and expertise (e.g. in relation to FGM, forced marriage or sexual violence) can and should play a leading role informing and equipping their colleagues working in non-specialist services. Lastly, research–practice partnerships can help to build and share knowledge about areas of excellence and specialism, as well as identify areas where work and attention is acutely needed. Effective partnerships can involve the sharing of resources and knowledge, enabling cross-pollination of ideas and new ways of working. This took place in the Daphne and Breaking the Taboo projects shared by Bridget Penhale, two studies that explored the perspectives of older female survivors of IPV, whose voices and needs are so often overlooked.

Clearly, there can be tensions and challenges working across organisational and disciplinary lines that can be ideological, practical and resource-orientated. These barriers can be particularly influential when it comes to brokering new relationships and all too often, it is victim-survivors who are negatively affected by inconsistency and uncertainty in service responses [4, 5]. However, given the gains of working collaboratively and forging new partnerships, the question this collection poses is: can we afford not to work together?

17.5   Reflecting on Some of the Gaps in the Book

Committed to developing a book that was led by survivors and practitioners, the collection highlights some of the unique and more common issues that health and social work practitioners face in relation to gender based violence. Each chapter encourages readers to reflect on the implications of theses insights for their own work and area of practice. Nevertheless, we recognise that the majority of contributors come from high-income countries and are engaged in research and practice in areas that have developed systems of health and social work/care. These systems also carry with them legacies, as well as contemporary problems, relating to prejudicial and discriminatory biases that affect the type of care and support offered to victim-survivors. However, they tend to benefit from resources and institutional stability in a way that is not consistently comparable with equivalent services in low- and middle-income countries. Clearly, there are other potentially important differences to consider, such as gender norms, social disadvantage and poverty, that can affect shape a country or region's responses to gender-based violence. This means that the collection is likely to be most relevant for professionals working in high-income countrie. We nevertheless hope there are insights and practices that colleagues from across the globe will find relevant and transferrable.

We recognise that this collection is not exhaustive and that there are expressions of gendered violence that are not covered in detail. For example, early and forced marriage, trafficking and its links with commercial sexual exploitation and so-called 'honour' based violence, to name but a few. The omission of contributions on these issues speaks to the complex and various forms of gender-based violence and some of the inevitable limitations of a single collection. It is vital that professionals learning about gender-based violence access a range of resources beyond this book in addition to their ongoing education and training. There are also some important gaps in terms of the voices and perspectives that are privileged within this book. There are no dedicated chapters, for example on the experiences of men and boys affected by violence and abuse, or the unique and additional dimensions of interpersonal violence and help-seeking for people within same-sex relationships, who identify as transgender and who identify as being from minoritised racial or ethnic groups. Whilst the unique experiences and needs of these groups are highlighted within a number of chapters and the relevance of broadly survivor-led and specifically feminist approaches are outlined, there is a clear need for greater exploration of the specific issues that some groups of victim-survivors face.

17.6   Concluding Thoughts

We have greatly enjoyed the process of editing this book. It has afforded us the happy opportunity to reflect on the innovations and alliances that are developing across disciplines, drawn together in their common work to tackle forms of gendered violence and inequality. Our motivation throughout this process was to curate a useful resource that spoke directly to health and social work professionals, taking into account their work and training and, in some cases, their concerns and frustrations. We also wanted to make clear to readers that, for those new to the field, they are entering an area with a rich intellectual, political and practice history—often led by people outside of their professions. As several of the contributors highlight, eliminating gender-based violence requires nothing short of transformation in our laws, economies and social structures. The need for this work is as pressing as ever. The ongoing coronavirus pandemic has laid bare pre-existing inequalities (and their evident interconnections), heightened the pressures and disadvantages under which many live, and compromised access and quality of care provided by health and social services. These are just some of the factors affecting the rise in IPV and sexual violence, mainly directed towards women and girls, reported across the globe [6]. The pandemic has also sparked a wave of activism and campaigning for equal rights and civil justice and led to renewed calls for transformative social change from a growing coalition of interests. Ending gender-based violence can and should be a priority in efforts to re-imagine and rebuild societies, economies and public and voluntary sector services. Health and social workers can play a critical role in ensuring that gender-based violence remains a core, mainstream issue—not a marginal one—during the crisis and its aftermath and recovery.

References

1. United Nations Women. COVID-19 and ending violence against women and girls. 2020. https:// www.unwomen.org/-/media/headquarters/attachments/sections/library/publications/2020/ issue-brief-covid-19-and-ending-violence-against-women-and-girls-en.pdf?la=en&vs=5006.
2. Abrar S, Lovenduski J, Margetts H. Feminist ideas and domestic violence policy change. Polit Stud. 2000;48(2):239–62.
3. Coy M. Joining the dots on sexual exploitation of children and women: a way forward for UK policy responses. Crit Soc Policy. 2016;36(4):572–91.
4. Hester M. The three planet model: towards an understanding of contradictions in approaches to women and children's safety in contexts of domestic violence. Br J Soc Work. 2011;41(5):837–53.
5. Holt S. Domestic violence and the paradox of post-separation mothering. Br J Soc Work. 2017;47(7):2049–67.
6. Cousins S. COVID-19 has "devastating" effect on women and girls. Lancet. 2020;396(10247):301–2.